Charting

made

Incredibly Easy!®

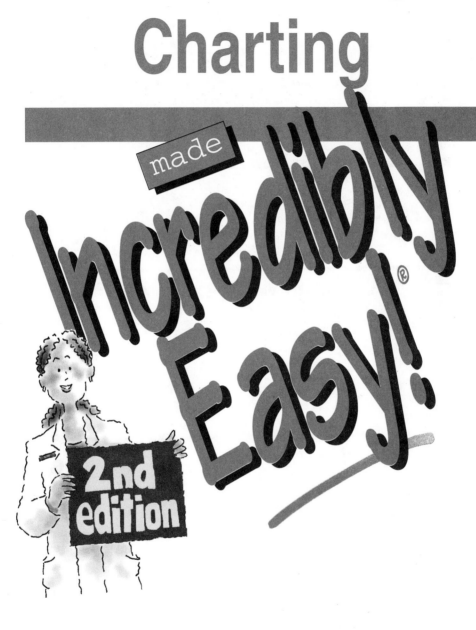

2nd edition

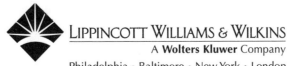

LIPPINCOTT WILLIAMS & WILKINS
A **Wolters Kluwer** Company

Philadelphia • Baltimore • New York • London
Buenos Aires • Hong Kong • Sydney • Tokyo

Staff

Publisher
Judith A. Schilling McCann, RN, MSN

Editorial Director
David Moreau

Clinical Director
Joan M. Robinson, RN, MSN, CCRN

Clinical Editors
Collette Bishop Hendler, RN, CCRN (clinical project manager); Pamela Kovach, RN, BSN; Jana L. Sciarra, RN, MSN, CRNP

Editors
Jaime L. Stockslager (senior associate editor), Cheryl Duksta, Ty Eggenberger, Stacey Ann Follin, Kevin Haworth, Brenna H. Mayer, Kirk Robinson

Copy Editors
Peggy Williams (supervisor), Virginia Baskerville, Kimberly Bilotta, Heather Ditch, Amy Furman, Shana Harrington, Dona Hightower, Marcia Ryan, Dorothy P. Terry, Pamela Wingrod

Designers
Arlene Putterman (senior art director), Mary Ludwicki (art director)

Illustrators
Scott Thorn Barrows, Barbara Cousins, John Cymerman, Mark Lefkowitz, Judy Newhouse, Bot Roda, Mary Stangl, Nina Wallace, Larry Ward

Electronic Production Services
Diane Paluba (manager), Joyce Rossi Biletz

Manufacturing
Patricia Dorshaw (senior manager), Beth Janae Orr

Associate Editor (Electronic)
Liz Schaeffer

Editorial Assistants
Danielle J. Barsky, Beverly Lane, Linda Ruhf

Indexer
Karen C. Comerford

Printed in the United States of America.
IECH2–D N O S A J J M A M F
04 03 02   10 9 8 7 6 5 4 3 2 1

FOCUS CHARTING is a registered trademark of Creative Healthcare Management, Inc.

Library of Congress Cataloging-in-Publication Data

Charting made incredibly easy!. — 2nd ed.
   p. ; cm.
   Includes index.
   Nursing records.
   [DNLM: 1. Nursing Records. 2. Documentation — Nurses' Instruction. 3. Nursing Process. WY 100.5 C486 2002] I. Lippincott Williams & Wilkins.
   RT50 .C483 2002
   610.73 — dc21
ISBN 1-58255-164-2 (alk. paper)   2001057633

Contents

Contributors and consultants

Debra Aucoin-Ratcliff, RN, MN
Nursing Program Director
Western Career College
Sacramento, Calif.

Athena A. Foreman, RN, MSN
Nursing Coordinator
Stanley Community College
Albemarle, N.C.

Lisa A. Salamon, RN,C, MSN
Clinical Nurse Specialist
Cleveland Clinic Foundation

Lourdes "Cindy" Santoni-Reddy, RN, MSN, MEd, CPP, FAAPM, NP-C
Pain Management Practitioner
Researcher
CRNP Associates, P.C.
Yardley, Pa.

Pamela B. Simmons, RN, PhD
Assistant Hospital Administrator for Patient Care
Services
LSU Health Sciences Center
Shreveport, La.

Marilyn Smith-Stoner, RN, PhD
Adjunct Faculty
University of Phoenix (Ariz.)
Home Care Consultant
Ontario, Calif.

Catherine Ultrino, RN, MSN, OCN
Nurse Manager
Boston Medical Center

Marilyn J. Vontz, RN, PhD
Nurse Educator
Bryan Hospital School of Nursing
Lincoln, Nebr.

Suzanne P. Weaver, RN, RHIT, CPHQ
Director of Nursing
Neshaminy Manor
Warrington, Pa.

The publisher would like to extend special thanks to the following people, who contributed to the first edition:

Dorothy T. Arnold, RN, BSN
Nancy Cirone, RN,C, MSN, CDE
Marie S. DeStefano, RN, MS, OCN
Elizabeth Heum, RN, BA, BS
Cynthia Lange Ingham, RN, BSN
Virginia Lee, RN, MS, MBA
Robert Rauch

Foreword

You probably didn't become a nurse in order to master the art of charting. You probably didn't get into the field to prevent a malpractice claim from occurring. I'm almost certain that you don't spend your waking hours fantasizing about charting. In fact, charting has probably become just one more thing that stands between you and your precious time with the patient. Sometimes, it may seem like a burdensome task that's necessary only to meet the demands of your supervisor and JCAHO.

How could you possibly *want* to chart, let alone enjoy it, when it keeps you from doing what you love most — patient care? I would like you to consider a different way of thinking about charting. Consider this: Charting isn't just another dull activity that removes you from patient care — in fact, charting *is* patient care.

Think of how many different health care providers the patient sees in 1 day — not to mention over an extended period. When these providers interview or examine the patient, they depend on your documentation to inform them about the patient's condition and responses to treatment. The patient trusts you to communicate what you know about his condition to other providers through thorough documentation. Establishing continuity of care depends on the quality of your documentation.

Charting Made Incredibly Easy, Second Edition, can help by providing information that's useful as well as delightful to read.

Part I discusses charting basics — including the medical record, the nursing process, and legal and professional requirements — in easy-to-understand terms. After covering these fundamentals, you'll find information on how to develop solid plans of care and document using several commonly used charting systems.

Part II covers charting in special health care settings, such as acute care, home care, and long-term care and rehabilitation.

Part III provides guidelines for enhancing your charting skills, for avoiding legal pitfalls that can place you and your facility in jeopardy, and for documenting patient care procedures.

Charting Made Incredibly Easy, Second Edition, can change your attitude about documentation drudgery with special features that will enhance your understanding, expedite your charting, and make learning enjoyable:

> Charting is essential to providing quality patient care.

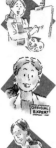

Art of the chart identifies filled-in forms with key points clearly highlighted to help you understand exactly how to chart in a wide variety of clinical settings.

Advice from the experts offers pointers, tips, and guidelines galore. Learn how to make your charting precise, patient focused, and litigation proof.

Cheat sheets summarize key points for quick review.

As in all *Incredibly Easy* books, a *Quick quiz* at the end of each chapter helps you assess what you've learned. Cartoon characters throughout the book provide comic relief but also reiterate important points. *Practice makes perfect* also helps reinforce learning by offering 40 questions and answers at the end of the book.

Completely revised and updated, this latest edition also includes up-to-date information on important charting changes related to such topics as JCAHO standards, computerized charting, and special patient care procedures. *Charting Made Incredibly Easy* will help you keep abreast of these changes; perform charting tasks with ease, accuracy, and speed; and, most of all, do what you do best—help you help your patients.

Ann Helm, RN, BSN, MS, JD
Nurse-attorney
Plaintiffs Medical Legal Consulting
Lafayette, Ore.

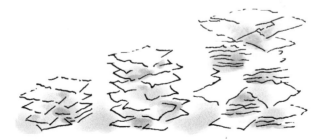

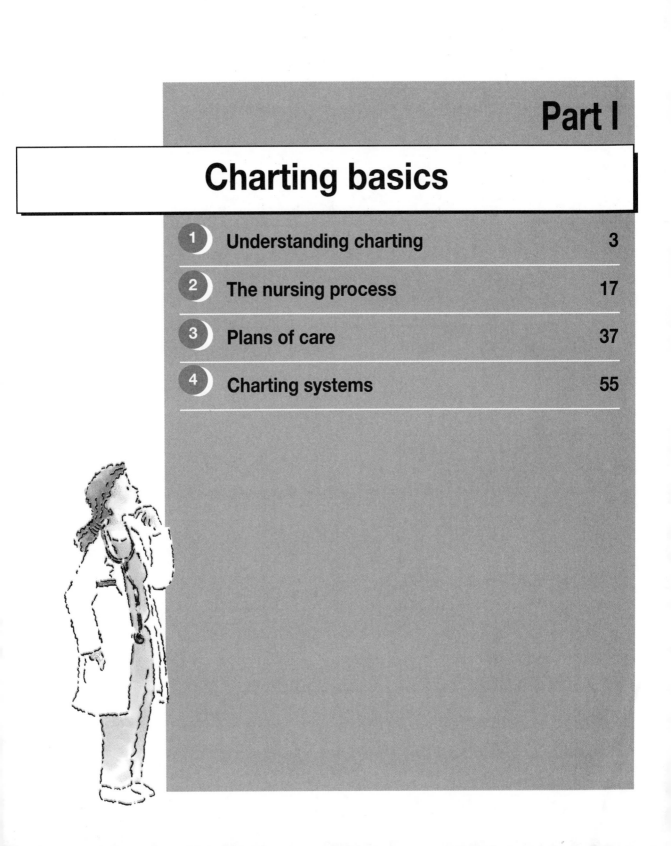

Part I

Charting basics

Understanding charting

Just the facts

In this chapter, you'll learn:

♦ why charting matters

♦ how a medical record is organized

♦ the benefits of computer charting.

A look at charting

Charting—or documentation—is the process of preparing a complete record of a patient's care. Accurate, detailed charting shows the extent and quality of the care you've provided, the outcome of that care, and treatment and education that the patient still needs.

Charting is a vital tool for communication among health care team members. Frequently, decisions, actions, and revisions related to the patient's care are based on charting from various team members. A well-prepared medical record shows the high degree of collaboration among health care team members.

You reach a wide audience

The information that's documented by team members must be easily retrievable and readable because a patient's medical record may be read by a wide audience, including:
• other members of the health care team
• reviewers from accrediting, certifying, and licensing organizations
• performance-improvement monitors
• peer reviewers
• Medicare and insurance company reviewers
• researchers and teachers
• lawyers and judges.

Proper charting is important for other reasons. One of the most compelling reasons for you to develop good charting prac-

tices is to establish your professional responsibility and accountability.

A short history of charting

In the past, charting consisted of cursory observations, such as
patient ate well or *patient slept well*. The chief purpose of these
documents was to show that the doctor's orders and the facility's
policies had been followed and that the patient had received the
proper care.

In the 19th century, the British nurse Florence Nightingale
paved the way for modern nursing documentation. In the book,
Notes on Nursing, she stressed the importance of training nurses
to gather patient information in a clear, concise, organized manner. As her theories gained acceptance, nurses' perceptions and
observations about patient care gained credence and respect.
More than a century later, in the 1970s, nurses began creating their
own vocabulary for documentation based on nursing diagnoses.

> The history
> of charting
> dates back to
> Florence
> Nightingale.

Role of charting

Accurate nursing documentation is important for many reasons,
including the following nine:

It's a mode of communication among health care professionals.

It's checked in health care evaluations.

It's legal evidence that protects you.

It's used to aid research and education.

It helps facilities obtain accreditation and licensure.

It's used to justify reimbursement requests.

It's used to develop improvements in the quality of care.

It indicates compliance with your nurse practice act.

It establishes professional accountability.

Communication

Patients are cared for by many people who work different shifts,
and these various caregivers may speak with each other infre-
quently. The medical record is the main source of information and
communication among nurses, doctors, physical therapists, social

workers, and other caregivers. Today, nurses are often considered managers of care as well as practitioners, and nurses usually document the most information. Everyone's notes are important, however, because together they present a complete picture of the patient's care.

A growing team

As health care facilities continue to streamline and redesign care delivery systems, tasks that were historically performed by nurses are now being assigned to multiskilled workers. To deliver highly specialized care, each caregiver must provide accurate, thorough information and be able to interpret what others have written about a patient. Then each can use this information to plan future patient care.

Health care evaluation

When health care is evaluated by other members of the health care team — reviewers, insurance companies, Medicare representatives, lawyers, or judges — accurate documentation is one way to prove that you're providing high-quality care. Complete documentation is both a record of what you do for your patient and written evidence that this care is necessary. It's also a record of your patient's response to your care and any changes you make in his plan of care.

Legal protection

On the legal side, accurate documentation shows that the care you provide meets the patient's needs and expressed wishes. It also proves that you're following the accepted standards of nursing care mandated by the law, your profession, and your health care facility.

The evidence speaks for itself

Proper documentation communicates crucial clinical information to caregivers so they make fewer errors. How and what you document can determine whether you or your employer wins or loses a legal dispute. Medical records are used as evidence in cases involving disability, personal injury, and mental competency. Poor documentation is the pivotal issue in many malpractice cases.

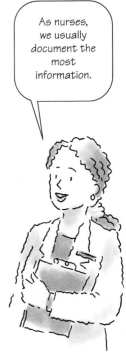

As nurses, we usually document the most information.

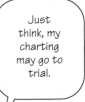

Just think, my charting may go to trial.

Research and education

Documentation also provides data for research and continuing education. For example, researchers and nurse-educators may study medical records to determine the effectiveness of nursing care. They may also be used to gauge how patient teaching affects compliance; the patient's educational level and barriers to learning are noted, as is an assessment of how well he followed the treatment regimen.

A reciprocal relationship

Just as documentation is used in research, research studies can be used to improve charting practices. For example, studies may uncover charting errors in the medical record, thereby pointing out the need for continuing education programs for health care providers.

Accreditation and licensure

For a facility to remain accredited, caregivers must document care that reflects the care standards set by national organizations, such as the American Nurses Association and the Joint Commission on Accreditation of Healthcare Organizations (JCAHO). Some states also require facilities to be licensed; licensing laws, in turn, require each facility to establish policies and procedures for operation.

A facility's accreditation and licensure may be jeopardized by substandard documentation. When a facility is cited for having poor documentation or for not meeting set standards, a warning is given and a target date is set for the facility to make necessary changes and corrections. A facility may lose its license if this isn't accomplished.

Quality is key

In effect, accreditation is evidence that a facility provides quality care and is qualified to receive federal funds. The federal government works with state accrediting organizations to make sure facilities are eligible to receive Medicare reimbursement. Accreditation and reimbursement eligibility require documentation that accurately reflects the care provided to patients. Good charting demonstrates that facility and state nursing policies were followed.

Getting what they deserve

How do officials of accrediting organizations decide if a facility should be accredited? They look at the facility's structure and function. They also conduct surveys and audits of patient records and medical records to see if care meets the required standards.

Quality and consistency

Officials review charts and files to ensure good charting. For example, in a case where physical restraints were used, officials may ask, "Is there a form for charting the need for restraints and their correct use?" and "Does the documentation in the charts show that restraints were used correctly?" Proper charting reflects the quality of care provided and the facility's accountability.

Accrediting organizations also regularly survey and audit records to make sure the standard of care is consistent throughout a facility. For example, a woman who is recovering from anesthesia after a cesarean birth should expect to receive the same monitoring in the labor and delivery suite as she would in the postanesthesia care unit. JCAHO inspectors review the documentation of both departments to ensure that a uniform standard of care is given and documented. Most accrediting organizations have similar standards for documentation. (See *What's in a medical record?*)

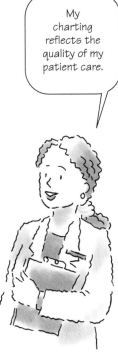

My charting reflects the quality of my patient care.

What's in a medical record?

Accrediting organizations require many of the same standards for documentation. For example, each patient's medical record must contain:
• identification data
• the medical history, which includes the patient's reason for seeking care; details of his present illness; relevant past, social, and family histories; and a body system assessment
• a summary of the patient's psychosocial needs as appropriate for the patient's age
• a report of relevant physical examination findings
• a statement of the impressions drawn from the admission history and physical examination
• the plan of care
• diagnostic and therapeutic orders
• evidence of informed consent
• clinical observations, including the effects of treatment

• progress notes
• consultation reports, if applicable
• reports of operative and other invasive procedures, tests, and their results, if appropriate
• reports of diagnostic and therapeutic procedures, such as radiology and nuclear medicine examinations
• records of donation and receipt of transplants or implants, if applicable
• a final diagnosis
• discharge summaries and instructions
• results of autopsy, when performed.

Reimbursement

Reimbursement from Medicare and insurance companies depends heavily on accurate nursing documentation. For example, many hospitals today use elaborate electronic dispensing carts to keep track of supplies. Nursing documentation has to justify the use of these supplies to be reimbursed for them.

It's payback time...or is it?

Charting is also used to determine the amount of reimbursement a facility receives. The federal government, for example, uses a prospective payment system based on diagnosis-related groups (DRGs) to determine Medicare reimbursements. In other words, they pay a fixed amount for a particular diagnosis. For a facility to receive payment, the patient's medical record at discharge must contain the correct DRG codes and show that he received the proper care, including appropriate patient teaching and discharge planning.

Most insurance companies likewise base reimbursements on a prospective payment system, and they usually don't reimburse for unskilled nursing care. They pay for skilled medical and nursing care only. For example, they compensate nurse practitioners and home health care nurses for skilled care, which includes assessing a patient's condition, creating a plan of care, and following a strict treatment regimen.

> Your charting also helps determine your facility's reimbursement.

Examinations aren't just for patients

Before reimbursing, an examiner studies the patient's medical record to decide whether he needed and received skilled nursing care. The examiner may request copies of the patient's monthly bills and look at documented progress notes, especially if the intensity, frequency, and cost of the care increased.

Examiners also check for inconsistencies in charting, such as a discrepancy between the treatment ordered and the one provided. If the discrepancy isn't explained adequately, the insurer may deny payment.

Keeping the proper care going

In addition to keeping a facility from getting reimbursed, faulty documentation can keep patients from getting the care they need. For example, an insurer might deny payment to a home health care agency if the nurse's charting doesn't prove that home visits were necessary. If that happens, home health care may be discontinued prematurely.

Performance improvement

Individual states and JCAHO require all health care facilities to regularly monitor, evaluate, and seek ways to improve the quality of care for their patients. In each facility, a committee of doctors, nurses, pharmacists, administrators, and other employees gets together to develop performance improvement measures. Committee members then implement the measures, analyze the improvements, and report their findings to the facility's board of trustees.

Multidisciplinary committee members also develop methods to assess the structure, process, and outcome of patient care. One way to implement these methods is to monitor and evaluate the content of medical records.

Up to snuff?

What if the care described in a medical record doesn't meet an established standard? Performance improvement committee members must then decide how to correct this problem. They may assign a focus group to investigate ways to do this.

The focus group may recommend changes in the facility's policies, procedures, or documentation forms in an effort to improve patient care. For example, many facilities have been cited in court for lack of documentation when physical restraints were used. As a result, some facilities have developed forms to document restraint orders from doctors, which may be used in court as proof that the facility's policy was followed and that restraints were needed.

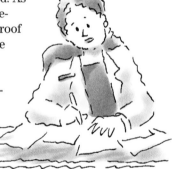

My charting may be monitored and evaluated by performance improvement committee members.

Nurse practice acts

Nurse practice acts are state laws spelling out what duties nurses can perform in that state. State nurse practice acts are revised frequently; when nurse practice acts change, charting requirements often change as well. With laws and regulations in a constant state of flux, you must be especially meticulous about charting your care to show compliance with standards.

Accountability

Accurate nursing documentation is evidence that you acted as required or ordered. Accountability means you comply with the charting requirements of your health care facility, professional organizations, and state law.

Types of medical records

Medical records are kept for virtually every person who steps through the door of a health care facility. That's a lot of assessment forms, flow sheets, and lists to fill out. How do you deal with this?

An insightful record

Many nurses try to create order in medical records by organizing patient data by category. However, this emphasizes form instead of content. *Remember:* A medical record isn't just a summary of illness and recovery. It's an insightful record of a patient's care and potential patient care problems.

Forms are your friends

You can think of the medical record as an ally in your organization efforts. It's a place to organize your thoughts about patient care and to record your actions. Used properly, it can help you save time, identify problem areas, plan better patient care, and avoid litigation. (See *Tips for fast, faultless charting.*)

Although every medical record provides evidence of the quality of patient care, not all records are alike. Some are organized by a source-oriented narrative method, some by a problem-oriented method, and others by variations of these two.

Source-oriented narrative method

With the source-oriented narrative method, caregivers (the source) from each discipline record information in a separate section of the medical record.

Missing the complete picture?

This traditional method of documentation has several serious drawbacks: Because charting is done in various parts of the record, information is disjointed, topics aren't always clearly identified, and information is difficult to retrieve. This keeps team members from getting a complete picture of the patient's care and causes breakdowns in communication.

Get on the same page

Collaborations among team members who use source-oriented narrative charting are more easily documented if everyone writes on the same progress notes. For example, doctors', nurses', and respiratory therapists' progress notes can be combined into what may be called patient progress notes. These notes serve as the pri-

---

Tips for fast, faultless charting

When you document, you must record information quickly without sacrificing accuracy. Here are some actions you can take to help you accomplish these two goals:
• Follow the nursing process.
• Use nursing diagnoses.
• Use flow sheets.
• Document at the bedside.
• Individualize your charting.
• Don't repeat information (this could lead to errors).
• Sign off with your name and credentials.
• Don't document for other caregivers.
• Use computerized documentation.

Art of the chart

Got a problem?

The chart below shows a nursing problem list for a patient with acute pancreatitis.

#	Date	Problem statement	Initials	Resolved
1	11/4/02	Deficient fluid volume related to vomiting	C.B.	
2	11/4/02	Acute pain related to physiologic factors	C.B.	
3	11/4/02	Imbalanced nutrition: Less than body requirements related to inability to digest nutrients	C.B.	
4	11/4/02	Ineffective tissue perfusion (GI) related to decreased cellular exchange	C.B.	
5	11/6/02	Ineffective coping related to situational crisis	B.A.	

mary source of reference and communication among health care team members.

Problem-oriented method

A problem-oriented medical record contains baseline data obtained from all departments involved in a patient's care. The problem-oriented charting method is based on the patient's reason for seeking care. Data include:
• the patient's health history, including his medical, social, and emotional status
• other initial assessment findings
• diagnostic test results.
   The problem-oriented record also contains:
• a problem list
• a plan of care for each problem
• progress notes.
   The problem list is distilled from baseline data and used to construct a plan of care. (See *Got a problem?*)

Whatever format you use, charting should reflect the quality of nursing care you deliver.

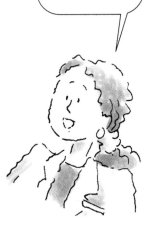

Focusing on each problem

The plan of care in a problem-oriented medical record addresses each of the patient's problems, which are routinely updated both in the plan and in the progress notes. (See *A close look at a medical record.*)

A close look at a medical record

Although each health care facility has its own system for keeping medical records, most records contain the documents described here:
- face sheet—first page of the medical record; contains the patient's name, birth date, social security number, address, marital status, closest relative or guardian, food or drug allergies, admitting diagnosis, and attending doctor
- medical history and physical examination—completed by the doctor; contains the initial medical examination and evaluation data
- doctor's order sheet—a record of the doctor's medical orders
- initial nursing assessment form—contains nursing data, including health history and physical assessment findings
- integrated assessment form—assessment form used by all members of the health care team
- problem or nursing diagnosis list—lists the patient's problems; used with problem-oriented medical records
- nursing plan of care—based on information gathered during the patient assessment; specifies patient's care needs, planned interventions, and the patient's progress toward meeting goals and objectives
- graphic form—flow sheet that tracks the patient's temperature, pulse, respiratory rate, blood pressure and, possibly, daily weight; also may record skin care, blood glucose levels, urinalysis results, neurologic assessment data, and patient intake and output; the nurse dates, initials, or checks off the appropriate column to show a task was completed
- medication administration record—lists medications a patient receives, including dosage, administration route, site, date, and time.
- nurses' progress notes—details patient care information, nursing interventions, and patient responses
- doctors' progress notes—contains doctors' observations, notes on the patient's progress, and treatment data
- diagnostic findings—contains diagnostic and laboratory data
- health care team records—includes information from physical therapist, respiratory therapist, social worker, and other team members
- consultation sheets—includes evaluations by specialists consulted for diagnostic and treatment recommendations
- discharge plan and summary—presents a brief account of the patient's time in the facility and plans of care after discharge.

Other medical record formats

Some facilities modify the source-oriented or problem-oriented method of documentation to suit their needs. If your facility does this, you're in a position to influence the type and style of documentation you use in medical records.

Designer documentation

For example, home health care nurses have created many specialized documentation forms—including an initial assessment form, problem list, day-visit sheet, and discharge summary—to reflect the unique services and the essential quality of care they provide. These forms meet their charting needs while complying with state and federal laws and other regulations. (See *Specialized forms*, page 14.)

Computerized charting

Computerized charting is popular for completing medical records from admission through discharge. Some of the benefits of computerized documentation are listed here:
- It promotes standardization.
- Legibility problems that accompany handwritten entries are eliminated.
- Fewer errors may be made.
- It leads to decreased recording time and costs.
- Communication among team members is aided.
- It allows easier access to medical data for education, research, and performance improvement.

They even have good bedside manner

Information filed on computers includes nursing plans of care, progress notes, medication records, records of vital signs, intake and output sheets, and patient classifications. Some facilities even have bedside computers for quick data entry and access. (See *Super-successful automated charting.*)

One of the drawbacks of computerized charting is the potential for unauthorized personnel to access confidential medical records.

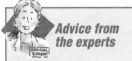

Advice from the experts

Super-successful automated charting

To be effective, an automated charting system must be able to:
- record and send data to the appropriate department
- adapt easily to the health care facility's needs
- display highly selective information on command
- provide easy access and retrieval for all trained personnel.

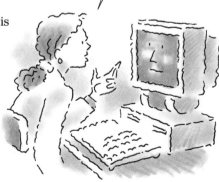

Now, you're supposed to make charting easier.

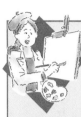

Art of the chart

Specialized forms

The form shown below is an example of a specialized form that may be developed by registered nurses, licensed practical nurses, and mental health technicians to target the essential elements of charting on their unit.

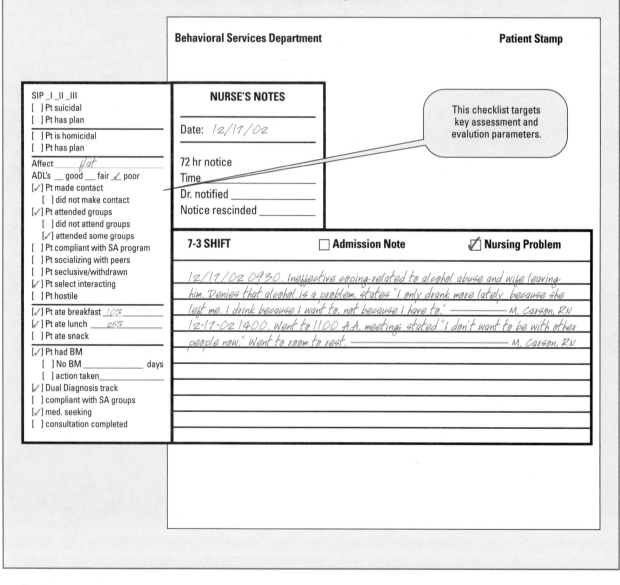

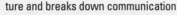

Cheat sheet

Charting fundamentals

Roles of charting
• Is the medium of communication for the health care team
• Can be used in health care evaluations
• Serves as legal evidence
• Can be used to aid research and education
• Helps facilities obtain accreditation and licensure
• Provides justification for reimbursement
• Is used to develop improvements in the quality of care
• Indicates compliance with your nurse practice act
• Establishes professional accountability

Types of records
• Source-oriented—has separate sections for each discipline's documentation, which keeps team members from getting the complete picture and breaks down communication
• Problem-oriented—is based on the patient's reason for seeking care and contains baseline data from all departments

Computerized charting
• Promotes standardization
• Eliminates legibility problems
• Leads to decreased recording time and costs
• Aids team communication
• Allows easier access to medical data

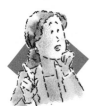

Quick quiz

1. The main drawback to source-oriented narrative records is:
    A. they're problem oriented.
    B. that a baseline assessment is needed.
    C. each discipline records information on a separate section of the record.

    Answer: C. This type of charting causes communication breakdowns because information is disjointed and hard to retrieve, topics aren't always clearly identified, and team members can't easily get a complete picture of the patient's care.

2. Which of the following choices is *not* a benefit of computer-ized charting?

   A.   There are fewer forms to fill out.
   B.   It promotes standardization.
   C.   Legibility is improved.

Answer: A. Computers can decrease the use of bulky paper files because they store information permanently for easy access and retrieval. However, you still have to complete all the required forms.

3. JCAHO regulates standards of care to:

   A.   make sure that all nurses use the same charting system.
   B.   ensure quality patient care.
   C.   ensure subjective documentation.

Answer: B. To meet JCAHO standards, facilities must uphold certain levels of quality in patient care.

4. Nursing documentation as we know it today was first used in what time period?

   A.   1970s
   B.   19th century
   C.   18th century

Answer: B. Florence Nightingale established modern nursing documentation in the 19th century.

5. Which part of the medical record can be used as evidence in court?

   A.   The plan of care
   B.   The medical orders
   C.   The entire record

Answer: C. The entire medical record is a legal document that's admissible in court.

Scoring

☆☆☆   If you answered all five items correctly, fantastic! You're clear, concise, and consistent—a charting champion!

☆☆   If you answered three or four items correctly, dandy! Your documentation definitely deserves to be accredited.

☆   If you answered fewer than three items correctly, don't worry. With a little review, your recording will reap regular reimbursement!

2

The nursing process

Just the facts

In this chapter, you'll learn:

♦ how to perform an assessment based on the nursing process

♦ how to formulate a nursing diagnosis

♦ how to write a nursing plan of care with expected outcomes and appropriate interventions

♦ how to evaluate and document your results.

A look at the nursing process

The nursing process is a problem-solving approach to nursing care. It's a systematic method for determining the patient's health problems, devising a plan of care to address them, implementing the plan, and evaluating the effectiveness of the care.

The nursing process emerged in the 1960s, as team health care came into wider practice and nurses were increasingly called on to define their specific roles. The roots of the nursing process can be traced to World War II, however, when technology, medical advances, and a growing need for nurses began to change the nursing profession.

Going through the phases

The nursing process consists of six distinct phases:

🖐 assessment

✌ nursing diagnosis

☝ outcome identification

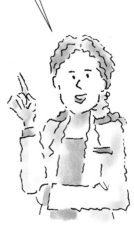

The nursing process is a six-step path from assessment to evaluation.

planning

implementation

evaluation.

These six phases are dynamic and flexible and they often overlap. Together, they resemble the steps that many other professions take to identify and correct problems.

Assessment

The first step in the nursing process — assessment — begins when you first see a patient. Assessment continues throughout the patient's hospitalization as you obtain more information about his changing condition.

Getting the whole picture

During assessment, you collect relevant information from various sources and analyze it to form a complete picture of your patient. As you collect this information, you need to document it accurately for two reasons:
• It guides you through the rest of the nursing process, helping you formulate nursing diagnoses, expected outcomes, and nursing interventions.
• It serves as a vital communication tool for other team members and as a baseline for evaluating a patient's progress.

The information that you gather at the first patient contact may indicate that the patient needs a broader or more detailed assessment such as a nutritional assessment. (See *Assessing nutritional status.*)

Further assessment depends on:
• patient's diagnosis
• care setting
• patient's consent to treatment
• care the patient is seeking
• patient's response to previous care.

First impressions

In your initial assessment, take into account the patient's immediate and emerging needs, including not only his physical needs but also his psychological, spiritual, and social concerns. The initial assessment helps you determine what care the patient needs and

> The assessment data I collect establish the basis for the rest of the nursing process.

sets the stage for further assessments. Remember that a patient's family, culture, and religion are important factors in the patient's response to illness and treatment.

Begin your assessment by collecting a health history and conducting a physical examination.

Health history

The health history includes physical, psychological, cultural, spiritual, and psychosocial data. It's the main source of information about the patient's health status and guides the physical examination that follows.

A nursing history is different from a medical history. A medical history guides diagnosis and treatment of illness; a nursing history focuses holistically on the human response to illness.

The nursing history you collect helps you to:
- plan health care
- assess the impact of illness on the patient and members of his family
- evaluate the patient's health education needs
- initiate discharge planning.

Getting started

Although nurses conduct health histories in different ways, all interviews must progress in a logical sequence and be an organized record of the patient's response.

Before conducting the health history, consider the patient's ability to participate. If he's sedated, confused, hostile, angry, dyspneic, or in pain, ask only the most essential questions. Then perform an in-depth interview later. In the meantime, ask family members or close friends to provide some information.

Get off on the right foot by finding a quiet, private space where the patient feels as comfortable and relaxed as possible. Ask another nurse to cover your other patients so you won't be interrupted. This reassures the patient that you're interested in what he says and that you'll keep the information confidential. (See *Health history lessons*, page 20.)

Making the most of your time

Finding time to conduct a thorough patient history can be hard. However, a few strategies can help you keep interview time to a minimum without sacrificing quality. (See *Health history in a hurry*, page 21.)

Sometimes an interview isn't even necessary — you can simply ask the patient to complete a questionnaire about his past and present health status. Then you can quickly and easily document the

Assessing nutritional status

As part of the admission assessment, the answers to some questions automatically call for another discipline to be consulted. An example is in the nutrition section.

With the following questions, one "no" requires a nutritional consult:
- Do you have sufficient funds to buy food?
- Do you have access to a food market?
- Are you able to shop, cook, and feed yourself?

With the following questions, one "yes" requires a nutritional consult:
- Do you have an illness or condition that made you change the amount or kind of food you eat?
- Do you have dental or mouth problems that make it difficult for you to chew or swallow food?
- Do you need help getting to a food market?
- Have you lost or gained 10 lb within the last 6 months without trying?

Health history lessons

Conduct a health history with class; when you show the patient that you're interested and empathetic, you elicit more accurate and complete answers.

Do

Here are some interviewing do's:

• *Use general leads.* Broad opening questions encourage the patient to discuss what's most important to him.

• *Ask open-ended questions.* Questions that require more than a yes-or-no answer encourage the patient to express himself.

• *Restate information.* Summarize the patient's comments and then give him a chance to clarify them.

Don't

These are some things you don't want to do in your interview:

• *Ask judgmental or threatening questions.* Saying "Why did you do that?" or "Explain your behavior" forces the patient to justify his feelings and might alienate him. He might even invent an appropriate answer just to satisfy you.

• *Ask persistent questions or probe.* Make one or two attempts to get information and then back off. Respect the patient's right to privacy.

• *Offer advice or false reassurance.* Giving advice implies that you know what's best for the patient. Instead, encourage him to participate in health care decisions. Saying "You'll be all right" devalues his feelings. But saying "You seem worried" encourages him to speak candidly.

patient's health history by reviewing the information on the questionnaire and filing it in the patient's chart.

This method is most successful for patients who are to undergo short or elective procedures. The questionnaire can be completed before the patient's admission, which can save you time.

In some acute care settings, modified questionnaires are used to evaluate any language and reading problems the patient may have. The nurse then reviews sections that are completed by the patient.

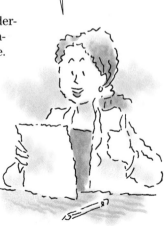

If a questionnaire saves time, I'm all for it!

Physical examination

The second half of the assessment process is performing a physical examination. Use the following techniques to conduct the examination:

Advice from the experts

Health history in a hurry

When you're pressed for time, use the following tips to speed up health history documentation:

• Before the interview, fill in as much information as you can from admission forms, transfer summaries, and the medical history. This avoids duplication of effort. If some information isn't clear, ask the patient for more details. For instance, you might say, "You told Dr. Brown that you sometimes feel like you can't catch your breath. Can you tell me more about when this happens?"

• Check your facility's policy on who may gather assessment data. Maybe you can have an unlicensed nursing assistant or technician collect routine information, such as allergies and past hospitalizations. Remember, however, that reviewing and verifying the information is your responsibility.

• Begin by asking about the patient's reason for seeking medical care. Then, even if the interview is interrupted, you'll still be able to write a plan of care.

• Use your facility's nursing assessment documentation form only as a guide to organize information. Ask your patient only pertinent questions from the form.

• Take only brief notes during the interview, so you don't interrupt the flow of conversation. Write detailed notes as soon as possible after the interview. You can always go back to the patient if you need to clarify or verify information.

• Record your findings in concise, specific phrases. Use only approved abbreviations.

• inspection
• palpation
• percussion
• auscultation.

The objective data you gather during the physical examination may be used to confirm or rule out health problems that were suggested or suspected during the health history. You rely on these findings when you develop a plan of care and when you deliver patient teaching. For example, if the patient's blood pressure is high, he may need a sodium-restricted diet and instruction on how to control hypertension.

It's in the details

How detailed should your examination be? That depends on the patient's condition, the clinical setting, and the policies and procedures established by your health care facility. The main components of the physical examination include:

• height
• weight
• vital signs

Advice from the experts

Rapid review of the physical assessment

During a physical examination, your main task is to record the patient's height, weight, and vital signs and review the major body systems. Here's a typical body system review for an adult patient.

Respiratory system
Note the rate and rhythm of respirations, and auscultate the lung fields. Inspect the lips, mucous membranes, and nail beds. Also inspect the sputum, noting color, consistency, and other characteristics.

Cardiovascular system
Note the color and temperature of the extremities, and assess the peripheral pulses. Check for edema and hair loss on the extremities. Inspect the neck veins and auscultate for heart sounds.

Neurologic system
Assess the patient's level of consciousness, noting his orientation to person, place, and time and his ability to follow commands. Also assess pupillary reactions. Check the extremities for movement and sensation.

Eyes, ears, nose, and throat
Assess the patient's ability to see objects with and without corrective lenses. Assess his ability to hear spoken words clearly. Inspect the eyes and ears for discharge and the nasal mucous

membranes for dryness, irritation, and blood. Inspect the teeth, gums, and condition of the oral mucous membranes and palpate the lymph nodes in the neck.

GI system
Auscultate for bowel sounds in all quadrants. Note abdominal distention or ascites. Gently palpate the abdomen for tenderness. Assess the condition of the mucous membranes around the anus.

Musculoskeletal system
Assess the range of motion of major joints. Look for swelling at the joints and for contractures, muscle atrophy, or obvious deformity. Assess muscle strength of the trunk and extremities.

Genitourinary and reproductive systems
Note any bladder distention or incontinence. If indicated, inspect the genitalia for rashes, edema, or deformity. (Inspection of the genitalia may be waived at the patient's request or if no dysfunction was reported during the interview.) If indicated, inspect the genitalia for sexual maturity. Also examine the breasts, noting any abnormalities.

Integumentary system
Note any sores, lesions, scars, pressure ulcers, rashes, bruises, or petechiae. Also note the patient's skin turgor.

• review of the major body systems. (See *Rapid review of the physical assessment.*)

JCAHO standards

Under the standards of the Joint Commission on Accreditation of Healthcare Organizations (JCAHO), your initial assessment of the patient should take into consideration:
• physical factors
• psychological and social factors
• environmental factors

- self-care capabilities
- learning needs
- discharge planning needs
- input from the patient's family and friends when appropriate.

Physical factors

Physical factors include the physical examination findings from your review of the patient's major body systems.

Psychological and social factors

The patient's fears, anxieties, and other concerns about hospitalization are psychological and social factors.

Family matters

Find out what support systems the patient has by asking questions such as, "How does being in the hospital affect your home situation?" A patient who is worried about his family might be less able or willing to comply with treatment.

Environmental factors

The patient's home environment affects care needs during hospitalization and after discharge. Factors to ask about may include:
- where he lives; whether it's a house or an apartment
- whether he has adequate heat, ventilation, hot water, and bathroom facilities
- how many flights of stairs he has to climb; whether the layout of his home poses any hazards
- whether his home is convenient to stores and doctors' offices.

Is the patient well-equipped?

In addition, ask if he uses equipment that isn't available in the hospital when he performs activities of daily living (ADLs) at home. Tailor your questions to his condition.

Self-care capabilities

A patient's ability to perform ADLs affects how well he complies with therapy before and after discharge. Assess your patient's ability to eat, wash, dress, use the bathroom, turn in bed, get out of bed, and get around.

Some facilities use an ADL checklist to indicate if a patient can perform these tasks independently or if he needs assistance.

Learning needs

Deciding early what your patient needs to know about his condition leads to effective patient teaching. During the initial assessment, evaluate your patient's knowledge of the disease process, self-care, diet, medications, lifestyle changes, treatment measures, and limitations caused by the disease or treatment.

No yes-or-no answers, please

One way to evaluate your patient's learning needs is to ask open-ended questions such as "What do you know about the medicine you take?" His response will tell you if he understands and complies with his medication regimen or if he needs more teaching.

Learning obstacles

You also should assess factors that can hinder learning, which can result from:
- the nature of the patient's illness or injury
- the patient's health beliefs
- the patient's religious beliefs
- the patient's educational level
- sensory deficits such as hearing problems
- language barriers
- the patient's stress level
- the patient's age
- pain or discomfort.

Discharge planning needs

Discharge planning also should start as soon as possible (in some cases, even before admission), especially if the patient needs help after discharge. Find out where the patient will go after discharge. Is follow-up care accessible? Is there a caregiver who will be available to assist the patient? Are community resources—such as visiting nurse services and Meals On Wheels—available where he lives? If not, you need time to help the patient make other arrangements. (See *Discharge assessment questions.*)

Prioritize, prioritize, prioritize

Because inpatient lengths of stay have become shorter and patient care has become increasingly complex, nurses need to prioritize their assessment data. (See *Establishing priorities for patient assessment.*)

Input from family and friends

Another JCAHO requirement is that you obtain assessment information from the patient's family and friends, when appropriate.

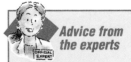

Advice from the experts

Establishing priorities for patient assessment

After completion of an initial assessment, the Joint Commission on Accreditation of Healthcare Organizations requires nurses to use the gathered information in prioritizing their care decisions. To systematically set priorities, follow these steps:
- Identify the patient's problems.
- Identify the patient's risk of injury.
- Identify the patient's need for help with self-care, both in the hospital and following discharge.
- Identify the education needs of the patient and members of his family.

Art of the chart

Discharge assessment questions

The sample discharge assessment form below is one section of the nursing admission assessment form.

Discharge planning needs

Living arrangements (caregiver): _____ Sara Smith (patient's daughter) _____

Type of dwelling: Apartment _____ House ✔ Nursing home _____ Boarding home _____ Other _____

Physical barriers in home: No _____ Yes ✔ Explain: ___ 12 step flight of stairs to bathroom and bedroom ___

Access to follow-up medical care: Yes ✔ No _____ Explain: _____

Ability to carry out ADLs: Self-care _____ Partial assistance _____ Total assistance ✔

Needs help with: Bathing ✔ Eating ✔ Ambulation ✔

Other_____

Anticipated discharge destination: Home _____ Rehab _____ Nursing home ✔ Skilled nursing facility _____

Boarding home _____ Other _____

When you interview someone other than the patient, be sure to document the nature of the relationship. If the interviewee isn't a family member, ask about and record the length of time the person has known the patient.

Nursing diagnosis

Your assessment findings form the basis for the next step in the nursing process: the nursing diagnosis. According to the North American Nursing Diagnosis Association, a nursing diagnosis is a clinical judgment about individual, family, or community responses to actual or potential health problems or life processes. Nursing diagnoses are used in selecting nursing interventions to achieve outcomes for which the nurse is accountable.

Diagnosing a diagnosis

Each nursing diagnosis describes an actual or potential health problem that a nurse can legally manage. A diagnosis usually has three components:

the human response or problem—an actual or potential problem that can be affected by nursing care

related factors—factors that may precede, contribute to, or be associated with the human response

signs and symptoms—defining characteristics that lead to the diagnosis.

One patient, two types of treatment

When you become familiar with nursing diagnoses, you'll clearly see how nursing practice and medical practice differ. Although problems are identified in both nursing and medicine, medical and nursing treatment approaches are very different.

The main difference is that doctors are licensed to diagnose and treat illnesses, and nurses are licensed to diagnose and treat the patient's *response* to illness. Nurses also can diagnose the

---

Maslow's pyramid

To formulate nursing diagnoses, you must know your patient's needs and values. Of course, physiologic needs—represented by the base of the pyramid in the diagram below—must be met first.

Self-actualization
Recognition and realization of one's potential, growth, health, and autonomy

Self-esteem
Sense of self-worth, self-respect, independence, dignity, privacy, self-reliance

Love and belonging
Affiliation, affection, intimacy, support, reassurance

Safety and security
Safety from physiologic and psychological threat, protection, continuity, stability, lack of danger

Physiologic needs
Oxygen, food, elimination, temperature control, sex, movement, rest, comfort

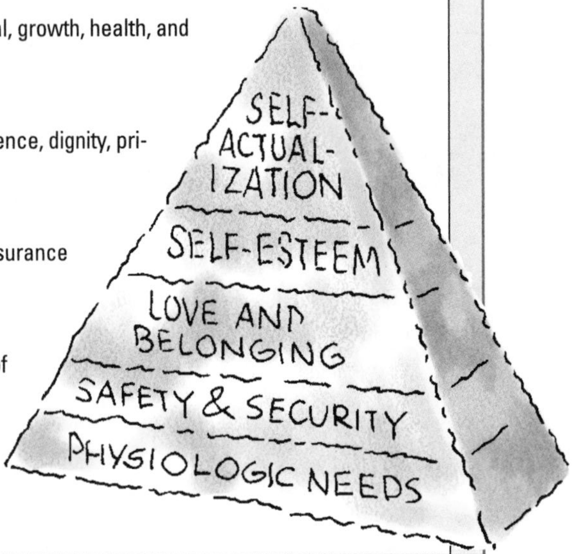

SELF-ACTUALIZATION
SELF-ESTEEM
LOVE AND BELONGING
SAFETY & SECURITY
PHYSIOLOGIC NEEDS

need for patient education, offer comfort and counsel to patients and families, and care for patients until they're physically and emotionally ready to provide self-care.

Emergencies get top billing

Whenever you develop nursing diagnoses, you must prioritize them. Then begin your plan of care with the highest priority. High-priority diagnoses involve emergency or immediate physical care needs.

Intermediate-priority diagnoses involve nonemergency needs, and low-priority diagnoses involve peripheral needs or those related to enhanced functioning or wellness. Maslow's hierarchy of needs can help you set priorities in your plan of care. (See *Maslow's pyramid.*)

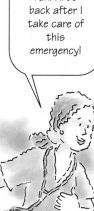

Gotta run! I'll be back after I take care of this emergency!

Outcome identification

The goal of your nursing care is to help your patient reach his highest functional level with minimal risk and problems. If he can't recover completely, your care should help him cope physically and emotionally with his impaired or declining health.

Keeping it real

With this in mind, you should identify realistic, measurable expected outcomes and corresponding target dates for your patient. Expected outcomes are goals the patient should reach as a result of planned nursing interventions. Sometimes, a nursing diagnosis requires more than one expected outcome.

An outcome can specify an improvement in the patient's ability to function, for example, an increase in the distance he can walk. Or it can specify the correction of a problem such as a reduction of pain. In either case, each outcome calls for the maximum realistic improvement for a particular patient.

These guidelines will help you write great outcome statements.

Four-part format

An outcome statement consists of four parts:

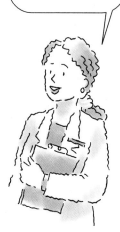

the specific behavior that shows the patient has reached his goal

criteria for measuring that behavior

the conditions under which the behavior should occur

when the behavior should occur. (See *Components of an outcome statement,* page 28.)

Components of an outcome statement

An outcome statement consists of four elements: behavior, measure, condition, and time.

 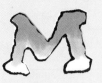 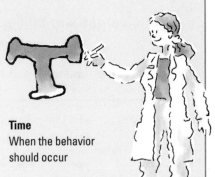

Behavior
A desired behavior for the patient; must be observable

Measure
Criteria for measuring the behavior; should specify how much, how long, how far, and so on

Condition
The conditions under which the behavior should occur

Time
When the behavior should occur

As indicated, the two outcome statements below have these four components.

Ambulate	one flight of stairs	unassisted	by 11/12/02
Demonstrate	measuring radial pulse	before exercising	by 11/12/02

Writing outcome statements

Save time when writing outcome statements by choosing your words carefully and being clear and concise. (See *Writing excellent outcome statements.*)

Here are some tips for writing efficient outcome statements:

• *Avoid unnecessary words.* For example, instead of writing *Pt will demonstrate correct wound-care technique by 11/1*, drop the first two words. Everyone knows you're talking about the patient.

• *Use accepted abbreviations.* Refer to your facility's approved abbreviation list. If it uses relative dates (describes the patient's stay in day-long intervals), use abbreviations like *HD1* for hospital day 1 or *POD 2* for postoperative day 2.

• *Make your statements specific. Understand relaxation techniques* doesn't tell you much; how do you observe a patient's understanding? Instead, *Practice progressive muscle relaxation techniques unassisted for 15 minutes daily by 4/9* tells you exactly what to look for when assessing the patient's progress.

Advice from the experts

Writing excellent outcome statements

The following tips will help you write clear, precise outcome statements:

• When writing expected outcomes in your plan of care, always start with a specific action verb that focuses on your patient's behavior. By telling your reader how your patient should *look, walk, eat, drink, turn, cough, speak, or stand,* for example, you give a clear picture of how to evaluate progress.

• Avoid starting expected outcome statements with *allow, let, enable,* or similar verbs. Such words focus attention on your own and other health team members' behavior—not on the patient's.

• With many documentation formats, you won't need to include the phrase *The patient will…* with each expected outcome statement. You will, however, have to specify which person the goals refer to when family, friends, or others are directly concerned.

• *Focus on the patient.* Outcome statements should reflect the patient's behavior, not your intervention. *Medication brings chest pain relief* doesn't say anything about behavior. A correct statement would be *Express relief of chest pain within 1 hour of receiving medication.*

• *Let the patient help you.* A patient who helps write his outcome statements is more motivated to achieve his goals. His input, along with his family members', can help you set realistic goals.

• *Consider medical orders.* Don't write outcome statements that ignore or contradict medical orders. For example, before writing *Ambulate 10' unassisted twice a day by 11/9,* make sure that the medical orders don't call for more restricted activity such as bedrest.

• *Adapt the outcome to the circumstances.* Consider the patient's coping ability, age, education, cultural influences, family support, living conditions, socioeconomic status, and anticipated length of stay. Also consider the health care setting. For example, *Ambulates outdoors with assistance for 20 minutes t.i.d. by 11/9* is probably unrealistic in a large city hospital.

Planning care

The fourth step of the nursing process is planning. The nursing plan of care is a written plan of action designed to help you deliver quality patient care. The plan of care is based on problems identified during the patient's admission interview. The plan consists of:

- nursing diagnoses
- expected outcomes
- nursing interventions.

The plan of care becomes a permanent part of the patient's record and is used by all members of the nursing team. *Remember:* Patients' problems and needs change, so review your plan of care often and modify it if necessary.

Take three giant steps

Writing a plan of care involves these three steps:

assigning priorities to the nursing diagnoses

Advice from the experts

Tips for top-notch plans of care

Use either a traditional or standardized method for recording your plan of care. A traditional plan of care is written from scratch for each patient. A standardized plan of care saves time because it's predetermined, based on the patient's diagnosis.

No matter which method you use, follow these tips to write a plan that's accurate and useful:

- Write in ink and sign your name.
- Use clear, concise language, not vague terms or generalities.
- Use standard abbreviations to avoid confusion.
- Review all your assessment data *before* selecting an approach for each problem. If you can't complete the initial assessment, immediately write *insufficient information* on your records.
- Write an expected outcome and a target date for each problem you identify.
- Set realistic initial goals.
- When writing nursing interventions, consider what to watch for and how often, what nursing measures to take and how to perform them, and what to teach the patient and family before discharge.
- Make each nursing intervention specific.
- Make sure your interventions match the resources and capabilities of the staff.
- Be creative; include a drawing or an innovative procedure if this makes your directions more specific.
- Record all of the patient's problems and concerns so they won't be forgotten.
- Make sure your plan is implemented correctly.
- Evaluate the results of your plan and discontinue nursing diagnoses that have been resolved. Select new approaches, if necessary, for problems that haven't been resolved.

✌ selecting appropriate nursing interventions to accomplish expected outcomes

✌ documenting the nursing diagnoses, expected outcomes, nursing interventions, and evaluations. (See *Tips for top-notch plans of care.*)

Implementation

Now you're ready to select interventions and implement them, the fifth step of the nursing process. Nursing interventions are actions that you and your patient agree will help him reach the expected outcomes. Base these interventions on the second part of your nursing diagnosis, the related factors.

For example, with a nursing diagnosis of *Impaired physical mobility related to arthritic morning stiffness*, select interventions that reduce or eliminate the patient's stiffness, such as mild stretching exercises. Write at least one intervention for each outcome statement.

Divine intervention

How do you come up with interventions? There are several ways. First, consider interventions that you or your patient have successfully tried before. For example, if the patient is having trouble sleeping in the hospital and he tells you that a glass of warm milk helps him get to sleep at home, this could work as an intervention for the expected outcome *Sleep through the night without medication by 11/9*.

You can also pick interventions from standardized plans of care, ask other nurses about interventions they have used successfully, or check nursing journals for ideas. If these methods don't work, try brainstorming with other nurses.

> When writing interventions, clearly state the necessary action.

Writing interventions

To help you write interventions clearly and correctly, follow these guidelines:

• *Clearly state the necessary action.* Note how and when to perform the intervention, and include special instructions. *Promote comfort* doesn't say what specific action to take, but *Administer ordered analgesic ½ hour before dressing change* says exactly what to do and when to do it.

- *Make interventions fit the patient.* Consider the patient's age, condition, developmental level, environment, and values. For instance, if he's a vegetarian, don't write an intervention that requires him to eat lean meat to gain extra protein for healing.
- *Keep the patient's safety in mind.* Consider the patient's physical and mental limitations. For instance, before teaching a patient how to give himself medication, be sure he's physically able to do it and that he can remember and follow the regimen.
- *Follow your facility's rules.* For example, if your facility allows only nurses to administer medications, don't write an intervention calling for the patient to *Administer hemorrhoidal suppositories as needed.*
- *Consider other health care activities.* Adjust your interventions when other activities interfere with them. For example, you might want your patient to get plenty of rest on a day when he has several diagnostic tests scheduled.
- *Use available resources.* If your patient needs to learn about his cardiac problem, use your facility's education department, literature from the American Heart Association, and local support groups. Write your intervention to reflect the use of these resources.

Charting interventions

Once you have performed an intervention, record the nature of the intervention, the time you performed it, and the patient's response. Also record other interventions that you performed based on his response and the reasons you performed them. This makes your documentation outcome-oriented.

Tailor your style (and format) to policy

Where do you document interventions? That depends on your facility's policy. You can document them on graphic records, on a patient care flow sheet that integrates all nurses' notes for a 1-day period, on integrated or separate nurses' progress notes, and on other specialized documentation forms such as the medication administration record.

Your facility's policies also dictate the style and format of your documentation. You should record interventions when you give routine care, give emergency care, observe changes in the patient's condition, and administer medications.

Evaluation

The current emphasis on evaluating your interventions has changed documentation. Traditional documentation didn't always reflect the end results of nursing care. But today, your progress notes must include an evaluation of your patient's progress toward the expected outcomes you have established in the plan of care.

Charting changes

The most commonly used charting method is expected outcomes and evaluation documentation. It focuses on the patient's response to nursing care and helps you provide high quality, cost-effective care. It's replacing narrative charting and lengthy, hand-written plans of care. (See *Effective evaluation statements.*)

A tough transition

The transition to outcome documentation has been difficult for some nurses. In outcome documentation, the nurse is expected to record nursing judgments, not just nursing interventions. Unfortunately, nurses have traditionally been trained not to make judgments. Today, nurses are being asked to gather and interpret data, refer and prioritize care, and document their findings.

The belief that hands-on care is more important than documentation is one reason nurses commonly focus more on nursing interventions than on documenting patient responses. Outcomes and evaluation documentation compels nurses to focus on patient responses. When you evaluate the results of your interventions, you help ensure that your plan is working.

The value of evaluation

Evaluation of care gives you a chance to:
- determine if your original assessment findings still apply
- uncover complications
- analyze patterns or trends in the patient's care and his response to it
- assess the patient's response to all aspects of his care, including medications, changes in diet or activity, procedures, unusual incidents or problems, and teaching
- determine how closely care conforms to established standards
- measure how well you have cared for the patient
- assess the performance of other members of the health care team
- identify opportunities to improve the quality of your care.

Effective evaluation statements

The evaluation statements below clearly describe common outcomes. Note that they include specific details of the care provided and objective evidence of the patient's response to care.

- *Able to describe the signs and symptoms of hyperglycemia.* (response to patient education)
- *States leg pain decreased from 9 to 6 (on a scale of 1 to 10) 30 minutes after receiving I.M. meperidine.* (response to pain medication within 1 hour of administration)
- *Able to ambulate to chair with a steady gait, approximately 10', unassisted.* (tolerance of change or increase in activity)
- *Unable to tolerate removal of O_2; became dyspneic on room air even at rest.* (tolerance of treatments).

Whenever within sight

Evaluation itself is an ongoing process that takes place whenever you see your patient. However, how often you're required to make evaluations depends on several factors, including where you work.

If you work in an acute care setting, your facility's policy may require you to review plans of care every 24 hours. But if you work in a long-term care facility, the required interval between evaluations may be up to 30 days. In either case, you should evaluate and revise the plan of care more often if warranted.

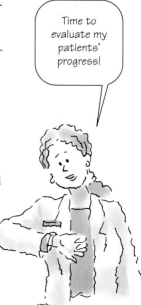

Time to evaluate my patients' progress!

Evaluating expected outcomes

Evaluation includes gathering reassessment data, comparing findings with the outcome criteria, determining the extent of outcome achievement (whether the outcome was met, partially met, or not met), writing evaluation statements, and revising the plan of care.

Not resolved? Revise...

Revision starts with determining whether the patient has achieved the outcomes. If they haven't been fully met and you decide that the problem is resolved, the plan can be discontinued. If the problem persists, continue the plan with new target dates until the desired status is achieved. If outcomes are partially met or unmet, identify interfering factors, such as misinterpreted information or a change in the patient's status, and revise the plan accordingly.

Revision may involve:
- clarifying or amending the database to reflect new information
- reexamining and correcting nursing diagnoses
- establishing outcome criteria that reflect new information and new or amended nursing strategies
- adding the revised nursing plan of care to the original document
- recording the rationale for the revision in the nurses' progress notes.

Documenting evaluation

Evaluation statements should indicate whether expected outcomes were achieved and should list evidence supporting this conclusion. Base these statements on outcome criteria from the plan of care, and use action verbs, such as *demonstrate* or *ambulate*.

Get specific

Include the patient's response to specific treatments, such as medication administration or physical therapy, and describe the condition under which the response occurred or failed to occur. Document patient teaching and palliative or preventive care as well.

After evaluating the outcome, be sure to record it in the patient's chart with clear statements that demonstrate his progress toward meeting the expected outcomes.

Cheat sheet

Notes on the nursing process

Assessment
• Guides the nursing process and communicates information to the health care team about the patient's condition
• Begins with a health history and physical examination
• Should follow JCAHO standards
 – physical factors
 – psychological and social factors
 – environmental factors
 – self-care capabilities
 – learning needs
 – discharge planning needs

Nursing diagnosis
• Consists of the human response or problem, related factors, and signs and symptoms
• Must be formulated, prioritized, and then used to guide the plan of care

Outcome identification
• Consists of four parts: behavior, measure, condition, and time
• Should be concise, specific, realistic, measurable, and patient focused

Plan of care
• May be traditional or standardized
• Consists of nursing diagnoses, expected outcomes, and nursing interventions
• Is used by all members of the health care team

• Involves assigning priorities, selecting nursing interventions, and documenting diagnoses, outcomes, interventions, and evaluations
• May need to be modified if your patient's condition changes

Implementation
• Involves interventions, which help the patient reach his expected outcomes and should be formulated with the patient's input
• Should be documented properly—involves writing interventions that clearly state the action, are individualized, address patient safety, adhere to facility policy, consider other heath care activities, and use available resources

Evaluation
• Consists of outcomes that include specific details about patient care and evidence of the patient's response to this care
• Includes gathering reassessment data, comparing findings, determining outcome achievement, writing evaluation statements, and revising plan of care, if necessary

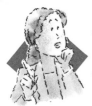

Quick quiz

1. The nursing health history is most accurately described as:
A.   a tool to guide diagnosis and treatment of the illness.
B.   a follow-up to the medical history.
C.   an interview that focuses holistically on the human response to illness.

Answer: C. This is how the nursing health history differs from a medical health history, which focuses on diagnosis and treatment.

2. Which of the following is the primary source of assessment information?
A.   The patient
B.   Past medical records
C.   The patient's family members

Answer: A. However, if the patient is sedated, confused, hostile, angry, dyspneic, or in pain, you may have to rely initially on family members or close friends to supply information.

3. Expected outcomes are defined as:
A.   goals the patient should reach as a result of planned nursing interventions.
B.   what the patient and family ask you to accomplish.
C.   goals a little higher than what the patient can realistically reach to help motivate him.

Answer: A. Expected outcomes are realistic, measurable goals and their target dates.

4. A good way to come up with interventions is by:
A.   asking the doctor.
B.   asking the patient what has worked for him before.
C.   reviewing past medical records.

Answer: B. You can also ask other nurses, check nursing journals, pick interventions from standardized plans of care, or brainstorm.

Scoring

☆☆☆   If you answered all four items correctly, chalk one up to success! You're an avid assessment aficionado!

☆☆   If you answered three items correctly, document your diligence! You're a dedicated diagnosis devotee!

☆   If you answered fewer than three items correctly, keep striving for excellence! Soon you'll be an expert evaluation enthusiast!

3

Plans of care

Just the facts

In this chapter, you'll learn:

♦ reasons for writing a plan of care

♦ differences between traditional and standardized plans of care

♦ parts of a patient-teaching plan and how to formulate one

♦ about critical pathways and how to use them.

A look at the nursing plan of care

The nursing plan of care is a vital part of documentation. To the health care team, the nursing plan of care is a principal source of information about the patient's problems, needs, and goals. It contains detailed instructions for achieving the goals established for the patient and is used to direct care. It also includes suggestions for solving the patient's problems and dealing with unexpected complications.

There are five aspects to writing the plan of care:

establishing care priorities based on assessment data

identifying expected outcomes

developing nursing interventions to attain these outcomes

evaluating the patient's responses

documenting the plan in the format required by your facility.

Now a part of the permanent record

Until 1991, the plan of care wasn't a required part of the patient's permanent record. It was used by the nursing staff and, in some facilities, it was discarded when the patient was discharged. Now, the Joint Commission on Accreditation of Healthcare Organizations (JCAHO) requires that the plan of care be permanently integrated into the medical record by written or electronic means.

JCAHO policy changes have also led to greater flexibility when writing plans of care. The commission no longer specifies the format for documenting patient care, so new methods have emerged that can make planning faster and easier.

Types of plans of care

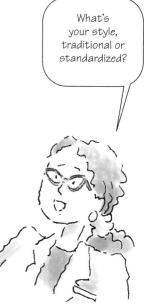

What's your style, traditional or standardized?

You may write your plans of care in one of two styles, *traditional* or *standardized*. Whatever approach you use, your plan of care should cover all nursing care from admission to discharge.

Traditional plan of care

Also called an *individually developed plan of care*, the traditional plan is written from scratch for each patient. After you analyze your assessment data for a patient, you either write the plan by hand or enter it into a computer. (See *It's traditional.*)

Good form

The basic form for the traditional plan of care varies, depending on the function of this important document in your facility or department. Most forms have four main columns:
• one for nursing diagnoses
• a second for expected outcomes
• a third for interventions
• a fourth for outcome evaluations.

There may be other columns for the dates when you initiated the plans of care, target dates for expected outcomes, and the dates for review, revisions, and resolutions. Most forms also have a place for you to sign or initial whenever you make an entry or a revision.

Looking toward an outcome

What should you include on the forms? This varies, too. Because shorter hospital stays are more common today, in most health care facilities, you're expected to write only short-term outcomes that the patient can reach by the time he's discharged.

However, some facilities—especially long-term care facilities—also want you to chart long-term outcomes for the patient's maximum functioning level. These facilities commonly provide forms with separate spaces for short- and long-term outcomes.

Art of the chart

It's traditional

Here's an example of a traditional plan of care. It shows how these forms are typically organized. Remember that a traditional plan is written from scratch for each patient.

Date	Nursing diagnosis	Expected outcomes	Interventions	Outcomes evaluation (initials and date)
2/15/02	Ineffective breathing pattern R/T pain as evidenced by c/o pain with deep breaths or coughing	Respiratory rate stays within 5 of baseline ABG levels remain normal Achieves comfort without depressing respirations Demonstrates correct use of incentive spirometry Auscultation reveals no adventitious breath sounds States understanding of the importance of taking deep breaths periodically Reports ability to breathe comfortably	Assess and record respiratory status q4h. Assess for pain q3h. Give pain medication as ordered p.r.n. Assist the patient to a comfortable position. Assist the patient in using incentive spirometry. Teach the patient how to splint chest while coughing. Perform chest physiotherapy to aid in mobilizing and removing secretions. Provide rest periods. Encourage the patient to use incentive spirometry. Provide oxygen as ordered.	

> Nursing diagnoses, expected outcomes, interventions, and outcomes evaluations are key elements of traditional plans of care.

Review dates		
Date	**Signature**	**Initials**
2/16/02	M. Hopper, RN	MH

Personal, visual, clear

The traditional method has several advantages:
• It provides a personalized plan for each patient.
• The format allows health care team members and the patient to easily visualize the plan.

- Columns for outcomes evaluations are clearly delineated.

Time isn't on its side

The main disadvantage of the traditional method is that it's time-consuming to read and write because it requires lengthy documentation.

Standardized plan of care

The standardized plan of care is commonly used today. A standardized plan eliminates the problems associated with the traditional plan by using preprinted information. This saves documentation time. (See *Why stand on tradition? Use a standardized plan.*)

Some standardized plans are classified by medical diagnoses or diagnosis-related groups (DRGs); others, by nursing diagnoses. The preprinted information included in a standardized plan of care includes interventions for patients with similar diagnoses and, usually, root outcome statements.

Insist on individuality

Early versions of standardized plans of care didn't allow for differences in patients' needs. However, current versions require you to explain how you have individualized the plan for each patient by adding the following information:

- *"related to" (R/T) statements and signs and symptoms for a nursing diagnosis.* If the form provides a root diagnosis — such as "Acute pain R/T _____" — you might fill in *inflammation, as exhibited by grimacing and other expressions of pain.*
- *time limits for the outcomes.* To a root statement of the goal *Perform postural drainage without assistance,* you might add *for 15 minutes immediately upon awakening in the morning, by 11/12.*
- *frequency of interventions.* To an intervention such as *Perform passive range-of-motion exercises,* you might add *twice per day: once in the morning and in the evening.*
- *specific instructions for interventions.* For the standard intervention *Elevate the patient's head,* you might specify *before sleep, on three pillows.*

Each patient has unique needs.

We sure do. I need dessert.

Art of the chart

Why stand on tradition? Use a standardized plan

The standardized plan of care below is for a patient with a nursing diagnosis of *Impaired tissue integrity*. To customize it to your patient, complete the diagnosis—including signs and symptoms—and fill in the expected outcomes.

> There's a lot less writing with standardized plans.

Date _2/15/02_

Nursing diagnosis

Impaired tissue integrity related to arterial insufficiency

Target date _2/17/02_

Expected outcomes

Attains relief from immediate symptoms: _pain, ulcers, edema_

Voices intent to change aggravating behavior: _will stop smoking immediately_

Maintains collateral circulation: _palpable peripheral pulses, extremities warm and pink with good capillary refill_

Voices intent to follow specific management routines after discharge: _foot care guidelines, exercise regimen as specified by physical therapy department_

Date _2/15/02_

Interventions

- Provide foot care. Administer and monitor treatments according to facility protocols.
- Encourage adherence to an exercise regimen as tolerated.
- Educate the patient about risk factors and prevention of injury. Refer the patient to a stop-smoking program.
- Maintain adequate hydration. Monitor I/O _q8h._
- To increase arterial blood supply to the extremities, elevate head of bed _6" to 8"._
- Additional interventions: _inspect skin integrity q8h._

Date _____

Outcomes evaluation

Attained relief of immediate symptoms: _____

Voiced intent to change aggravating behavior: _____

Maintained collateral circulation: _____

Voiced intent to follow specific management routines after discharge: _____

Computers make combos less cumbersome

When a patient has more than one diagnosis, you have to combine standardized plans of care, which can make records long and cumbersome. However, if your facility uses computerized plans, you can extract only the parts you need from each plan and then combine them to make one manageable plan. Some computer programs provide a checklist of interventions from which you can select to build your own plan.

Although standardized plans usually include only essential information, most provide space for you to write additional nursing diagnoses, expected outcomes, interventions, and outcomes evaluations.

These advantages come standard

Standardized plans of care offer many advantages because they:
- require far less writing than traditional plans
- are more legible
- are easier to duplicate
- make compliance with a facility's policy easier for all members of the health care team, including experts, novices, and ancillary staff
- guide you in creating the plan and allow you the freedom to adapt it to your patient.

Is it individualized?

This method has one main drawback: If you simply check off items on a list or fill in the blanks, you might not individualize the patient's care or document your findings adequately.

Patient-teaching plan

A patient-teaching plan serves several important functions:
- It pinpoints what the patient needs to learn and how he'll be taught.
- It sets criteria for evaluating how well the patient learns.
- It helps all caregivers coordinate their teaching.
- It serves as legal proof that the patient received appropriate instruction and satisfies the requirements of regulatory agencies such as JCAHO.

Pointers for the perfect plan

To make sure that your teaching plan is as effective as possible, consider carefully what the patient needs to learn, how you'll teach him, and how you'll measure the results. Work closely with the patient, members of his family, and other health care team members to create realistic and attainable goals for your plan. Also provide for follow-up teaching at home, if appropriate.

Be sure to keep your plan flexible. Allow for factors that may interfere with effective teaching, such as a patient's unreceptiveness because of a poor night's sleep or your own daily time constraints.

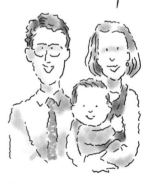

Make sure that you include us in your teaching plan.

Parts of the teaching plan

The patient-teaching plan is divided into five sections:

- the patient's learning needs
- expected learning outcomes
- teaching content
- teaching methods
- teaching tools.

Learning needs

The first step in developing a teaching plan is to identify what your patient needs to learn. Consider what you, the doctor, and other health care team members expect him to learn as well as what he expects to learn.

Learning outcomes

After you identify the patient's learning needs, you can establish expected learning outcomes, sometimes called *learning objectives*. Beginning with your assessment findings, list the topics and strategies that the patient needs to learn to reach the maximum level of health and self-care.

An integrated approach

Like other patient care outcomes, expected learning outcomes should focus on the patient and be easy to measure. Learning behaviors and the outcomes you develop fall into three categories:

- cognitive — relating to understanding
- affective — dealing with attitudes and feelings
- psychomotor — involving manual skills.

For example, for a patient who is learning to give himself subcutaneous injections, identifying an injection site is a *cognitive outcome*, coping with the need for injections is an *affective outcome*, and giving the injection is a *psychomotor outcome*. (See *Penning precise learning outcomes*, page 44.)

Which evaluation techniques are most valuable?

To develop precise, measurable outcomes, decide which evaluation techniques best reveal the patient's progress. For cognitive

Penning precise learning outcomes

Learning behaviors fall into three categories: cognitive, psychomotor, and affective. Keeping these categories in mind will help you to write clear, concise learning outcomes. Remember that your outcomes should clarify what you plan to teach, what behavior you expect to see, and what criteria you'll use for evaluating the patient's learning.

Compare the following two sets of learning outcomes.

Well-phrased learning outcomes	Poorly phrased learning outcomes
Cognitive domain	
The patient with heart failure will be able to: • state when to take each prescribed drug • describe symptoms of heart failure.	The patient with heart failure will be able to: • remember his medication schedule • recognize when his respiratory rate is increased.
Affective domain	
The patient with heart failure will be able to: • report feeling comfortable when breathing • demonstrate willingness to comply with therapy by keeping scheduled doctor appointments.	The patient with heart failure will be able to: • adjust successfully to limitations of disease • realize the importance of seeing his doctor.
Psychomotor domain	
The patient with heart failure will be able to: • demonstrate diaphragmatic pursed-lip breathing • demonstrate skill in conserving energy while carrying out activities.	The patient with heart failure will be able to: • take his respiratory rate • bring in a sputum specimen for laboratory studies.

learning, you might use questions and answers; for psychomotor learning, you might use return demonstration.

To measure affective learning — which can be difficult because changes in attitude develop slowly — you can use several evaluation techniques. For example, to determine whether a patient has overcome his anxiety about giving himself an injection, try asking him if he still feels anxious. You also can assess his willingness to perform the procedure and observe whether he hesitates or shows other signs of stress while doing it.

Then write the outcome statement based on the selected evaluation technique. For example, if you select return demonstration as your evaluation technique, an appropriate outcome statement might be *Patient demonstrates skill in giving a subcutaneous injection.*

Content

Next, select what to teach the patient to help him achieve the expected outcomes. Be sure to consult with the patient, members of his family, and other caregivers before deciding what to teach. Even if the patient is learning to care for himself, you still should teach a family member how to provide physical and emotional support or how to help the patient remember his care.

Start simple

Once you have decided what to teach, organize your instruction to begin with the simplest concepts and work toward the more complex ones. This is especially helpful when teaching a patient with little education or one with a learning disability.

Methods

Now, select the appropriate teaching methods. Most of your teaching probably can be done one-on-one. This allows you to learn about your patient, build a relationship with him, and individualize your teaching to his needs.

Taking different paths to learning

Many different teaching methods work well along with, or instead of, one-on-one teaching. For instance, try incorporating demonstration, practice, and return demonstration in your teaching plan. Role playing can increase your patient's involvement in the plan, as can case studies, which require him to evaluate how someone else with his disorder responds to different situations.

Other methods include self-monitoring, which requires the patient to assess his situation and to determine which aspects of his environment or behavior need correction. You also can conduct group lectures and discussions if several patients require similar instruction, such as with childbirth or diabetes education.

Tools

Finally, decide what teaching tools will help enhance patient education. When choosing your tools, focus on what will work best for your patient. For instance, if your patient learns best by watching how something is done, use a videotape of a procedure or a closed-circuit television demonstration. (See *Tools for tuning up teaching*, page 46.)

If the patient prefers a hands-on approach, let him handle the equipment he'll use. If he likes to work interactively at his own pace, try an interactive, computerized patient-teaching program. If he learns best by reading, provide written materials.

Tracking down teaching tools

To get the tools you need, consult the staff-development instructors on your unit, your facility's librarian, or staff specialists. If you can't find what you need, call pharmaceutical and medical supply companies in your community. Also, contact national associations and foundations such as the American Cancer Society. These organizations usually have many patient education materials written for the layperson. They also provide pamphlets and brochures in several languages.

Keep the patient's abilities and limitations in mind as you choose teaching tools. For example, before giving him written materials, such as brochures and pamphlets, make sure that he can read and understand them. Keep in mind that the average adult reads at only a seventh-grade level.

Break down language barriers

Likewise, make sure you're aware of any language barriers between you and your patient. Use translators and bilingual aids — such as cards and pamphlets — to overcome these barriers.

Documenting the patient-teaching plan

The patient-teaching plan is a key part of the patient's plan of care. By reading it, health care team members can see at a glance what the patient learned and what he still needs to learn. It's also needed by the health care facility to show what quality improvement measures are in progress.

Give it time...and thought

Constructing individual teaching plans requires time and thought. Fortunately, some facilities have patient education departments that develop and implement standard teaching plans for many common disorders.

Forms, forms, and more forms

There are several different forms for documenting your patient-teaching plan. Many of these incorporate the nursing process as it applies to patient education. (See *Go with the flow sheet*.)

Just your type

Patient-teaching plans also come in two basic types that are similar to traditional and standardized plans of care. The traditional type begins with the nursing diagnosis statement *deficient knowl-*

Tools for tuning up teaching

This list includes teaching materials and methods you can use to optimize your patient's learning.

Teaching materials
Teaching materials include:
• brochures and pamphlets
• videotapes
• closed-circuit television
• computers
• equipment being used for patient care (for example, syringes, needles, and pumps).

Teaching methods
Teaching methods include:
• role playing
• return demonstration
• student-to-student instruction, if appropriate.

Art of the chart

Go with the flow sheet

Below is the first page of a patient-teaching flow sheet. Flow sheets like this one let you quickly and easily individualize your teaching plan to fit your patient's needs.

PATIENT-TEACHING FLOW SHEET

ASTHMA

Problems affecting learning

☐ None   ☐ Cognitive or sensory impairment   ☐ Lack of motivation

☑ Fatigue or pain   ☐ Physical disability   Other_____

☐ Communication problem

> This form provides standard learning outcomes for patients with asthma.

LEARNING OUTCOMES	INITIAL TEACHING						REINFORCEMENT					
	Date	Time	Learner	Techniques and tools	Evaluation	Initials	Date	Time	Learner	Techniques and tools	Evaluation	Initials
Basic knowledge												
• Define asthma.	3/9/02	1100	P	E,W	Dv	CB	3/10/02	1100	P	E,W	S	CB
• List two symptoms of asthma.	3/9/02	1100	P	E,W	Dv	CB	3/10/02	1100	P	E,W	S	CB
Medication												
• State the action of theophylline and its effects on the body.	3/9/02	1100	P	E,W	S	CB						
• Name the two inhalers used. Give their onsets, peaks, and durations.	3/9/02	1100	P	E,W,V	Dv	CB						
• Demonstrate the ability to use the inhalers using correct technique.	3/9/02	1100	P	E,W	S	CB						

KEY	**Learner**	**Teaching techniques**	**Evaluation**
	P = patient	D = demonstration	S = states understanding
	S = spouse	E = explanation	D = demonstrates understanding
	M = mother	R = role playing	Dp = demonstrates understanding
	F = father	**Teaching tools**	with physical coaching
	D1 = daughter 1_____	F = filmstrip	Dv = demonstrates understanding
	D2 = daughter 2_____	P = physical model	with verbal coaching
	S1 = son 1 _____	S = slide	T = passes written test
	S2 = son 2 _____	V = videotape	N = no indication of learning
	O = other_____	W = written material	NE = not evaluated

edge and an individualized *related to* statement — for example, *Deficient knowledge related to low-sodium diet*. It provides only the format and requires you to come up with the plan.

The standardized type allows you to check off or date steps as you complete them and add or delete information to individualize the plan. It's best suited for patients who need extensive teaching.

Some plans include space for documenting problems that could hinder learning, for comments and evaluations, and for dates and signatures. Or you may need to include this information in your progress notes. No matter which teaching plan you use, this information becomes a permanent part of the patient's medical record.

Critical pathways

A critical pathway is an interdisciplinary plan of care that describes assessment criteria, interventions, treatments, and outcomes for specific health-related conditions (usually based on a DRG) across a designated time line.

Accomplished a goal? Check it off!

Think of the pathway as a predetermined checklist describing the tasks you and the patient need to accomplish. In this way, it's similar to a standardized plan of care. However, unlike a plan of care, its focus is multidisciplinary, covering all of the patient's problems, not just those identified during a nursing assessment.

Critical pathways go by many different names: clinical pathways, critical paths, interdisciplinary plans, anticipated recovery plans, care maps, interdisciplinary action plans, and action plans.

A collaborative effort

Members of the health care team involved in providing care should collaborate to develop each critical pathway. The goals of the critical pathway include:
• achieving expected patient and family outcomes
• promoting professional collaborative practice and care
• ensuring continuity of care
• ensuring appropriate use of resources
• reducing the cost and length of stay
• establishing a framework for instituting and monitoring continuous quality improvement.

Practical when predictable

Critical pathways are most useful in specific types of patient care situations. They work well with high-volume cases (meaning the facility cares for a lot of patients with this particular problem) and in situations that have relatively predictable outcomes. Complex situations with unpredictable outcomes normally aren't managed with critical pathways.

It's simple: A critical pathway is a critical tool...

A critical pathway is a permanent part of the medical record. It provides a consistent assessment and documentation tool for third-party payers. It's also used to compare the diagnoses of patients and determine their needs.

Critical pathways cover the key events that must occur before the patient's target discharge date. These events include:
- consultations
- diagnostic tests
- treatments
- medications
- procedures
- activities
- diet
- patient teaching
- discharge planning
- achievement of anticipated outcomes.

I predict that you'll achieve your outcomes.

Charting the path

A critical pathway is usually organized according to categories, such as activity, diet, treatments, medications, patient teaching, and discharge planning. Appropriate categories are determined based on the patient's medical diagnosis. The medical diagnosis also dictates expected length of stay, daily care guidelines, and expected outcomes. Care guidelines are listed under appropriate categories.

The structure of a critical pathway and the categories it contains vary among facilities. Within a facility, the structure and content of critical pathways may vary depending on the specific DRG. (See *Take the critical pathway,* page 50.)

Some facilities use nursing diagnoses as the basis for critical pathways, but this is controversial. Critics argue that this format interferes with communication and the coordination of care among nonnursing members of the health care team.

A bundle of benefits

For the most part, critical pathways are a benefit to nurses. Here's why:
- They eliminate duplicate charting. The only time you need to write narrative notes is when a standard on the pathway remains

(Text continues on page 52.)

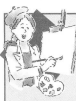

Art of the chart

Take the critical pathway

At any point in a treatment course, a glance at the critical pathway allows you to compare the patient's progress and your performance as a caregiver with standards.

The standard critical pathway below outlines care for a patient with a colon resection.

CRITICAL PATHWAY: COLON RESECTION WITHOUT COLOSTOMY				
	Patient visit	**Presurgery day 1**	**Day 0 O.R. day**	**Postoperative day 1**
Assessments	History and physical with breast, rectal, and pelvic examinations Nursing assessment	Nursing admission assessment	Nursing admission assessment on TBA patients in holding area Postoperative review of systems assessment*	Review of systems assessment*
Consults	Social service consult Physical therapy consult	Notify referring doctor of impending admission		
Labs and diagnostics	Complete blood count (CBC) PT/PTT Electrocardiogram Chest X-ray (CXR) Chemistry profile CT scan ABD w/wo contrast CT scan pelvis Urinalysis Barium enema and flexible sigmoidoscopy or colonoscopy Biopsy report	Type and screen for patients with Hg level < 10	Type and screen for patients in holding area with Hg level < 10	CBC
Interventions	Many or all of the above labs and diagnostics will have already been done. Check all results and fax to the surgeon's	Admit by 8 a.m. Check for bowel preparation orders Bowel preparation* Antiembolism stockings Incentive spirometry Ankle exercises* I.V. access* Routine VS* Pneumatic inflation boots	Shave and prepare in operating room NG tube maintenance* I/O VS per routine* Foley care* Incentive spirometry* Ankle exercises* I.V. site care* HOB 30° Safety measures* Wound care* Mouth care*	NG tube maintenance* I/O* VS per routine* Foley care* Incentive spirometry* Ankle exercises* I.V. site care* HOB 30°* Safety measures* Wound care* Mouth care* Antiembolism stockings
I.V.s		I.V. fluids, D5½ NSS	I.V. fluids, D5LR	I.V. fluids, D5LR
Medication	Prescribe GoLYTELY or NuLYTELY 10a-2p Neomycin @ 2p, 3p, and 10p Erythromycin @ 2p, 3p, and 10p	GoLYTELY or NuLYTELY 10a-2p Erythromycin @ 2p, 3p, and 10p Neomycin @ 2p, 3p, and 10p	Preoperative ABX in holding area Postoperative ABX × 2 doses PCA (basal rate 0.5 mg) S.C. heparin	
Diet/GI	Clears presurgery day NPO after midnight	Clears presurgery day NPO after midnight	NPO/NG tube	
Activity			4 hours after surgery ambulate with abdominal binder* D/C pneumatic inflation boots once patient ambulates	Ambulate t.i.d. with abdominal binder* May shower Physical therapy b.i.d.
KEY: *NSG Activities **V = Variance** **N = No Var.** **NSG care performed:** **Signatures:**	V V V N N N ☑ ☑ ☑ 1. _C. Malloy, RN_ 2. _____ 3. _____	V V V N N N ☑ ☑ ☑ 1. _M Connel, RN_ 2. _____ 3. _____	V V V N N N ☑ ☑ ☑ 1. _L. Singer, RN_ 2. _J. Smith, RN_ 3. _P. Joseph, RN_	V V V N N N ☑ ☑ ☑ 1. _L. Singer, RN_ 2. _J. Smith, RN_ 3. _P. Joseph, RN_

The pathway designates a specific time frame for patient care activities.

The pathway is organized into categories based on the patient's medical diagnosis.

The pathway lists tasks that the patient and caregivers need to accomplish.

Take the critical pathway (continued)

CRITICAL PATHWAY: COLON RESECTION WITHOUT COLOSTOMY

	Postoperative day 2	Postoperative day 3	Postoperative day 4	Postoperative day 5
Assessments	Review of systems assessment*	Review of systems assessment*	Review of systems assessment	Review of systems assessment*
Consults		Dietary consult		Oncology consult if indicated (Dukes B2 or C or high risk lesion) (or to be done as outpatient)
Labs and diagnostics	Electrolyte 7 (EL-7) CXR	CBC EL-7	Pathology results on chart	CBC EL-7
Interventions	D/C nasogastric (NG) tube if possible* (per guidelines) Intake and output (I/O)* VS per routine* D/C Foley* Ambulating* Incentive spirometry* Ankle exercises* I.V. site care* Head of bed (HOB) 30°* Safety measures* Wound care* Mouth care* Antiembolism stockings	I/O* VS per routine* Incentive spirometry* Ankle exercises* I.V. site care* Safety measures* Wound care* Antiembolism stockings	I/O* VS per routine* Incentive spirometry* Ankle exercises* I.V. site care* Safety measures* Wound care* Antiembolism stockings	Consider staple removal Replace with Steri-Strips Assess that patient has met D/C criteria* D/C saline lock
I.V.s	I.V. fluids $D_5\frac{1}{2}$ NSS+ MVI	I.V. convert to saline lock	Continue saline lock	D/C s
Medication	PCA (0.5 mg basal rate)	D/C PCA P.O. analgesia Resume routine home meds	P.O. analgesia Preoperative meds	P.O. analgesia Preoperative meds
Diet/GI	D/C NG tube per guidelines: (Clamp tube at 8 a.m. if no N/V and residual < 200 ml, D/C tube @ 12 noon)* (Check with doctor first)	Clears if+bm/flatus Advance to postoperative diet if tolerating clears (at least one tray of clears)	House	House
Activity	Ambulate q.i.d. with abdominal binder* May shower Physical therapy b.i.d.	Ambulate at least q.i.d. with abdominal binder* May shower Physical therapy b.i.d.	Ambulate at least q.i.d. with abdominal binder* May shower Physical therapy b.i.d.	
Teaching	Reinforce preoperative teaching* Patient and family education p.r.n.* Re: family screening	Reinforce preoperative teaching* Patient and family education p.r.n.* Re: family screening Begin D/C teaching	Reinforce preoperative teaching* Patient and family education p.r.n.* D/C teaching re: reportable s/s, follow-up, and wound care*	Review all D/C instructions and Rx including:* follow-up appointments: with surgeon within 3 weeks with oncologist within 1 month if
KEY: *NSG Activities **V = Variance** **N = No Var.** **NSG care performed:** **Signatures:**	V V V N N N ☑ ☑ ☑ 1. _A. McCarthy, RN_ 2. _R. Mayer, RN_ 3. ____	V V V N N N ☑ ☑ ☑ 1. _A. McCarthy, RN_ 2. _R. Mayer, RN_ 3. ____	V V V N N N ☑ ☑ ☑ 1. _L. Singer, RN_ 2. _J. Smith, RN_ 3. _P. Joseph, RN_	V V V N N N ☑ ☑ ☑ 1. _L. Singer, RN_ 2. _J. Smith, RN_ 3. _P. Joseph, RN_

> The pathway lists key events that must occur before the patient's discharge date.

unmet or when the patient needs different care than what's written on the form. Most pathways provide a place to document alterations in care.

• With standardized orders or protocols, you can advance the patient's activity level, diet, and treatment regimen without waiting for a doctor's order. Nurses have more freedom to make care decisions.

• Communication improves between members of the health care team because everyone works from the same plan. That's why problems are called *collaborative problems*. The goal is for all members of the team to work together to achieve the desired outcome.

• Quality of care improves because of shared accountability for patient outcomes.

• Patient teaching and discharge planning improves. In facilities where critical pathways are adapted and given to patients, they feel less anxious and are more cooperative because they know what to expect and what's expected of them. Some patients even recover and go home sooner than anticipated.

Yippee! Critical pathways improve my performance!

Here's where it gets complicated...

A significant disadvantage of critical pathways is that they're less effective for patients who have several diagnoses or who have complications. Establishing a time line for these patients is more difficult.

For example, treatment progress is usually predictable for a patient who has a cholecystectomy and is otherwise healthy. However, if a patient has diabetes and coronary artery disease, the treatment course is fairly unpredictable, and the plan of care is likely to change, resulting in lengthy and fragmented documentation.

Priorities in the pathway

Just as you prioritize your nursing diagnoses, you must set priorities for the collaborative problems in the critical pathway. For example, if your patient needs whirlpool treatments by the physical therapy department and nebulizer treatments from a respiratory therapist, you must coordinate these activities according to the patient's current status and needs.

If everyone on the health care team plans carefully and pays attention to the patient's response to treatments, you should be able to carry out your respective activities for the patient's benefit.

Cheat sheet

Plans of care review

Five aspects to writing plans of care
- Establishing care priorities
- Identifying expected outcomes
- Developing nursing interventions to attain these outcomes
- Evaluating the patient's response
- Documenting

Types of plans
Traditional
- Provides a personalized plan for each patient
- Allows the health care team and patient to visualize the plan
- Is clearly organized
BUT
- Is time-consuming to read and write

Standardized
- Uses preprinted information organized by diagnosis, which saves documentation time and facilitates adherence to facility standards
- Requires less writing, which makes it easier to read
- Is easier to duplicate
- Guides care while allowing adaptability
BUT
- May not be individualized properly if the nurse overlooks this important step

Patient-teaching plan
Functions
- To pinpoint what the patient needs to learn and how he'll be taught
- To establish criteria for patient-learning evaluation
- To help caregivers coordinate teaching
- To prove that the patient received appropriate instruction

Five sections
- Patient's learning needs
- Expected learning outcomes
- Teaching content

- Teaching methods
- Teaching tools

Critical pathway
Basics
- Includes a predetermined checklist of tasks you and your patient must accomplish
- Provides daily care guidelines and expected outcomes
- Dictates the length of stay

Goals
- To achieve expected patient and family outcomes
- To promote professional collaborative practice and care
- To ensure continuity of care
- To ensure appropriate use of resources
- To reduce the cost and length of stay
- To establish a framework for instituting and monitoring continuous quality improvement

Benefits
- Eliminates duplicate charting
- Gives nurses more freedom in making care decisions
- Improves communication between members of the health care team
- Improves quality of care
- Improves patient teaching and discharge planning

Disadvantage
- Is less effective for patients with multiple diagnoses and those who experience complications

Don't move on to the next chapter until you've reviewed this information on plans of care.

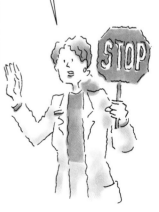

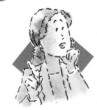

Quick quiz

1. Before 1991, the nursing plan of care was commonly:
   A. discarded when the patient was discharged.
   B. part of the patient's permanent record.
   C. used by doctors as well as nurses.

Answer: A. In 1991, JCAHO began requiring that the plan of care be permanently integrated into the patient's medical record.

2. People with access to the plan of care include:
   A. all caregivers, the patient, and members of his family.
   B. the nursing staff only.
   C. just nurses and doctors.

Answer: A. In addition to caregivers, the patient and members of his family should use the plan of care and make recommendations and evaluations.

3. Compared with a standardized plan of care, a traditional plan of care is:
   A. easier to duplicate.
   B. easier to adapt to recent policy changes by the JCAHO.
   C. easier to adapt to the individual patient.

Answer: C. The traditional plan of care is written from scratch to meet the needs of an individual patient. Standardized plans are preprinted and based on interventions for patients with similar diagnoses.

Scoring

☆☆☆ If you answered all three items correctly, wow! You might be nominated for the Pulitzer Prize in Outstanding Outcomes!

☆☆ If you answered two items correctly, wonderful! Your plans are more than precise, they're poetic. You excel in traditional, standardized, and free-verse formats.

☆ If you answered only one item correctly, practice more planning! The critics will soon be raving about your crafted critical pathways!

Charting systems

Just the facts

In this chapter, you'll learn:

♦ about different types of charting systems, including computerized charting, and how to use them

♦ advantages and disadvantages of each type of system

♦ how to choose a charting system.

A look at charting systems

Different health care facilities set their own requirements for documentation and evaluation, but all must comply with legal, accreditation, and professional standards. A nursing department also may select a documentation system, as long as it adheres to those standards.

Narrative or alternative?

Depending on your facility's policy, you'll use one or more documentation systems to record your nursing interventions and evaluations and the patient's response. Some facilities use traditional narrative charting systems. Others choose alternative systems.

Each documentation system includes specific policies and procedures for charting, so make sure you understand the documentation requirements for the system your facility uses. Understanding and adhering to these requirements will help you to document care systematically and accurately. (See *Comparing charting systems*, page 56.)

Comparing charting systems

The table below compares elements of the different charting systems used today. Note that the second column provides information on which systems work best in which settings.

System	Useful settings	Parts of record	Assessment	Plan of care	Outcomes and evaluation	Progress notes format
Narrative	• Acute care • Long-term care • Home care • Ambulatory care	• Progress notes • Flow sheets to supplement plan of care	• Initial: history and admission form • Ongoing: progress notes	• Plan of care	• Progress notes • Discharge summaries	• Narration at time of entry
Problem-oriented medical record (POMR)	• Acute care • Long-term care • Home care • Rehabilitation • Mental health facilities	• Database • Plan of care • Problem list • Progress notes • Discharge summary	• Initial: Database and plan of care • Ongoing: progress notes	• Database • Nursing plan of care based on problem list	• Progress notes (section E of SOAPIE and SOAPIER)	• SOAP, SOAPIE, SOAPIER
Problem-intervention-evaluation (PIE)	• Acute care	• Assessment flow sheets • Progress notes • Problem list	• Initial: Assessment form • Ongoing: assessment form every shift	• None; included in progress notes (section P)	• Progress notes (section E)	• Problem • Intervention • Evaluation
FOCUS	• Acute care • Long-term care	• Progress notes • Flow sheets • Checklists	• Initial: patient history and admission assessment • Ongoing: assessment form	• Nursing plan of care based on problems or nursing diagnoses	• Progress notes (section R)	• Data • Action • Response
Charting by exception (CBE)	• Acute care • Long-term care	• Plan of care • Flow sheets, including patient-teaching records and patient discharge notes • Graphic record • Progress notes	• Initial: database assessment sheet • Ongoing: nursing and medical order flow sheets	• Nursing plan of care based on nursing diagnoses	• Progress notes (section E)	• SOAPIE or SOAPIER
Flow sheet, assessment, concise, timely (FACT)	• Acute care • Long-term care	• Assessment sheet • Flow sheets • Progress notes	• Initial: baseline assessment • Ongoing: flow sheets and progress notes	• Nursing plan of care based on nursing diagnoses	• Flow sheets (section R)	• Data • Action • Response
Core (with DAE)	• Acute care • Long-term care	• Kardex • Flow sheets • Progress notes	• Initial: baseline assessment • Ongoing: progress notes	• Plan of care	• Progress notes (section E)	• Data • Action • Evaluation
Computerized	• Acute care • Long-term care • Home care • Ambulatory care	• Progress notes • Flow sheets • Nursing plan of care • Database • Teaching plan	• Initial: baseline assessment • Ongoing: progress notes	• Database • Plan of care	• Outcome-based plan of care	• Evaluative statements • Expected outcomes • Learning outcomes

Traditional narrative

Narrative charting is a chronological account of:
- the patient's status
- the nursing interventions performed
- the patient's responses.

No longer going it alone

Today, few facilities rely on this system alone. Instead, they combine it with other systems, especially the source-oriented record.

Using narrative charting

In the traditional narrative system, the nurse usually records data as progress notes, with flow sheets supplementing the narrative notes. Knowing when and what to document and how to organize the data are the key elements of effective narrative charting in the progress notes. (See *The full story on narrative charting,* page 58.)

The Joint Commission on Accreditation of Healthcare Organizations (JCAHO) requires all health care facilities to establish policies on the frequency of patient reassessment. So assess your patient at least as often as required by your facility's policy, and then document your findings.

Documentation mania!

If you find yourself writing repetitious, meaningless notes, you may be documenting too often. If so, double-check your facility's policy. You may be following a time-consuming, unwritten standard initiated by staff members, not by your facility. To guard against this, review the policy at least every 6 months.

Observe and take note

In addition to documenting according to facility policy, be sure to write specific and descriptive narrative in the progress notes whenever you observe:
- a change in the patient's condition, such as progression, regression, or new problems. For example, write *The patient can ambulate with a walker for 3 minutes before feeling tired.*
- a patient's response to a treatment or medication. For example, write *The patient states that abdominal pain is relieved 1 hour after receiving medication. He's smiling and able to turn in bed without difficulty.*

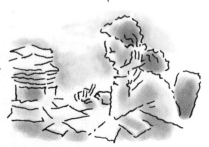

This is beginning to look all too familiar, not to mention meaningless. Am I documenting too much?

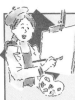

Art of the chart

The full story on narrative charting

This progress note is one example of narrative charting.

Date	Time	Notes
5/26/02	2245	Pt 4 hours postoperative: awakens easily; oriented x 3 but groggy. Incision site in front of ⓛ ear extending down and around ear and into neck - approximately 6" in length - without dressing. No swelling or bleeding, bluish discoloration below ⓛ ear noted, sutures intact. Jackson Pratt drain in ⓛ neck below ear with 20 ml bloody drainage measured. Drain remains secured in place with suture and anchored to ⓛ anterior chest wall with tape. Pt denied pain but stated she felt nauseated and promptly vomited 100 ml of clear fluid. Pt attempted to get OOB to ambulate to bathroom with assistance but felt dizzy upon standing. Assisted to lie down in bed. Voided 200 ml clear, yellow urine in bedpan. Pt encouraged to deep-breathe and cough q/h and turn frequently in bed. Antiembolism pads applied to both lower extremities. Explanations given re: these preventive measures. Pt verbalized understanding. —————————— Bridget Smith, RN
5/26/02	2255	Pt continues to feel nauseated. Compazine 10 mg I.M. given in R gluteus maximus. —————————— Bridget Smith, RN
5/26/02	2335	Pt states she is no longer nauseated, remains pain free. No further vomiting. Pt demonstrated taking deep breaths and coughing effectively. —— Bridget Smith, RN

> Be sure to record the date and time of each entry.

> Entries should be in chronological order.

> Remember to sign each entry.

• a lack of improvement in the patient's condition. For example, write *No change in size or condition of sacral decubitus ulcer after 6 days of treatment. Dimensions and condition remain as stated in 11/20/02 note.*

• a patient's or family member's response to teaching. For example, write *The patient was able to demonstrate walking with crutches using the proper technique.*

One thought leads to another

Before you write anything, organize your thoughts so your paragraphs flow smoothly. If you have trouble deciding what to write, refer to the patient's plan of care to review:

• unresolved problems
• prescribed interventions
• expected outcomes.

Then write down your observations of the patient's progress in these areas. (See *Put your thoughts in order.*)

A narrative with a happy story

Narrative charting has a lot going for it. After all, this charting format:

• is the most flexible of all the charting systems and is suitable in any clinical setting
• strongly conveys your nursing interventions and your patients' responses
• is ideal for presenting information that's collected over a long period
• combines well with other documentation devices, such as flow sheets, which cuts down on charting time

Advice from the experts

Put your thoughts in order

If you have trouble organizing your thoughts, use this sequence of questions to order your entry:
• How did I first become aware of the problem?
• What has the patient said about the problem that's significant?
• What have I observed that's related to the problem?
• What is my plan for dealing with the problem?
• What steps have I taken to intervene?
• How has the patient responded to my interventions?

A paragraph for each problem
To make your notes as coherent as possible, discuss each of the patient's problems in a separate paragraph; don't lump them together. Alternatively, use a head-to-toe approach to organize your information.

Doctor's orders
Be sure to notify the doctor of significant changes that you observe. Then document this communication, the doctor's responses, and any new orders to be implemented.

AIR: A fresh narrative format

A charting format called AIR may help you to organize and simplify your narrative charting. AIR is an acronym for:
• **A**ssessment
• **I**ntervention
• **R**esponse.

The AIR format synthesizes major nursing events and avoids repetition of information found elsewhere in the medical record. Combined with nursing flow sheets and the nursing plan of care, the AIR format can be used to document the care you provide clearly and concisely.

Here's how AIR is used to document nursing care.

Assessment

Summarize your physical assessment findings. Begin by specifying each issue that you address, such as nursing diagnosis, admission note, and discharge planning. Rather than simply describing the patient's current condition, document trends and record your impression of the problem.

Intervention

Summarize your actions and those of other caregivers in response to the assessment data. The summary may include a condensed nursing plan of care or plans for additional patient monitoring.

Response

Summarize the outcome or the patient's response to the nursing interventions. Because a response may not be evident for hours or even days, this documentation may not immediately follow the entries. In fact, it may be recorded by another nurse, which is why titling each of your assessments and interventions is so important.

• uses narration, the most common form of writing, so training new staff members can usually be done quickly
• places its narrative notes in chronological order, so other team members can review the patient's progress daily.

The narrative takes a turn for the worse...

On the other hand, narrative charting has the following things working against it:
• You have to read the entire record to find the patient outcome. Even then, you may have trouble determining the outcome of a problem because the same information may not be consistently documented.
• For the same reason, you may have trouble tracking problems and identifying trends in the patient's progress.
• Narrative charting offers no inherent guide to what's important to document, so nurses often document everything, resulting in a lengthy, repetitive record.

- Narrative charting doesn't always reflect the nursing process.
- Narratives may contain vague or inaccurate language, such as "appears to be bleeding" or "small amount."

You may be able to avoid some disadvantages of narrative charting by organizing the information you record. (See *AIR: A fresh narrative format.*)

Problem-oriented medical record

The problem-oriented medical record (POMR) focuses on specific patient problems and aids communication among team members. It was originally developed by doctors and later adapted by nurses. The POMR is most effective in acute care or long-term care settings.

A multidiscipline approach

In this charting system, you describe each problem in multidisciplinary patient progress notes (not on progress notes with only nursing information).

Five-part format

The POMR is divided into five parts:

database

problem list

initial plan

progress notes

discharge summary.

A five-star knowledge

In POMR charting, you record your interventions and evaluations in the progress notes and discharge summary only. But to really understand POMR, review all five parts.

Database

Usually completed by a nurse, the database, or initial assessment, is the foundation for the patient's plan of care. A collection of subjective and objective information about the patient, the database includes the reason for hospitalization, medical history, allergies, medication regimen, physical and psychosocial findings, self-care abilities, educational needs, and other discharge planning concerns. The database is the basis for a problem list.

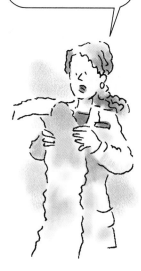

My database forms the basis for a problem list.

Problem list

After analyzing the database, various caregivers list the patient's current problems in chronological order according to the date when each is identified—not in the order of acuteness or priority. This list provides an overview of the patient's health status.

Dividing the diagnoses

Originally, POMR called for one interdisciplinary problem list. Although this may still be done, nurses and doctors usually keep separate lists with problems stated as either nursing diagnoses or medical diagnoses.

It's as easy as 1, 2, 3, 4, 5...

As you list the patient's problems, number them so they correspond to the problems in the rest of the POMR. Have every entry on the patient's initial plan, progress notes, and discharge summary correspond to a number. File the numbered problem list at the front of the patient's chart. Keep the list current by adding new numbers as new problems arise. When writing notes, be sure to identify the problem you're discussing by the appropriate number.

Once you have resolved a problem, draw a line through it, or show that it's inactive by retiring the problem number and highlighting the problem with a colored felt-tip pen. Don't use the number again for the same patient.

Initial plan

After constructing the problem list, write an initial plan for each problem. This plan includes:
• expected outcomes
• plans for further data collection, if needed
• patient care
• teaching plans.

Plan on patient participation

Involve the patient in goal setting as you construct the initial plan. This fosters the patient's compliance and is essential to the effectiveness of your interventions.

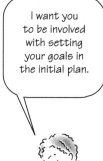

I want you to be involved with setting your goals in the initial plan.

Progress notes

One of the most prominent features of the POMR is the structured way that narrative progress notes are written by all team members using the SOAP, SOAPIE, or SOAPIER format. (See *SOAP, SOAPIE, SOAPIER charting,* page 64.)

Usually, you must write a complete note in one of these formats every 24 hours whenever a problem is unresolved or the patient's condition changes.

A clean SOAP or SOAPIE component

You don't need to write an entry for each SOAP or SOAPIE component every time you document. If you have nothing to record for a component, either omit the letter from the note or leave a blank space after it, depending on your facility's policy. (See *Problem-oriented progress notes,* page 65.)

Discharge summary

The discharge summary—the last part of POMR—covers each problem on the list and notes whether or not it was resolved. This is the place in your SOAP or SOAPIE note to discuss any unresolved problems and to outline your plan for dealing with the problem after discharge. Also, record communications with other facilities, home health agencies, and the patient.

POMR pros...

The POMR charting system has several advantages:
• Information about each problem is organized into specific categories that all caregivers can understand. This eases data retrieval and communication between disciplines.
• Continuity of care is shown by combining the plan of care and progress notes into a complete record of care that's planned and care that's delivered. The caregiver addresses each problem or nursing diagnosis in the nurses' notes.
• It encourages nurses to document the nursing process, to chart more consistently, and to chart only essential data.
• It can be used effectively with standardized plans of care and is an integrated medical record.

...and cons

The POMR system also has some disadvantages. For example:
• The emphasis on the chronology of problems, rather than their priority, may cause caregivers to disagree about which problems to list.
• Trends may be hard to analyze if information is buried in the daily narrative.

SOAP, SOAPIE, SOAPIER charting

To use the SOAP format in POMR charting, document the following information for each problem:
- **S**ubjective data: Information the patient or family members tell you, such as the chief complaint and other impressions.
- **O**bjective data: Factual, measurable data you gather during assessment, such as observed signs and symptoms, vital signs, and laboratory test values.
- **A**ssessment data: Conclusions based on the collected subjective and objective data and formulated as patient problems or nursing diagnoses. This dynamic and ongoing process changes as more or different subjective and objective information becomes known.
- **P**lan: Your strategy for relieving the patient's problem. This plan should include both immediate or short-term actions and long-term measures.

It's getting SOAPIE.
Some facilities use the SOAPIE format, adding the following to SOAP:
- **I**ntervention: Measures you take to achieve an expected outcome. As the patient's health status changes, you may need to modify your interventions. Be sure to document the patient's understanding and acceptance of the initial plan in this section of your notes.
- **E**valuation: An analysis of the effectiveness of your interventions.

It's even SOAPIER.
The SOAPIER format adds a revision section for the documentation of alternative interventions. If your patient's outcomes fall short of expectations, use the evaluation process called for in SOAPIE as a basis for developing revised interventions, then document these changes:
- **R**evision: Document any changes from the original plan of care in this section. Interventions, outcomes, or target dates may need to be adjusted to reach a previous goal.

- Assessments and interventions apply to more than one problem, so charting of these findings is repetitious, especially with the SOAPIE format. This makes documentation time-consuming to perform and to read.
- The format emphasizes problems, so routine care may be left undocumented unless flow sheets are used.
- The format doesn't work well in settings with rapid patient turnover, such as a postanesthesia care unit, a short procedure unit, or an emergency department.
- Problems may arise if caregivers don't keep the problem list current or if they're confused about which problems to list.
- Considerable time and cost are needed to train people to use the SOAP, SOAPIE, and SOAPIER method.

Art of the chart

Problem-oriented progress notes

The table below is an example of progress notes as they appear in a problem-oriented medical record.

> No problem!

> Number each problem for easy reference.

> Progress notes are in SOAPIE format.

Date	Time	Notes
2/1/02	0645	#1 Acute pain
		S: Pt states, "I am having severe back pain again and I'm nauseated."
		O: Pt states pain is #9 on 1 to 10 scale; skin is warm, pale, moist. Pt is restless, pacing in room, holding R flank area with his hand.
		A: Pt in severe pain, needs medication for relief.
		P: Check orders for analgesia; check for any allergies; take VS; if within normal limits, give analgesia as ordered. Recheck pt in 30 minutes for response. Monitor pt for adverse reactions to drug. Observe pt for pain frequently; offer medication as ordered before pain becomes severe. ———— Ann Davis, RN
2/1/02	0651	#1 Acute pain
		S: Pt states, "The pain is less and I'm not nauseated."
		O: Pt states his pain is now a #2 on 1 to 10 scale. Skin warm, dry, color normal. Pt sitting on bed, watching the news.
		A: Pt has improved.
		P: Continue to monitor for pain and other symptoms.
		I: BP 158/84, P 104, RR 24 — morphine 4 mg I.V.
		E: Medication was effective. ———— Ann Davis, RN
2/1/02	0130	#2 Anxiety
		S: Pt states, "I am worried about the surgery and being out of work."
		O: Pt wringing his hands, eyes downcast.
		A: Pt is anxious regarding upcoming surgery and its impact on his job.
		P: Encourage verbalization of feelings and concerns. Offer emotional support. Involve family to discuss his concerns if agreeable to pt. ———— Ann Davis, RN
2/1/02	0130	#3 Deficient knowledge
		S: Pt states, "I never had surgery before."
		O: Pt is unsure about what to expect.
		A: Pt needs preoperative and postoperative education.
		P: Teach pt about events before and after surgery; for example, I.V. insertion; teach about the need for coughing and deep breathing, moving frequently in bed, and early ambulation after surgery. Explain why these are important. Evaluate pt's response to the teaching, and document. ———— Ann Davis, RN

Problem-intervention-evaluation system

The problem-intervention-evaluation (PIE) system organizes information according to patients' problems and was devised to simplify the documentation process.

This system requires you to keep a daily patient assessment flow sheet and to write structured progress notes. Integrating the plan of care into the nurses' progress notes eliminates the need for a separate plan of care. The idea is to provide a concise, efficient record of patient care that has a nursing focus. (See *Easy as PIE.*)

Using the PIE system

To use the PIE system, first assess the patient and document your findings on a daily patient assessment flow sheet.

Pieces of PIE

The daily assessment flow sheet lists defined assessment terms under major categories (such as respiration) along with routine care and monitoring measures (such as providing ventilation and monitoring breath sounds). The flow sheet generally includes space to record pertinent treatments.

On the flow sheet, initial only the assessment terms that apply to your patient and mark abnormal findings with an asterisk. Record detailed information in your progress notes.

Next, chart:

- the patient's problems

- your interventions

- your evaluations of the patient's responses.

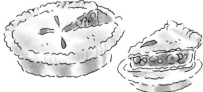

Problem

After performing and documenting an initial assessment, use the collected data to identify pertinent nursing diagnoses. These form the *problem* piece of PIE. Use the list of nursing diagnoses accepted by your facility, which usually corresponds to the diagnoses approved by the North American Nursing Diagnosis Association (NANDA).

Got a problem with that?

If you can't find a nursing diagnosis on an approved list, write the problem statement yourself using accepted criteria. Make sure you don't use medical diagnoses.

Keeping track

In the progress notes, document all nursing diagnoses or problems, labeling each as *P* and numbering it. For example, the first nursing diagnosis is labeled *P#1*. This way, you can later refer to a specific problem by its label only, without having to redocument the problem statement. Some facilities also use a separate problem-list form to keep a convenient running account of the nursing diagnoses for each patient.

> Number each problem for future reference.

Intervention

To chart the *intervention* piece of PIE, document the nursing actions you take for each nursing diagnosis. Write them on the progress sheet, labeling each as *I* and assigning the appropriate

---

Art of the chart

Easy as PIE

This sample chart shows how to write progress notes using the problem-intervention-evaluation (PIE) system.

Date	Time	Notes
2/20/02	1300	~~P#1: Sudden onset of generalized itching and hives possibly related to an allergic reaction.~~
		IP#1: Note extent of symptoms; take VS; assess breath sounds for wheezing. Notify doctor immediately.
		Administer medications as ordered, including I.V. access. Reassure pt.
		EP#1: Symptoms abate; pt maintains adequate respiratory and hemodynamic status; pt verbalized under-
		standing of treatments and need to report further symptoms. ———————— Mary Smith, RN
2/20/02	1300	~~P#2: Ineffective breathing pattern related to possible allergic reaction.~~
		IP#2: Take VS frequently and monitor breath sounds and pulse oximetry. Notify doctor for abnormal pulse
		oximetry or wheezing. Give medications as ordered. Teach pt signs of respiratory distress and the need to
		report these immediately. ———————— Mary Smith, RN
		EP#2: Pt will have no wheezing or dyspnea; pt verbalized understanding of need to notify nurse of
		changes in breathing patterns. ———————— Mary Smith, RN

> This stands for evaluation of problem # 1.

> After a problem is resolved, draw a line through it to indicate that it's no longer current.

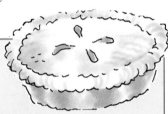

problem number. For example, to refer to an intervention for the first nursing diagnosis, write *IP#1*.

Evaluation

After charting your interventions, document the patient's responses in your progress notes. These form the *evaluation* piece of PIE. Use the label *E* followed by the assigned problem number. For example, to identify each evaluation write *EP#1*.

Reevaluate and review

Make sure that you, or another nurse, evaluate each problem at least once every 8 hours. After every three shifts, review the notes from the previous 24 hours to identify the patient's current problems and responses to interventions.

Document continuing problems daily, along with relevant interventions and evaluations. Cross out resolved problems from the daily documentation.

Reasons to give PIE a try

The PIE format has many attractive features, including:
• ensuring that your documentation includes all the necessary pieces: nursing diagnoses (problems), related interventions, and evaluations
• providing ongoing documentation of current problems
• encouraging you to meet JCAHO requirements by providing an organized framework for your thoughts and writing
• simplifying documentation by combining the plan of care and progress notes and by using the flow sheet for assessment and patient care data
• improving the quality of your progress notes by highlighting interventions and requiring a written evaluation of the patient's response to them.

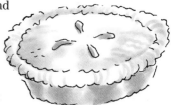

Problems with PIE

Don't take a "pie-in-the-sky" attitude to this charting system. Here's why:
• Staff members may need in-depth training before they can use it.
• It requires you to reevaluate each problem once every shift, which is time-consuming, often unnecessary, and leads to repetitive entries.
• It omits documentation of the planning step in the nursing process. This step, which addresses expected outcomes, is essential in evaluating the patient's responses.
• It doesn't incorporate multidisciplinary charting.
• It isn't suitable for long-term care patients.

FOCUS system

Nurses who found the SOAP format awkward developed the FOCUS system of charting. This system is organized into patient-centered topics, or *foci*. It encourages you to use assessment data to evaluate these concerns. FOCUS charting works best in acute care settings and on units where the same care and procedures are repeated frequently.

Coming into FOCUS

To implement FOCUS documentation, you use a progress sheet with columns for the date, time, focus, and progress notes. You can identify the foci by reviewing your assessment data. (See *Focus on FOCUS charting*, page 70.)

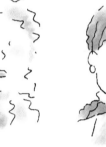

In FOCUS charting, you typically write each focus as a nursing diagnosis, such as *Risk for infection* or *Deficient fluid volume*. However, the focus also may refer to:

- a sign or symptom — such as purulent drainage or chest pain
- a patient behavior — such as an inability to ambulate
- a special need — such as a discharge need
- an acute change in the patient's condition — such as loss of consciousness or increase in blood pressure
- a significant event — such as surgery.

Writing FOCUS progress notes

In the progress notes column, identify and divide the information into three categories:

data (D), which include subjective and objective information describing the focus

action (A), which includes immediate and future nursing actions based on your assessment of the patient's condition as well as changes to the plan of care as necessary, based on your evaluation

response (R), which describes the patient's response to nursing or medical care.

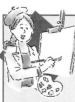

Art of the chart

Focus on FOCUS charting

The table below is an example of progress notes when using the FOCUS system.

> Progress notes are divided into data, action, and response.

Date	Time	Focus	Progress notes
8/3/02	1000	Deficient knowledge R/T diagnosis	D: Pt states she does not understand what her diagnosis means.
			A: Illness explained to pt according to her level of understanding. Pt taught symptoms she may expect and why she is having current symptoms. Treatments and procedures explained. Questions answered. Pt encouraged to verbalize need for further instruction or information.
			R: Pt verbalized better understanding of her illness. ————————— Donna Jones, RN
	1000	Risk for deficient fluid volume	D: Pt states her period just began and she is passing a large amount of clots.
			A: Amount of bleeding assessed. Pt saturated 2 sanitary napkins in the past hour, currently large amount of bright red clots noted. BP 114/70 P 98 RR 20. Pt status reported to doctor. Orders received. 20G IV catheter started, labs drawn; 1,000 ml NSS hung; macro tubing at 100 ml/hr. Pt tolerated procedures well. Will continue to monitor vital signs and bleeding. Dr. Smith will be in to see pt. Pt taught how to assess amount of vaginal drainage.
			R: Pt verbalizes correct amount of drainage and type. Pt understands procedures. Donna Jones, RN
8/3/02	1000	Anxiety	D: Pt states, "I'm afraid of all this blood."
			A: Emotional support provided. Encouraged verbalization. Explanations given regarding treatments and procedures. Family in to provide support.
			R: Pt observed talking and laughing with family. States she feels less anxious. Donna Jones, RN

> This focus is written as a nursing diagnosis.

> The focus zooms in on the topics of major concern

Lights, camera, data, action, response!

Using all three categories guarantees complete documentation based on the nursing process. Be sure to record routine nursing tasks and assessment data on your flow sheets and checklists.

DAR-e to succeed?

FOCUS charting has several strong points:
• It's flexible enough to adapt to any clinical setting.
• It centers on the nursing process, and the data-action-response format encourages you to record in a process-oriented way.
• Information on a specific problem is easy to find because the FOCUS statement is separate from the progress note. This promotes communication between health care team members.

• It encourages regular documentation of patient responses to nursing and medical care and ensures adherence to JCAHO requirements.
• You can use this format to document many topics in addition to those on the problem list or plan of care.
• It helps you organize your thoughts and document succinctly and precisely.
• It helps you identify areas in the plan of care that need revising as you document each entry.

DAR downers

FOCUS charting also has weaknesses:
• Staff members — especially those who are used to other systems — may need in-depth training before they can use it.
• You need to use many flow sheets and checklists, which can cause inconsistent documentation and problems tracking a patient's problems.
• If you forget to include the patient's response to interventions, FOCUS charting resembles a long narrative, like that seen in progress notes.

Charting by exception

The system called charting by exception (CBE) was designed to eliminate lengthy and repetitive notes, poorly organized information, difficult-to-retrieve data, errors of omission, and other long-standing charting problems.

To avoid these pitfalls, the CBE format radically departs from traditional systems by requiring documentation of significant or abnormal findings only.

CBE guidelines

To use CBE effectively, you must adhere to established guidelines for nursing assessments and interventions and follow written standards of practice that identify the nurse's basic responsibilities. Facilities using CBE must have critical pathways or interdisciplinary plans of care that address every possible patient problem.

Document deviations

Guidelines for each body system are printed on CBE forms. For example, care standards for patient hygiene might specify a complete linen change every 3 days or sooner, if necessary.

This patient's condition is unchanged, EXCEPT she reports less pain!

Having the standards clearly and concisely written eliminates the need to chart routine nursing care or any other care outlined in the standards — all you document are deviations from the standards.

Get your guidelines here

Guidelines for interventions used in the CBE system come from these sources:
- *nursing diagnosis–based standardized plans of care.* These identify patient problems, desired outcomes, and interventions.
- *patient care guidelines.* These are standardized interventions created for specific patients, such as those with a nursing diagnosis of *Acute pain* or *Chronic pain*. These guidelines outline the nursing interventions, treatments, and time frame for repeated assessments.
- *doctor's orders.* These are prescribed medical interventions.
- *incidental orders.* These are usually one-time, miscellaneous nursing or medical orders or interdependent interventions related to a protocol or a piece of equipment.
- *standards of nursing practice.* These define the acceptable level of routine nursing care for all patients. They may describe the essential aspects of nursing practice for a specific unit or for all clinical areas.

CBE format

The CBE format includes a standardized plan of care based on the nursing diagnosis and several types of flow sheets. These flow sheets include:
- nursing and medical order flow sheet
- graphic form
- patient-teaching record
- patient discharge note.

Making progress?

Sometimes you may need to supplement your CBE documentation by using nurses' progress notes.

Standardized plans of care

When using the CBE format for charting, you fill out a preprinted plan of care for each nursing diagnosis.

Fill in the blanks

The preprinted plans of care have blank spaces so you can individualize them as needed. For example, include expected outcomes and major revisions in your plan of care. Place the completed forms in the nurses' progress notes section of the clinical record.

Nursing and medical order flow sheets

Use nursing and medical order flow sheets to document your assessments and interventions. Each flow sheet covers a 24-hour period of care for one patient.

The top part of the flow sheet contains the doctor's orders for assessments and interventions. Each nursing order includes a corresponding nursing diagnosis, labeled *ND#1*, *ND#2*, and so on; doctor's orders are labeled *DO*. (See *Using a nursing and medical order flow sheet*, page 74.)

Checks, asterisks, and arrows

In addition to the abbreviations, ND for nursing diagnosis and DO for doctor's orders, use these symbols when you record care on flow sheets:
• a check mark (✔) to indicate a completed medical order or nursing assessment with no abnormal findings
• an asterisk (✳) to indicate an abnormal finding on an assessment or an abnormal response to an intervention
• an arrow (➔) to indicate that the patient's status hasn't changed since the previous entry.

After completing an assessment, compare your findings with the printed guidelines on the back of the form. If a finding is within normal parameters, place a check mark in the appropriate box. If a finding isn't within the normal range, put an asterisk in the box. Then explain your findings in the comments section on the form.

Note normalcy

An assessment finding that isn't defined in the guidelines may be normal for a particular patient. For example, unclear speech may be normal in a patient with a long-standing tracheostomy. Reference this type of note by nursing diagnosis number or doctor's order and time. If the patient's condition hasn't changed from the last assessment, draw a horizontal arrow from the previous category box to the current one.

Make more marks

Document interventions similarly. Use a check mark to indicate a completed intervention and an expected patient response. Indicate significant findings or abnormal patient responses with an asterisk, and write an explanation in the comments section. When the patient's response is unchanged, use an arrow.

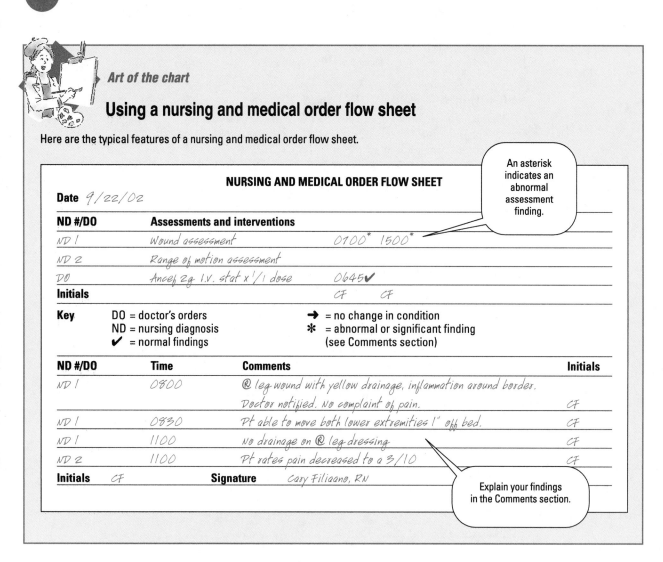

Art of the chart

Using a nursing and medical order flow sheet

Here are the typical features of a nursing and medical order flow sheet.

An asterisk indicates an abnormal assessment finding.

NURSING AND MEDICAL ORDER FLOW SHEET

Date 9/22/02

ND #/DO	Assessments and interventions		
ND 1	Wound assessment	0100*	1500*
ND 2	Range of motion assessment		
DO	Ancef 2g I.V. stat x 1/1 dose	0645✔	
Initials		CF	CF

Key   DO = doctor's orders   → = no change in condition
ND = nursing diagnosis   ✱ = abnormal or significant finding
✔ = normal findings   (see Comments section)

ND #/DO	Time	Comments	Initials
ND 1	0800	® leg wound with yellow drainage, inflammation around border. Doctor notified. No complaint of pain.	CF
ND 1	0830	Pt able to move both lower extremities 1" off bed.	CF
ND 1	1100	No drainage on ® leg dressing	CF
ND 2	1100	Pt rates pain decreased to a 3/10	CF
Initials CF		**Signature** Cary Filiaano, RN	

Explain your findings in the Comments section.

After you document an entire column in the assessments and interventions section, initial it at the bottom. Also initial all your entries in the comments section and sign the form at the bottom of the page.

Care-ful combinations

Some facilities use a special nursing care flow sheet that combines all the necessary forms, such as the graphic record, the daily activities checklist, and the patient care assessment section. (See *It flows together: Using a combined nursing care flow sheet*, pages 76 to 78.)

Graphic form

This section of a flow sheet is used to document trends in the patient's vital signs, weight, intake and output, and stool, urination, appetite, and activity levels.

More checks and asterisks

As with the nursing and medical order flow sheet, use check marks to indicate expected findings and asterisks to indicate abnormal ones. Record information about abnormalities in the nurses' progress notes or on the nursing and medical order flow sheet.

In the box labeled "routine standards," check off the established nursing care interventions you performed such as providing hygiene. Don't rewrite these standards as orders on the nursing and medical order flow sheet. Refer to the guidelines on the back of the graphic form for complete instructions.

Patient-teaching record

Use the patient-teaching form (or section) to identify the information, psychomotor skills, and social or behavioral measures that your patient or his caregiver must learn by a predetermined date.

A lot to learn? Use more forms...

This record includes teaching resources, dates of patient achievements, and other pertinent observations. If the patient has multiple learning needs, you can use more than one form.

Patient discharge note

Like other discharge forms, the patient discharge note is a flow sheet for documenting ongoing discharge planning. To chart discharge planning, follow the instructions printed on the back of the form. A typical discharge note includes patient instructions, appointments for follow-up care, medication and diet instructions, signs and symptoms to report, level of activity, wound care, and patient education.

Progress notes

Use the progress notes to document revisions in the plan of care and interventions that don't lend themselves to the nursing and medical order flow sheet. Because the CBE format allows you to document most assessments and interventions on the nursing and medical order flow sheet, your progress notes usually contain little assessment and intervention data.

(Text continues on page 79.)

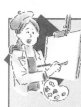

Art of the chart

It flows together: Using a combined nursing care flow sheet

This sample shows a portion of a nursing care flow sheet that combines a graphic record, a daily nursing care activities checklist, and a patient care assessment form.

> The graphic record makes it easy to spot trends.

Name _Maureen Gallen_

Date		2/29/02											
Hour		0700	0800	0900	1000	1100	1200	1300	1400	1500	1600	1700	1800
Temperature													
°C	°F												
40.6	105												
40	104												
39.4	103												
38.9	102												
37.8	100												
37.2	99												
36.7	98												
36.1	97												
35.6	96												
Pulse		84	80	82	78	76	78	78	82	84	82	80	78
Respiration		16	20	20	22	24	24	18	20	22	20	18	24
BP	Lying												
	Sitting	136/82	130/80	126/74	132/82	132/80	140/82	136/74	130/70	138/78	140/80	132/78	136/76
	Standing												
Intake	Oral	240						360					120
	Tube												
	I.V.												
	Blood												
8-hour total		600											
Output		400				450							
Other													
8-hour total		850											
Teaching		dressing changes, s/s of infection											
Signature		Mary Murphy, RN						Ann Burns, RN					
		0700 - 1500						1500 - 2300					

It flows together: Using a combined nursing care flow sheet *(continued)*

> This section allows for efficient documentation of daily activities.

	Hour		0800	0900	1000	1100	1200	1300	1400	1500	1600	1700
ACTIVITY	Bed								→	AB		→
	OOB											
	Ambulate (assist)											
	Ambulatory											
	Sleeping											
	Bathroom privileges											
	HOB elevated	MM							→	AB		→
	Cough, deep-breathe, turn		MM								AB	
	ROM ^{Active} _{Passive}		MM								AB	
HYGIENE	Bath		MM									
	Shave		MM									
	Oral		MM									
	Skin care											
	Peri care											
NUTRITION	Diet	House										
	% eating			15%			60%					15%
	Feeding											
	Supplemental											
	S-Self, A-Assist, F-Feed		A				A					A
BLADDER	Catheter	indwelling urinary #18 Fr.										
	Incontinent											
	Voiding	clear, yellow urine										
	Intermittent catheter											
BOWEL	Stools (occult blood + or -)											
	Incontinent											
	Normal	large formed brown stool										
	Enema											
SPECIAL TREATMENTS	Special mattress	Low-pressure airflow mattress applied 0900										
	Special bed											
	Heel and elbow pads											
	Antiembolism stockings											
	Traction: + = on, - = off											
	Isolation type											

(continued)

It flows together: Using a combined nursing care flow sheet (continued)

Findings marked by an asterisk need to be documented.

ASSESSMENT FINDINGS

KEY: ✓ = normal findings
✳ = significant findings

	Day	Evening	Night	
Neurologic	✳ MM	✓ AB		0800 Limited ROM Ⓡ shoulder. Pt. states, "I have arthritis and my shoulder is always stiff."
Cardiovascular(CV)	✓ MM	✓ AB		
Respiratory	✓ MM	✳ AB		1800 Shallow breathing with poor inspiratory effort at 1700.
GI	✓ MM	✓ AB		
Genitourinary (GU)	✓ MM	✓ AB		
Surgical dressing and incision	✳ MM	✓ AB		0930 Incision reddened; dime-sized area of serous sanguineous drainage on old dressing
Skin integrity	✓ MM	✓ AB		
Psychosocial	✓ MM	✓ AB		
Educational	✳ MM	✓ AB		0945 Taught pt incisional care and dressing change, and s/s of infection
Peripheral vascular	✓ MM	✓ AB		

NORMAL ASSESSMENT FINDINGS

Neurologic assessment:
- Alert and oriented to person, place, and time.
- Speech clear and understandable.
- Memory intact.
- Behavior appropriate to situation and accommodation.
- Active range of motion (ROM) of all extremities, symmetrically equal strength.
- No paresthesia.

Cardiovascular assessment:
- Regular apical pulse.
- Palpable bilateral peripheral pulses.
- No peripheral edema.
- No calf tenderness.

Pulmonary assessment:
- Resting respirations 10 to 20 per minute, quiet and regular.
- Clear sputum.
- Pink nailbeds and mucous membranes.

Gastrointestinal assessment:
- Abdomen soft and nondistended.
- Tolerates prescribed diet without nausea or vomiting.
- Bowel movements within own normal pattern and consistency (as described in Patient Profile).

Genitourinary assessment:
- No indwelling catheter in use.
- Urinates without pain.
- Undistended bladder after urination.
- Urine is clear, yellow to amber color.

Surgical dressing and incision assessment:
- Dressing dry and intact.
- No evidence of redness, increased temperature, or tenderness in surrounding tissue.
- Sutures, staples, or Steri-Strips intact.
- Wound edges well-approximated.
- No drainage present.

Skin integrity assessment:
- Skin color normal.
- Skin warm, dry, and intact.
- Moist mucous membranes.

Psychosocial assessment:
- Interacts and communicates in an appropriate manner with others (family, significant others, health care personnel).

Educational assessment:
- Patient or significant others communicate understanding of the patient's health status, plan of care, and expected response.
- Patient or significant others demonstrate ability to perform health-related procedures and behaviors as taught.
- Items taught and expected performance must be specifically described in Significant Findings Section.

Peripheral vascular assessment:
- Affected extremity is pink, warm, and movable within average ROM.
- Capillary refill time less than 3 seconds.
- Peripheral pulses palpable.
- No edema, sensation intact without numbness or paresthesia.
- No pain on passive stretch.

Advantages of CBE

The CBE format has several important benefits:
• It eliminates documentation of routine care through the use of nursing care standards. This stops redundancies and clearly identifies abnormal data.
• CBE is easily adapted to documentation on clinical pathways.
• Information that has already been recorded isn't repeated. For instance, you don't have to write a long entry each time you assess a patient whose condition has stayed the same.
• The use of well-defined guidelines and standards of care promotes uniform nursing practice.
• The flow sheets let you track trends easily.
• Guidelines are printed on the forms for ready reference. Abnormal findings are highlighted to help you quickly pinpoint significant changes and trends in a patient's condition.
• Patient data are immediately written on the permanent record. Because you don't need to keep temporary notes and then transcribe them in the patient's chart later, all caregivers always have access to the most current data, which decreases charting time.
• Assessments are standardized so all caregivers evaluate and document findings consistently.
• All flow sheets are kept at the patient's bedside, where they serve as a ready reference. This encourages immediate documentation.

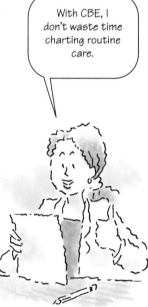

With CBE, I don't waste time charting routine care.

Disadvantages of CBE

Nothing is perfect, including the CBE system. Here are the drawbacks:
• The development of clear guidelines and standards of care is time-consuming. For legal reasons, these guidelines and standards must be written and understood by all nurses before the system can be implemented.
• This system takes a long time for people to learn, accept, and use correctly and consistently.
• Duplicate charting occurs with CBE; nursing diagnosis on a problem list are also written on the plan of care.
• Narrative notes and evaluations of patients' responses may be brief and sketchy in facilities that use multiple forms instead of one combination form.
• This system was developed for RNs. Before LPNs can use it, it must be evaluated and modified to meet their scope of practice.

FACT documentation system

The computer-ready FACT documentation system incorporates many CBE principles. It was developed to help caregivers avoid the documentation of irrelevant data, repetitive notes, and inconsistencies among departments and to reduce the amount of time spent charting.

Using the FACT system

In this system, you document only exceptions to the norm or significant information about the patient.

That's a FACT

The FACT format uses:
• an assessment and action flow sheet
• a frequent assessment flow sheet
• progress notes.
   The content of flow sheets and notes may be individualized to some extent. The flow sheets cover a 24- to 72-hour time span, and you'll need to date, time, and sign all entries. (See *Face facts with FACT charting.*)

Assessment and action flow sheet

Use the assessment and action flow sheet to document ongoing assessments and interventions. Normal assessment parameters for each body system are printed on the form, along with the planned interventions. You may individualize the flow sheet according to the patient's needs.

Frequent assessment flow sheet

The frequent assessment flow sheet is where you chart vital signs and frequent assessments. On a surgical unit, for example, this form would include a postoperative assessment section.

Progress notes

The FACT system requires an integrated progress record. Use narrative notes to document the patient's progress and any significant incidents. As in FOCUS charting, write narrative notes using the data-action-response method. Update progress notes related to patient outcomes every 48 hours.

Memory jogger

FACT is an acronym for the four key elements of this charting system. Here's how to remember these elements:

Flow sheets individualized to specific services

Assessment features standardized with baseline parameters

Concise, integrated progress notes and flow sheets documenting the patient's condition and responses

Timely entries recorded when care is given.

Art of the chart

Face facts with FACT charting

This sample shows portions of an assessment flow sheet and a postoperative flow sheet using the FACT format.

> Assessment parameters for each body system are on the form.

> Only document exceptions to the norm or significant information about the patient.

ASSESSMENT RECORD

	Date Time	8/18/02 0100	8/18/02 0500	8/18/02 0900
Neurologic Alert and oriented to time, place, and person. PERLA. Symmetry of strength in extremities. No difficulty with coordination. Behavior appropriate to situation. Sensation intact without numbness or paresthesia.		✓		✔
Orient patient.				
Refer to neurologic flow sheet.				
Pain No report of pain. If present, include patient statements about intensity (0 to 5 scale), location, description, duration, radiation, precipitating and alleviating factors.		5 - Neck pain	✓	1- Neck pain "It hurts."
Location		Cervical spine area		Cervical spine area
Relief measures		Pt repositioned		Percocet † p.o.
Pain relief: Yes/No		Y		Y
Cardiac Apical pulse 60 to 100. S_1 and S_2 present. Regular rhythm. Peripheral (radial, pedal) pulses present. No edema or calf tenderness. Extremities pink, warm, movable within patient's ROM.		✓	✔	✓
I.V. solution and rate		$D_5 \frac{1}{2}$ NSS @ KVO	$D_5 \frac{1}{2}$ NSS @ KVO	$D_5 \frac{1}{2}$ NSS @ KVO
Pulmonary Respiratory rate 12 to 20 at rest, quiet, regular and nonlabored. Lungs clear and aerated equally in all lobes. No SOB at rest. No abnormal lung sounds. Mucous membranes pink.		✓	✓	✔
O_2 therapy				
Taught coughing, deep breathing, incentive spirometer		✓	✓	✓
Musculoskeletal Extremities pink, warm, and without edema; sensation and motion present. Normal joint ROM, no swelling or tenderness. Steady gait without aids. Pedal, radial pulses present. Rapid capillary refill.		✓	✓	✔
Activity (describe)		bed rest	OOB in chair	bed rest
Nurse's signature and title		Jane Doe, RN	Jane Doe, RN	Jane Doe, RN

Key: ✓ Meets assessment criteria

Face facts with FACT charting (continued)

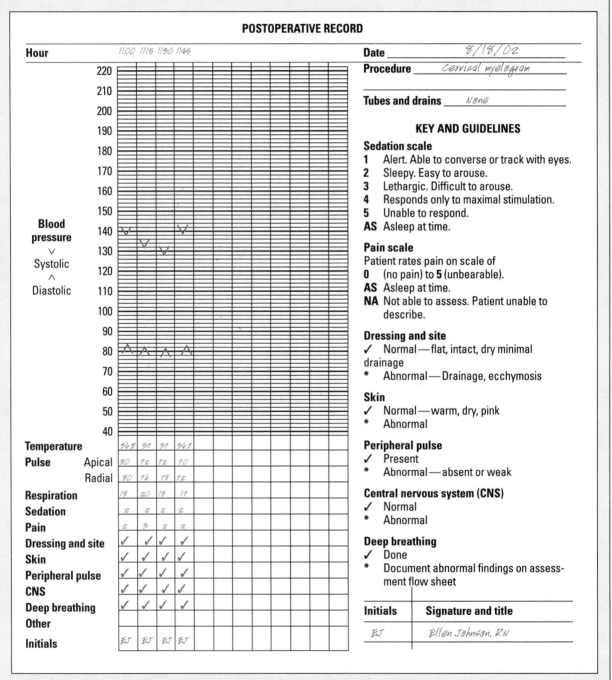

POSTOPERATIVE RECORD

Hour | 1100 1115 1130 1145

Date _8/18/02_

Procedure _Cervical myelogram_

Tubes and drains _None_

KEY AND GUIDELINES

Sedation scale
1 Alert. Able to converse or track with eyes.
2 Sleepy. Easy to arouse.
3 Lethargic. Difficult to arouse.
4 Responds only to maximal stimulation.
5 Unable to respond.
AS Asleep at time.

Pain scale
Patient rates pain on scale of
0 (no pain) to **5** (unbearable).
AS Asleep at time.
NA Not able to assess. Patient unable to describe.

Dressing and site
✓ Normal — flat, intact, dry minimal drainage
* Abnormal — Drainage, ecchymosis

Skin
✓ Normal — warm, dry, pink
* Abnormal

Peripheral pulse
✓ Present
* Abnormal — absent or weak

Central nervous system (CNS)
✓ Normal
* Abnormal

Deep breathing
✓ Done
* Document abnormal findings on assessment flow sheet

Blood pressure
∨ Systolic
∧ Diastolic

Blood pressure values (systolic ∨ / diastolic ∧):

Measure	1100	1115	1130	1145
Temperature	36.8	37	37	36.7
Pulse Apical	80	12	12	10
Radial	80	16	18	12
Respiration	18	20	18	17
Sedation	2	2	2	2
Pain	2	3	2	2
Dressing and site	✓	✓	✓	✓
Skin	✓	✓	✓	✓
Peripheral pulse	✓	✓	✓	✓
CNS	✓	✓	✓	✓
Deep breathing	✓	✓	✓	✓
Other				
Initials	EJ	EJ	EJ	EJ

Initials	Signature and title
EJ	Ellen Johnson, RN

Favorable FACTs

The FACT charting system has many good points. For example, this system:
• eliminates repetition and encourages consistent language and structure
• eliminates detailed charting of normal findings and incorporates each step of the nursing process
• is outcome oriented and communicates the patient's progress to all health care team members
• permits immediate recording of current data and is readily accessible at the patient's bedside
• eliminates the need for many different forms and reduces the time spent writing narrative notes
• is cost-effective.

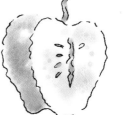

The FACT system eliminates repetitive charting? Thank goodness!

Finding fault with FACT

However, FACT charting does have some problems:
• Development of standards and implementation of a facility-wide system requires a major time commitment.
• Narrative notes may be sketchy, and the nurse's perspective on the patient may be overlooked.
• The nursing process framework may be difficult to identify.

Core charting system

The Core system focuses on the nursing process, which is the core of documentation. It's most useful in acute care and long-term care facilities.

Core framework

This system requires you to assess and record a patient's functional and cognitive status within 8 hours of admission. It consists of:
• database
• plan of care
• flow sheets
• progress notes
• discharge summary.

Database

The database (initial assessment form) focuses on the patient's body systems and activities of daily living. It includes a summary of his problems and appropriate nursing diagnoses. The nurse enters the completed database onto the patient's medical record card or Kardex.

Plan of care

The completed plan of care (like the database) goes on the patient's medical record card or Kardex.

Flow sheets

Use flow sheets to document the patient's activities and his response to nursing interventions, diagnostic procedures, and patient teaching.

Progress notes

On the progress notes sheet, record the DAE — that's data (D), action (A), and evaluation (E) or response — for each problem.

Discharge summary

The discharge summary includes information about the nursing diagnoses, patient teaching, and recommended follow-up care.

Core gets a high score

The Core with DAE charting system has several things going for it:
• It incorporates the entire nursing process.
• The DAE component helps to ensure complete documentation based on the nursing process.
• It encourages concise documenting with minimal repetition.
• It allows the daily recording of psychosocial information.

Core concerns

Oh no! Core with DAE has a worm (four worms, actually). They are:
• Staff members who are used to other documenting systems may need in-depth training.
• Development of forms may be costly and time-consuming.
• The DAE format doesn't always present information chronologically, making it difficult to quickly perceive the patient's progress.
• The progress notes may not always relate to the plan of care, so you need to monitor carefully to make sure the record shows high-quality care.

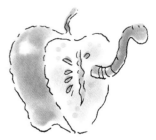

Computerized charting

Computerization can significantly reduce the time you spend on documentation and increase your accuracy. Computers can also be used to help you with other types of paperwork, such as:
- nurse management reports
- patient classification data
- staffing projections.

In addition, they can help you identify patient education needs and supply data for nursing research and education. Some bedside terminals can even measure vital signs.

Networking

In addition to having a mainframe computer, most health care facilities place personal computers or terminals at workstations throughout the facility so departmental staff will have quick access to vital information. Some facilities put terminals at patients' bedsides, making data even more accessible.

What's the secret code?

Before entering a patient's clinical record onto a computer, you must first enter a special code, which is usually your computer ID number. Some codes may specify the type of information that a particular team member has access to. For example, a dietitian may be assigned a code that allows her to see dietary orders and nutrition histories but not physical therapy information. These codes can help maintain a patient's privacy, unless they're misused.

Cybercharting

Here's how to use a computerized system for documentation: First, enter the special code, the patient's name, or his account number to bring the patient's electronic chart to the screen. Then choose the function you want to perform.

For example, you can enter new data on the nursing plan of care or progress notes or scan the record to compare data on vital signs or intake and output. Usually, you can obtain information more quickly with computers than with traditional documentation systems.

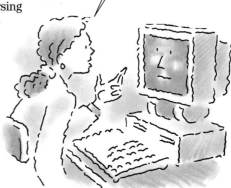

So, you're my new charting partner.

Computer systems and functions

Depending on which type of computer and software your facility has, you may access information by using your voice, a keyboard, light pen, touch-sensitive screen, or mouse.

Specialized nursing information systems can increase your efficiency in all phases of documentation. Most provide a menu of words or phrases you can choose from to individualize your charting on standardized forms.

With a few phrases — narrative complete!

With some systems, you can use a series of phrases to quickly create a complete narrative note. Then you can elaborate on a problem or clarify flow sheet documentation in the comment section of a computerized form by entering standardized phrases or typing in comments. Important developments in computer systems include specialized nursing information systems (NISs), the nursing minimum data set (NMDS), and voice-activated systems. (See *Computers speed up the nursing process.*)

Nursing information systems

Currently available NIS software programs allow you to record nursing actions in the electronic record, making documentation easier. These systems reflect most or all of the components of the nursing process so they can meet the standards of the American Nurses Association and JCAHO.

Furthermore, each NIS provides different features and can be customized to conform to a facility's documentation forms and formats. NIS can link nursing resources to educational applications.

Passive at present

At present, most NISs manage information passively. That is, they collect, transmit, organize, format, print, and display information that you can use to make a decision, but they don't suggest decisions for you. (See *Computerized give and take.*)

Nursing minimum data set

The NMDS program attempts to standardize nursing information. It contains three categories of data:

- nursing care, such as nursing diagnoses and interventions

- patient demographics, such as the patient's name, birth date, gender, race and ethnicity, and residence

- service elements such as length of hospitalization.

Computerized give and take

The most recent nursing information systems interact with you, prompting you with questions and suggestions about the information you enter. Ultimately, this computerized, sequential decision-making format should lead to more effective nursing care and documentation.

An interactive system requires you to enter only a brief narrative. The questions and suggestions the computer program provides make your documentation thorough and quick. The program also allows you to add or change information so that your documentation fits your patient.

Computers speed up the nursing process

A computer information system can either stand alone or be a subsystem of a larger hospital system. Nursing information systems (NISs) can increase efficiency and accuracy in all phases of the nursing process — assessment, nursing diagnosis, planning, implementation, and evaluation — and can help nurses meet the standards established by the American Nurses Association and the Joint Commission on Accreditation of Healthcare Organizations. In addition, an NIS can help you spend more time meeting the patient's needs. Consider the following uses of computers in the nursing process.

Assessment

Use the computer terminal to record admission information. As you collect data, enter further information as prompted by the computer's software program. Enter data about the patient's health status, history, chief complaint, and other assessment factors.

Some software programs prompt you to ask specific questions and then offer pathways to gather further information. In some systems, if you enter an assessment value that's outside the usual acceptable range, the computer will flag the entry to call your attention to it.

I'll help you increase efficiency and accuracy!

Nursing diagnosis

Most current programs list standard diagnoses with associated signs and symptoms as references. But you must still use clinical judgment to determine a nursing diagnosis for each patient. With this information, you can rapidly obtain diagnostic information.

For example, the computer can generate a list of possible diagnoses for a patient with selected signs and symptoms, or it may enable you to retrieve and review the patient's records according to the nursing diagnosis.

Planning

To help nurses begin writing a plan of care, newer computer programs display recommended expected outcomes and interventions for the selected diagnoses. Computers can also track outcomes for large patient populations.

You can use computers to compare large amounts of patient data, help identify outcomes the patient is likely to achieve based on individual problems and needs, and estimate the time frame for reaching outcome goals.

Implementation

Use the computer to record actual interventions and patient-processing information, such as transfer and discharge instructions, and to communicate this information to other departments. Computer-generated progress notes automatically sort and print out patient data — such as medication administration, treatments, and vital signs — making documentation more efficient and accurate.

Evaluation

During evaluation, use the computer to record and store observations, patient responses to nursing interventions, and your own evaluation statements. You may also use information from other members of the health care team to determine future actions and discharge planning. If a desired patient outcome has not been achieved, record new interventions taken to ensure desired outcomes. Then reevaluate the second set of interventions.

The ABCs of NMDS

The NMDS charting system allows you to collect nursing diagnoses and intervention data and identify the nursing needs of various patient populations. It lets you track patient outcomes and describe nursing care in different settings, including the patient's home. It also helps establish accurate estimates for nursing service costs and provides data about nursing care that may influence health care policy and decision making.

Comparing trends

In addition, you can compare nursing trends locally, regionally, and nationally and compare nursing data from various clinical settings, patient populations, and geographic areas.

Better care through better charting

The NMDS also helps you provide better patient care. For instance, examining the outcomes of patient populations will help you set realistic outcomes for an individual patient. This system also can help you develop accurate nursing diagnoses and plan interventions.

The standardized format encourages more consistent documentation. All data are coded, making documentation and information retrieval faster and easier. Currently, NANDA assigns numerical codes to all nursing diagnoses so they can be used with the NMDS.

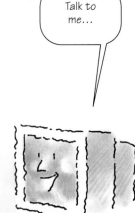

Talk to me...

Voice-activated systems

Some facilities have voice-activated nursing documentation systems. These are most useful in departments that have a high volume of structured reports, such as the operating room.

This system uses a specialized knowledge base of nursing words, phrases, and report forms combined with automated speech recognition technology. You can record nurses' notes by voice, promptly and completely. The system requires little or no keyboard use—you simply speak into a telephone handset, and the text appears on the computer screen.

Triggering text

The software program includes information on the nursing process, nursing theory, nursing standards of practice, and report forms in a logical format. Trigger phrases cue the system to display passages of report text. You can use the text displayed to design an individualized plan of care or to fill in standard hospital forms.

Although voice-activated systems work most efficiently with trigger phrases, word-for-word dictation and editing are possible.

The system increases the nurse's recording speed and decreases paperwork.

Pros of computerized charting

Most nurses have good things to say about computerized charting:
• It makes storing and retrieving information fast and easy.
• You can store data on patient populations that can help improve the quality of nursing care.
• You can efficiently and constantly update information and help link diverse sources of patient information.
• It uses standard terminology, which improves communication among health care disciplines and promotes more accurate comparisons.
• The charting is always legible.
• You can send request slips and patient information from one terminal to another quickly and efficiently, which helps ensure confidentiality.
• It facilitates individualized patient assessments and supports the use of the nursing process.

Cons of computerized charting

Some nurses also have gripes about computerized charting:
• If used incorrectly, the computer may scramble patient information.
• Computerized charting can threaten patient confidentiality if security measures are neglected.
• The use of standardized phrases and a limited vocabulary can make information inaccurate or incomplete.
• Some people have trouble adjusting to computers, thus increasing the margin for error.
• When the system is down, information is temporarily unavailable.
• Computerized charting can take extra time if too many nurses try to chart on too few terminals.
• Implementing a computerized system is expensive.
• Software that puts patient data into categories may cause important information to be omitted.

Choosing a charting system

What new charting system should I choose? Let's see, I need to consider the type of care my facility provides.

Health care facilities are always striving for greater efficiency and quality of care. A top-notch charting system can help a facility reach these goals.

Remember, documentation is often examined to make sure a facility meets the profession's minimum acceptable level of care. If efficiency and quality levels are low, your

Advice from the experts

Does your charting system measure up?

How useful is your current charting system? Is it incomplete, disorganized, or confusing? If so, it won't stand up to later scrutiny in case of a lawsuit or formal review.

To evaluate your charting system, ask yourself the following questions. If you answer "no" to any of them, you might recommend a closer evaluation of your system.

Documenting interventions and patient progress

• Does your current system reflect the patient's progress and the interventions based on recorded evaluations? Look for records that describe the patient's progress, actual interventions, and evaluations of provided care.

• Does the record include evidence of the patient's response to nursing care? For example, does it report the effectiveness of analgesics or the patient's response to I.V. medications? Does it show that care was modified according to the patient's response to treatment? For example, does it show what action was taken if the patient tolerated only half of a prescribed tube feeding?

• Does the record note continuity of care, or do unexplained gaps appear? If gaps appear, are notes entered later that document previous happenings? If late entries appear in the nurses' notes on subsequent days, do you have to check the entire record to validate care?

• Are daily activities documented? For example, do the notes include evidence that the patient bathed himself or indicate that the patient could independently transfer himself to a wheelchair?

Documenting the health care team's actions

• Does the record portray the nursing process clearly? Look for actual nursing diagnoses, written assessments, interventions, and evaluation of the patient's responses to them.

• Does the current documentation system facilitate and show communication among health care team members? Check for evidence that telephone calls were made, that doctors were paged and notified of changes in a patient's condition, and that actions reflected these communications.

• Is discharge planning clearly documented? Do the records show evidence of interdisciplinary coordination, team conferences, completed patient teaching, and discharge instructions?

• Does the record reflect current standards of care? Does it indicate that caregivers and administrators follow facility policies and procedures? If not, does the system provide for explanations of why a policy wasn't implemented or was implemented in a different way?

Checking for clarity and comprehensiveness

• Are all portions of the record complete? Are all flow sheets, checklists, and other forms completed according to facility policy? Are all necessary entries apparent on the medication forms? If not, does the record describe why a medication wasn't given as ordered and who was informed of the omission, if necessary?

• Does the documentation make sense? Can you track the patient's care and hospital course on this record alone?

charting system may need to be modified or replaced. (See *Does your charting system measure up?*)

Getting better and better

Continuous quality improvement programs are mandated by the state and JCAHO. Committees that set up these programs choose well-defined, objective, and easily measurable indicators that help them assess the structure, process, and outcome of patient care. They also use these indicators to monitor and evaluate the contents of a patient's medical record.

Does your charting measure up?

Shorter hospital stays and the requirement to verify the need for supplies and equipment have placed greater emphasis on nursing documentation as a yardstick for measuring the quality of patient care and determining if it was required and provided.

To verify that treatment was required and provided or that medical tests and supplies were used, the insurers (also called third-party payers) review nursing documentation carefully. As a result, nurses now need to document more information than ever before, including every I.V. needle used to start an infusion, each use of an I.V. pump to deliver a specific volume of medication, and every test that the patient undergoes.

Are you committed? Serve on a committee...

When changes are called for, you may be asked to serve on a committee that decides whether your charting system needs a simple revision or total overhaul. Before committing to a totally new system, your committee will discuss the possibility of revising the current system. This, of course, is easier than switching to a new system and changing the way information is collected, entered, and retrieved. (See *To change or not to change.*)

> Don't miss the review of charting systems on the next page.

To change or not to change

Whether you're selecting a new charting system or modifying an existing one, ponder the following questions:
• What are the specific positive features of our current charting system?
• What are the specific problems or limitations of our current system? How can they be resolved?
• How much time will we need to develop a new system, educate the staff, and implement the changes?
• Will a new system be cost-effective?
• How will changing the charting system affect other members of the health care team, including the business office staff and medical staff?
• How will we handle resistance to the proposed changes?

When choosing a new charting system, consider the type of care that's provided at your facility. For example, some systems work better in acute care than in long-term care settings.

Cost is another important factor to consider. Although computer systems are used in almost every care setting, the cost of a new system can be astronomical.

If a new charting system is selected, staff will require plenty of training. The system may be initiated on one unit at a time to make the transition easier.

Cheat sheet

Charting systems review

Narrative
• Flexible, easy-to-learn system that keeps notes in chronological order, making them accessible, but may be time-consuming, repetitive, and difficult to read and understand
• Requires the nurse to be descriptive and specific about patient progress

POMR
• Problem-oriented system that uses multidisciplinary progress notes and a five-part format (database, problem list, initial plan, progress notes, discharge summary)
• Conducive to use in acute and long-term care settings
• Facilitates communication between disciplines, which results in continuity of care
• Organization by problem makes assessments and interventions difficult to follow and allows routine care to go undocumented

PIE
• Nonmultidisciplinary system that uses daily assessment flow sheets and nursing-focused progress notes, eliminating the need for a separate plan of care
• Ensures that notes have necessary information: problems, interventions, and evaluation of the patient's response
• Elimination of planning step makes tracking patient evaluation difficult

FOCUS
• Adaptable system that typically uses nursing diagnosis–based foci to organize information
• Use of three categories (data, action, response) guarantees complete documentation that's based on the nursing process
• Use of many flow sheets can cause inconsistent documentation and problems tracking patient complications

CBE
• Timesaving system that was designed to eliminate repetitive notes, poor organization, and other charting problems by requiring that only significant or abnormal findings be documented
• Requires the nurse to adhere to established guidelines and follow written standards of practice
• Includes a standardized plan of care based on the nursing diagnosis and several types of flow sheets (nursing and medical order flow sheets, graphic form, patient-teaching record, patient discharge note)

FACT
• Computer-ready, outcome-oriented system that incorporates the CBE principles of documenting only significant or abnormal findings but that attempts to reduce charting time and costs
• Eliminates repetition and detailed charting of normal findings

Reviewing charting systems *(continued)*

• Development and implementation may be difficult and time-consuming

Core
• Nursing process–focused system that uses a database, plan of care, flow sheets, progress notes, and discharge summary
• Progress notes record the DAE—**d**ata, **a**c-tion, and **e**valuation
• Incorporates the entire nursing process, which ensures complete documentation but is not always presented chronologically, making evaluation difficult

Computerized charting
• Time-saving system that increases accuracy and legibility, organizes data, and supports the use of the nursing process
• Use of current technology improves commu-nication between disciplines but increases the likelihood of human error and, possibly, lack of patient confidentiality

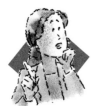

Quick quiz

1. The PIE charting format is useful in which setting?
   A. Acute care
   B. Long-term care
   C. Home care

Answer: A. Patients in long-term care and home care usually aren't acutely ill, so they don't need to be assessed every 8 hours, which the PIE system requires. Doing so would generate lengthy, repetitious notes.

2. A disadvantage of POMR documentation is its emphasis on:
   A. the priority of problems.
   B. the chronology of problems.
   C. SOAP notes.

Answer: B. When the emphasis is put on chronology instead of priority, teammates may disagree about which problems to list.

3. An advantage of narrative documentation is:
   A. it clearly tracks trends and problems.
   B. it's flexible in various clinical settings.
   C. it uses flow charts.

Answer: B. The most flexible of all charting systems, narrative charting suits any clinical setting and strongly conveys your nurs-ing interventions and your patients' responses.

4.   When deciding which charting system to use, give the least consideration to:
   A.   your geographic area.
   B.   legal issues.
   C.   professional standards.

Answer: A. Health care facilities also consider accrediting requirements when deciding which charting system would be the most effective.

Scoring

☆☆☆   If you answered all four items correctly, be careful. You're doing so much charting, you risk getting "narrative note elbow!"

☆☆   If you answered three items correctly, three cheers! You have an uncanny aptitude for filling in the blanks in a standardized plan of care!

☆   If you answered fewer than three items correctly, don't fret! You'll have plenty of opportunities to document your way to distinction, using narrative notes, POMR, the PIE system, FOCUS charting…

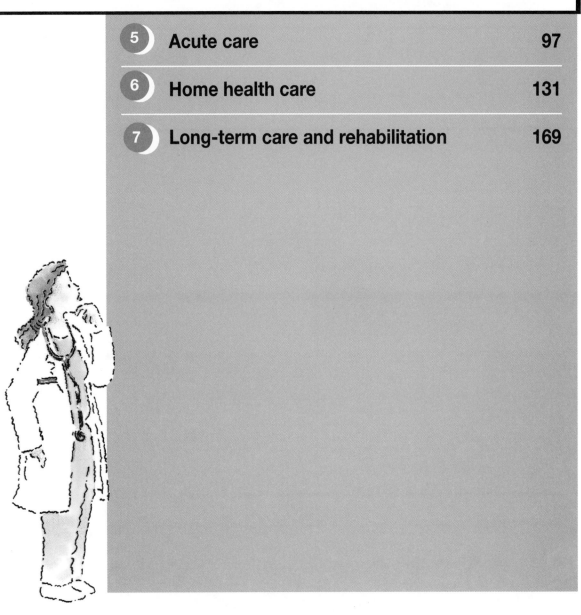

Part II

Charting in contemporary health care

Acute care

Just the facts

In this chapter, you'll learn:

♦ the medical record forms used in acute care settings

♦ the contents and organization of those forms

♦ the advantages and disadvantages of each form

♦ more detailed information about critical pathways.

A look at acute care

Like many nurses working in acute care settings, you may feel discouraged—even overwhelmed—by the amount of information you have to document each day. You may also be baffled by new methods of documentation, such as computer charting, flow sheets, and critical pathways. Ironically, formats that are meant to save time for nurses may actually end up costing time. Nurses accustomed to writing long, handwritten notes may be uncomfortable taking advantage of shortcuts offered by newer methods, especially given today's litigious environment, in which documentation is strongly linked to liability. The result: Many nurses end up double documenting, for example, recording the information with a check mark on a flow sheet and then documenting it again in longhand in progress notes.

Let familiarity (and this book) be your friend

To cope with the documentation chaos that characterizes contemporary nursing, your best weapon is familiarity with the variety of formats available, their advantages and disadvantages, and how you can use them to enhance your nursing practice.

> I'd hate to have to document all this information twice. That's what can happen when nurses are uncomfortable with newer methods of charting.

Forms, forms, and more forms

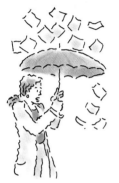

The following forms—commonly used to create medical records in acute care settings—are explained in this chapter:

- admission database or admission assessment forms
- nursing plans of care
- critical pathways
- patient care Kardexes
- graphic forms
- progress notes
- flow sheets
- discharge summary and patient discharge instruction forms.

Other forms include patient-teaching documents, dictated documentation, and patient self-documentation. Adapted or newly developed forms also may be used.

> I know another purpose for these forms—wrist exercise!

Yes, these forms do serve a purpose

A medical record with well-organized, completed forms serves three purposes:

    It helps you to communicate patient information to other members of the health care team.

    It protects you and your employer legally by providing evidence of the nature and quality of care the patient received.

    It's used by your facility to obtain accreditation and reimbursement for care.

In the long run, taking the time to carefully commit patient information to a standard, easy-to-use format frees you to spend more time on direct patient care.

Admission database form

The admission database form—also known as an admission assessment—is used to document your initial patient assessment. The scope of information documented at this stage is usually broad because you're establishing a comprehensive base of clinical information.

> A patient was just admitted? At the most, I have 24 hours to complete an admission assessment.

The clock is ticking

The Joint Commission on Accreditation of Healthcare Organizations (JCAHO) requires that the admission assessment—including a health history and physical examination—be completed within 24 hours of admission; some facilities require a shorter time frame. To complete the admission database form, you must collect relevant information from various sources and analyze it. The finished form portrays a complete picture of the patient at admission.

Finding form

The admission database form may be organized in different ways. Some facilities use a form organized by body system. Others use a format that groups information to reflect such principles of nursing practice as patient response patterns.

Get integrated! You'll be complimented for it

More and more facilities are using integrated admission database forms. On integrated admission database forms, nursing and medical assessments complement each other, reducing the need for repeated documentation. (See *Integrated admission database form*, pages 100 to 103.)

Charting with style

Regardless of how the form is organized, findings are documented in two basic styles:

☝ standardized, open-ended style, which comes with preprinted headings and questions

✌ standardized, closed-ended style, which has preprinted headings, checklists, and questions with specific responses (you simply check off the appropriate response). Most facilities use a combination of styles in one form.

As you complete the admission database form, keep in mind that the information you chart is used by JCAHO, quality improvement groups, and other parties to continue accreditation, justify requests for reimbursement, and maintain or improve patient care standards.

Form and function

A carefully completed admission database form is extremely valuable. It contains physiologic, psychosocial, and cultural information that's useful throughout the patient's stay in your facility. It contains:
• baseline data that's used later for comparison with the patient's progress
• important information about the patient's current health status as well as clues about actual and potential health problems (for example, your admission assessment may turn up facts about pre-

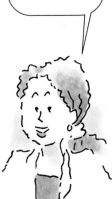

I feel like a million bucks! The wealth of information I gather during admission is invaluable.

(Text continues on page 104.)

▶ *Art of the chart*

Integrated admission database form

Most health care facilities use a multidisciplinary admission form. The sample form below has spaces that can be filled in by the nurse, the doctor, and other health care providers.

> Be time-efficient by asking technicians or nursing assistants to get some information, if your policy allows.

Name _Beatrice Perry_
Address _2 Clayton Street_
Dallas, Texas 55532
Admission Date _12_ / _21_ / _02_ Time _1345_
Admitted per: ____ Ambulatory
✔ Stretcher ____ Wheelchair
T _97_ P _92_ R _24_ BP _98_ / _52_
Ht. _5'2"_ Wt. _225 lb_
(estimated/actual)

**ORIENTATION TO ROOM/UNIT
POLICIES EXPLAINED**
✔ Call light
✔ Bed oper.
✔ Phone
✔ Television
✔ Meals
___ Advance directive explained
___ Living will

___ Living will on chart
___ Valuables form com
✔ Elec.
✔ Smoking
___ Side rails
✔ ID bracelet
___ Visiting hours

SECTION COMPLETED BY: _K. Crawford CAT_   **TIME:** _1350_

Name and phone numbers of two people to call if necessary:

NAME	RELATIONSHIP	PHONE #
Mary Ryan	daughter	665-2190
John Carr	son	665-4185

REASON FOR HOSPITALIZATION ___(patient quote:) _I go numb in my rt. arm and leg_
ANTICIPATED DATE OF DISCHARGE: _12/30/02_
PREVIOUS HOSPITALIZATIONS: SURGERY/ILLNESS   DATE
TIA   _11/4/91_

HEALTH PROBLEM	Yes	No	?
Arthritis		✔	
Blood problem (anemia, sickle cell, clotting, bleeding)		✔	
Cancer		✔	
Diabetes	✔		
Eye problems (cataracts, glaucoma)		✔	
Heart problem		✔	
Liver problem		✔	
Hiatal hernia		✔	
High blood pressure	✔		
HIV/AIDS		✔	
Kidney problem		✔	
Comments:			

HEALTH PROBLEM	Yes	No	?
Lung problem (Emphysema, Asthma, Bronchitis, TB, Pneumonia, Shortness of breath)	✔		
Stroke		✔	
Ulcers		✔	
Thyroid problem		✔	
Psychological disorder		✔	
Alcohol abuse		✔	
Drug abuse			
Drug(s)			
		✔	
Smoking	✔		
Other			

ALLERGIES: ☐ TAPE ☐ IODINE ☐ LATEX ☐ no known allergies
☐ FOOD:_____ ☑ DRUG: _Penicillin_
☐ BLOOD REACTION:_____ ☐ OTHER:_____

MEDICATIONS: _____
**HERBAL
PREPARATIONS:** _____

INFORMATION RECEIVED FROM: **SECTION COMPLETED BY:**

☑ Patient ☐ Relative_____ ☐ Friend_____ ☐ Other_____   _N. O'Meara, RN_ Date _12/21/02_ Time _1405_

Integrated admission database form *(continued)*

All assessment sections are to be completed by a professional nurse. Date __12/21/02__

> This diagram allows you to map any impairment in skin integrity.

GENERAL PHYSICAL APPEARANCE

✔ Clean _____ Disheveled

SKIN INTEGRITY: Indicate the location of any of the following on the chart to the right using the designated letter: a = rashes, b = lesions, c = significant bruises/abrasions, d = burns, e = pressure sores, f = recent scars, g = presence of tubes/appliances, h = other _____

Comments: ___b ischemic leg ulcer (2 cm – healing)_____

PRESSURE SORE POTENTIAL ASSESSMENT

PARAMETERS	0	1	2	3	Score
Mental status	(Alert)	Lethargic	Semicomatose	Comatose	0
			Count These Conditions As Double		
Activity	Ambulatory	(Needs help)	Chairfast	Bedfast	1
Mobility	Full	(Limited)	Very limited	Immobile	1
Incontinence	(None)	Occasional	Usually of urine	Total of urine and feces	0
Oral nutrition intake	Good	(Fair)	Poor	None	1
Oral fluid intake	(Good)	Fair	Poor	None	0
Predisposing diseases (diabetes, neuropathies, vascular disease, anemias)	Absent	Slight	Moderate	(Severe)	6
Patients with scores of 10 or above should be considered at risk.				Total	9

FALL-RISK ASSESSMENT

Impaired: ___sensory function ___general debility/weakness
___urinary/GI function ✔history of recent falls/dizziness/blackouts
___mobility function (automatically designates patient as prone-to-fall)
___mental status ✔prone-to-fall risk (indicated on nursing Kardex___✔___)

NEUROLOGICAL

___Dizziness ___Syncope ___Headache ___Blurred vision
___Recent seizure ✔Numbness/tingling location: _Rt. arm and leg_
LOC: ✔Alert ___Lethargic ___Semicomatose ___Comatose
Mental Status: ✔Oriented ___Confused ___Disoriented
Speech: ✔Clear ___Slurred ___Garbled ___Aphasic

Neurological Checklist								
	Right Arm	Right Leg	Right Pupil	Pupil Reaction	Coma Scale			
	Left Arm	Left Leg	Left Pupil		Eyes Open	Best Verbal Response	Best Motor Response	Total
12/14		12/14	5/6	+	4	5	6	15

Response	1	2	3	4	5	6
COMA SCALE CODE EYES OPEN	Never	To Pain	To Sound	Spontaneously		
VERBAL	None	Incomprehensible Sounds	Inappropriate words	Confused Conversation	Oriented	
MOTOR	None	Extension	Flexion Abnormal	Flexion Withdrawal	Localizes Pain	

+1:cannot move +3:move against gravity
+2:cannot move against gravity +4:move strongly against gravity

Extremities movement/strength
Pupil Reaction
- Reactive
- Nonreactive
D Dilated
C Constricted
> Greater than
< Less than
= Equal
= Sluggish

CODE
Pupils:
mm
1 ●
2 ●
3 ●
4 ●
5 ●
6 ⬤
7 ⬤

Comments: _numbness transient_ T. Jones, MD

> These circles will help you document pupil reaction accurately.

BEHAVIORAL

Behavior: ✔Cooperative ___Uncooperative ___Depressed
___Restless ___Other
___Combative ✔Anxious ___Unresponsive

Comments: _____
Religious/Spiritual beliefs: _Lutheran_
P. request to contact minister/priest/rabbi? ✔Y ___N
Name _Reverend Thomas Jones_ Phone # _555 4192_

PAIN

Pt. having pain at present? ___Y ✔N
Pt. had pain in last several months? ___Y ✔N
Rate pain on a scale of 0-10 (0 = no pain, 10 = severe pain) _____
Pain location_____ Quality_____

Radiation___Y ___N Duration_____
What aggravates pain?_____What alleviates pain_____
Effects on ADLs_____
Pt. pain goals _____

(continued)

Integrated admission database form *(continued)*

Addressograph   Date _12/27/02_

CARDIOVASCULAR

Skin Color: ____Normal ____Flushed ____Pale ✔Cyanotic
Apical Pulse: ____Regular ✔Irregular ____Pacemaker: Type _____ Rate _____
Peripheral Pulses: ✔Present ____Equal ✔Weak ____Absent Comments: _bilat. weak lower extremities_
Specify: R____radial ____pedal L ___radial ___pedal
Comments:_____
Edema: ____No ✔Yes _+1 bilat. pretibial_ Numbness: ____No ✔Yes Site:____Rt. arm and leg_____
Chest Pain: ✔No ___Yes____ P _____ Q _____ R _____ S _____ T _____
Family Cardiac History: ____No ✔Yes Telemetry Monitor: ____No ✔Yes rhythm _normal sinus_

PULMONARY

Respirations: ✔Regular ____Irregular ____Shortness of breath ____Dyspnea on exertion
O₂ use at home? ___Yes ✔No
Chest expansion: ✔Symmetrical ____Asymmetrical (explain: _____)
Breath sounds: ____Clear ____Crackles ____Rhonchi ✔Wheezing Location____bilat upper lobe, inspiratory____
Cough: None ✔Nonproductive ____Productive ____Describe _____
Comments: _pulse oximetry 98% on 2 L; sleeps with 2 pillows_

GASTROINTESTINAL

Stool: ✔Formed
____Loose
____Liquid
____Mucus
____Ostomy
____Incontinent
Color: ✔Brown
____Black
____Red tinged
____Bloody

Diarrhea ____
Constipation ____
Abdomen: ✔Soft
____Rigid
✔Nontender
____Tender
____(Location)
Bowel Sounds ✔Present
____Absent
____Hypoactive
____Hyperactive

Obese ✔
thin ____
emaciated ____
nourished ____

*NUTRITION:
✔Special Diet
1800 ADA
____Tube feeding
____Chewing problem
____Swallowing problems
____Nausea/vomiting
____Poor appetite
____Wt. loss/gain ____ lb

* Refer to dietitian if any ✔

GENITOURINARY/ REPRODUCTIVE

Color of Urine: ✔Yellow ____Amber ____Pink/Red tinged ____Brown ____Orange ____Clear ____Cloudy
____Ileo-Conduit ____Incontinent ____Catheter in place ____Frequency ____Urgency
____Difficulty in initiating stream ____Pain ____Burning ____Oliguria ____Anuria
____Dialysis Access site: _____ Date of last Dialysis: _____
Comments:_____
Date of LMP _1977_ Date of last PAP _5/01_ Breast self-exam ____Yes ✔No
Use of contraceptives: ____Yes (type _____) ____No ✔N/A
    Vaginal Discharge: ____Yes (describe _____) ✔No
    Bleeding: ____Yes (amount _____) ✔No
Pregnancies: Pregnant ____Yes ____Weeks gravida _____ Para _____ ✔No
Date of last Prostate Exam _____ Testicular self-exam ____Yes ____No
Comments: _____

ACTIVITY/ MOBILITY PATTERNS

____Ambulates independently ____Full ROM ____Limited ROM (explain: _____)
✔Ambulates with assistance (explain:_____) ✔cane ____walker ____crutches
____Gait steady/unsteady ____Mobility in bed (ability to turn self) _____
Musculoskeletal ____Pain____Weakness____Contractures____Joint swelling
____Paralysis____Deformity____Joint stiffness____Cast____Amputation
Describe: _____
Comments: _____

> Note that the form contains room for additional comments.

REST/ SLEEP PATTERNS

____Use of sleeping aids _____ Sleeps _6_ hr/day
Comments:_____
_____

Additional assessment comment: _On arrival, diaphoretic and (+) hand tremors, vital signs stable. Glucose 56 mg/dl._
Orange juice and lunch given to pt. 2 hr postprandial glucose 284. Symptoms subsided with juice. Nutrition and diabetes
educator consulted. —N. O'Meara, RN
MRI shows no cerebral lesions. Carotid doppler ultrasound pending. —T. Jones, MD

Integrated admission database form *(continued)*

> This final page deals with patient teaching and discharge planning.

EDUCATION/DISCHARGE SECTION
Instructions: Assessment sections must be completed within 8 hours of admission. Discharge planning and summary must be completed by day of discharge.

Addressograph

EDUCATIONAL ASSESSMENT

Yes	No	
✔		Patient understands current diagnosis
✔		Family/significant other understands diagnosis
✔		Patient able to read English
✔		Patient able to write English
✔		Patient able to communicate
	✔	Patient/family understands prehospital medication/treatment regimen

Yes	No	Emotional Factors:
✔		Patient appears to be coping
✔		Family appears to be coping*
	✔	Any suspicion of family violence
	✔	Any suspicion of family abuse
	✔	Any suspicion of family neglect

Comment: _diabetic teaching_

Language spoken, written, and read (other than English): _____
Interpreter services needed: ✔No ___Yes
Are there any barriers to learning (e.g., emotional, physical, cognitive)? _No_
Religious or cultural practices that may alter care or teaching needs? ___Yes ✔No Describe: _____
Is pt/family motivated to learn? ✔Yes ___No describe: _____

> This assessment form is multidisciplinary. In this example, both nurses and doctors provided information.

DISCHARGE ASSESSMENT

Living arrangements/caregiver (relationship): _lives alone_
Type of dwelling: ___Apartment ✔House ___ Nursing Home ___More than 1 floor? ✔Yes___No Describe: ___
___Boarding Home ___Other _____
Physical barriers in home: ✔No ___Yes (explain: _____
Access to follow-up medical care: ✔Yes ___ No (explain: _____
Ability to carry out ADL: ___Self-care ✔Partial assistance ___Total assistance
Needs help with: ✔Bathing ___Feeding ___Ambulation ___Other _____
Anticipated discharge destination: ___Home ___Rehab. ✔Nursing Home ___SNF ___Boarding Home
___Other _____
Currently receiving services from a community agency? ___Yes ___No
If yes, check which one ___visiting nurses ___Meals on Wheels
Concerned about returning home? ___Being alone ___Financial problems ___Homemaking ___Meal prep.
___Managing ADLs ___Other _____
Assessment completed by: _N. O'Meara, RN_ Date _12/27/02_ Time _1430_
Assessment completed by: _T. Jones, MD_ Date _12/27/02_ Time _1445_

DISCHARGE PLANNING

Resources notified:	Name	Date	Time	Signature
Social worker				
Home care coordinator	M. Murphy, RN	12/28/02	0900	
Other_____				

Equipment/Supplies needed: _stair chair_
Arranged for by: _M. Murphy, RN_ Date _12/28/02_ Time _0930_
Comment: _daughter to stay with pt at home_

DISCHARGE SUMMARY

Alterations in patterns: If yes, explain.	Yes	No	Explanation
Nutrition	✔		adherence to ADA diet regimen
Elimination		✔	
Self-care		✔	
Skin integrity		✔	
Mobility	✔		needs help with stairs
Comfort pain		✔	
Mental status/behavior		✔	
Vision/Hearing/Speech		✔	

Discharge instructions given (specify): _standard hosp. discharge instruction sheet_
Effects of illness on employment/lifestyle: _____
Central venous line removed: _N/A_ By whom: _____
Belongings sent with patient: ✔clothes ✔dentures ✔eyeglasses ___ hearing aid ___ prosthesis ___ valuables
✔prescriptions ✔other _cane_
Follow-up medical supervision to be provided by: _Dr. Gehran_
✔Patient/family instructed to call for follow-up appointment Discharge destination: _pt's home with daughter_
Section completed by: _C. Rafferty, RN_ Date _12/30/02_ Time _1215_

scription and over-the-counter drugs the patient takes; possible drug allergies also may be revealed)
- insight into the patient's ability to comply with therapy and his expectations for treatments
- details about the patient's lifestyle, family relationships, and cultural influences (during discharge planning, you'll need information about the patient's living arrangements, caregivers, resources, and support systems).

How to use the admission database form

Conduct the patient interview and record the information on the admission form or progress notes as soon as possible, noting the date and time of the entry.

Acute illness, short hospital stays, and staff shortages can make it difficult to conduct a thorough and accurate initial interview. In some cases, you can ask the patient to complete a questionnaire about his past and present health status and use this to document his health history.

Ready, willing, and able?

Before completing the admission database form, consider the patient's ability and readiness to participate. For example, if he's sedated, confused, hostile, angry, or having pain or breathing problems, ask only the most essential questions. You can perform an in-depth interview later, when his condition improves.

Turning to friends and family

If the patient can't provide information, consider seeking help from friends or family members. Be sure to document your sources.

During your interview, try to alleviate as much of the patient's discomfort and anxiety as possible. Also, try to create a quiet, private environment for your talk.

If the patient is too ill to be interviewed and family members aren't available, base your initial assessment on your observations and physical examination. *Be sure to document on the admission form why you couldn't obtain complete data and then obtain the rest of the information as soon as possible.*

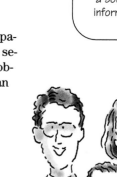

Don't forget that we can also be a source of information.

Potential problems

Admission database forms can present some difficulties. At times, through no fault of your own, you won't be able to complete some forms. The quality of recorded data depends in part on the ability of the patient or members of his family to provide accurate information.

Too many cooks...er, health care workers...can spoil the chart

Many other people will chart on the integrated admission database forms, increasing the risk of missing or incorrect information. You can't assume that colleagues collected the right information. You're responsible for verifying and correcting information gathered by nursing assistants and licensed practical nurses; likewise, the doctor is responsible for verifying information that you have collected. Remember, adding new information later may require you to revise the plan of care accordingly.

Plans of care and critical pathways

In acute care settings today, two different formats are being used to guide the process of care for a patient:

☞ the traditional plan of care

✌ the critical pathway.

Stick with the traditional? Let's take a critical look...

Both formats offer important advantages and disadvantages. The traditional plan of care, based on a nursing assessment and nursing diagnosis, provides a more precise account of the patient's individual nursing needs. The standardized critical pathway is a better tool for facilitating interdisciplinary communication and is perhaps more suited to the demands of the managed care environment.

Plans of care

The full nursing care needs of any patient are unlikely to be documented on a critical pathway. For this reason, some acute care facilities are continuing to rely on the traditional format of a plan of care as the chief mechanism for documenting each patient's nursing care.

As usual, there are requirements to meet

Although JCAHO no longer requires a specific care-planning format, the commission does require that the following information be included in plans of care in an acute care setting:
• ongoing assessments of the patient's illness and response to care, including patient needs, concerns, problems, capabilities, and limitations

• ongoing evaluation and modification of nursing diagnoses, interventions, and expected outcomes, based on identified patient needs and care priorities
• notation of nursing interventions, patient monitoring and surveillance, and patient responses
• reevaluation of patient progress compared with goals and the plan of care
• documentation of the inability to meet patient care goals and the reason for this. (For more information about plans of care, see chapter 3, Plans of care.)

Critical pathways

Many acute care facilities are abandoning the traditional plan of care in favor of a standardized critical pathway. Critical pathways are combinations of multidisciplinary plans of care.

A time of transition

The changeover from plan to pathway has thrown nursing documentation into a transitional state. You may find yourself working in a facility that uses both formats. Many nurses aren't yet comfortable with critical pathways and are double-documenting — copying information from a pathway into a plan of care.

Critical pathways are on the case

Critical pathways are used in health care facilities that employ case management systems for delivering care. In such a system, a registered nurse acting as case manager oversees a closely monitored and controlled system of multidisciplinary care.

Nurses, doctors, and other health care providers are responsible for establishing a care track, or case map, for each diagnosis-related group (DRG). A DRG is a way of classifying a patient according to his medical diagnosis for the purpose of obtaining reimbursement for hospital costs. The care track is used to determine a patient's daily care requirements and desired outcomes. The average length of stay for the patient's DRG is used in defining the care track. The case manager oversees achievement of outcomes, length of stay, and the use of equipment throughout the patient's illness.

Why take the pathway?

For acute care facilities, critical pathways work best with diagnoses that have fairly predictable outcomes, for example, hip replacement, cerebrovascular accident, myocardial infarction, or

> Critical pathways work best with diagnoses that have fairly predictable outcomes.

open heart surgery. The pathway is a way to standardize and organize care for routine conditions. It makes it easier for the case manager to track data needed to streamline use of materials and human resources, ensure that patients receive quality care, improve coordination of care, and reduce the cost of care.

Health care facilities have a financial incentive to switch to critical pathway documentation. Well-developed critical pathways with demonstrated cost reductions may provide the facility with an advantage when negotiating contracts with managed care organizations.

Precautions along the pathway

Using a critical pathway doesn't eliminate the need for nurses to diagnose and treat human responses to health problems. Patients are individuals and commonly require nursing intervention beyond that specified in the critical pathway.

For example, a patient enters the hospital for a hip replacement and can't communicate verbally because of a previous stroke. The critical pathway wouldn't include measures to assist this patient in making his needs known. Therefore, you would develop a nursing plan of care around the nursing diagnosis *Verbal communication impairment*. By using the critical pathway and developing a nursing plan of care based on the patient's individual nursing diagnoses, you can provide the best in collaborative care. (For more information about critical pathways, see chapter 3, Plans of care.)

Patient care Kardex

The patient care Kardex, sometimes called the nursing Kardex, gives a quick overview of basic patient care information. A Kardex can be computer-generated, or it may be a checklist on a large index card, on which the nurse can mark off items that apply to the patient. It also contains space for recording current orders for medications, patient care activities, treatments, and tests. (See *Considering the Kardex*, pages 108 and 109.)

A Kardex isn't a JCAHO requirement. Some facilities have eliminated Kardexes, incorporating the information they contain into the patient's plan of care.

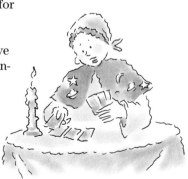

It's all in the Kardex

Refer to the Kardex during change-of-shift reports and throughout the day. The information it contains includes:
- patient's name, age, marital status, and religion
- medical diagnoses, listed by priority

(Text continues on page 110.)

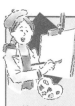

Art of the chart

Considering the Kardex

Here's an example of a patient care Kardex for a critical care unit. Remember that the categories, words, and phrases on a Kardex are brief and are intended to trigger images of special circumstances, procedures, activities, or patient conditions.

Care status
Self-care ☐
Partial care with assistance ☐
Complete care ☑
Shower with assistance ☑
Tub ☐
Active exercises ☐
Passive exercises ☐

Special Care
Back care ☑
Mouth care ☑
Foot care ☐
Perineal care ☑
Catheter care ☐
Tracheostomy care ☐
Other (specify)_____ ☐

Condition
Satisfactory ☐
Fair ☐
Guarded ☑
Critical ☐
No code ☐
Advance directive?
  Yes ☑
  No ☐
Date_11/12/02___

Prosthesis
Dentures
  upper ☑
  lower ☑
Contact lenses ☐
Glasses ☑
Hearing aid ☑
Other (specify)_____ ☐

Isolation
Strict ☐
Contact ☐
Airborne ☑
Neutropenic ☐
Droplet ☐
Other (specify)_____ ☐

Diet
Type: *low-fat, no conc. sweets*
Force fluids ☐
NPO ☐
Assist with feeding ☐
Isolation tray ☑
Calorie count ☐
Supplements_____

Tube feedings ☐
Type: _____
Rate: _____
Route: _____
  NG ☐
  G tube ☐
  J tube ☐

Admission
Height: *60"*
Weight: *145 lb (67 kg?)*
BP: *124/72*
TPR: *100.4 T.P.O. - 92-24*

Frequency
BP: *q1°*
TPR: *q1°*
Apical pulses:
Peripheral pulses: *q1°*
Weight:
Neuro check:
Monitor:
Strips:
Turn:
Cough: *q1°*
Deep breathe: *q1°*
Central venous
  pressure:
Other (specify)_____

GI tubes
Salem sump ☐
Levin tube ☐
Feeding tube ☐
Type (specify):_____
Other (specify):_____ ☐

Activity
Bed rest ☑
Chair t.i.d. ☐
Dangle ☐
Commode ☐
Commode with assist ☐
Ambulate ☐
BRP ☐
Fall-risk category (specify): ___ ☐
Other (specify):_____ ☐

Mode of transport
Wheelchair ☐
Stretcher ☑
With oxygen ☑

I.V. devices
Saline lock ☐
Peripheral I.V. ☐
Central line ☐
Triple-lumen CVP ☑
Hickman ☐
Jugular ☐
Peripherally inserted ☐
PICC ☐
Parenteral nutrition ☐
Irrigations:_____

Dressings
Type:
Change: *CVP*
  as needed

The check marks are intended to alert you to important patient care considerations.

Considering the Kardex (continued)

> You can quickly find the information you need with this format.

...rapy

- Liters/minute ☐
- Method
  - Nasal cannula ☐
  - Face mask ☐
  - Venturi (Venti) mask ☐
  - Nonrebreather mask ☐
  - Trach collar ☐
- Nebulizer ☐
- Chest PT ☐
- Incentive spirometry ☐
- T-piece ☐
- Ventilator ☑
  - Type: ☐
  - Settings: ☐
- Other (specify)_____ ☐

Drains
Type: _____
Number: _____
Location: _____

Urine Output
- I&O ☑
- Strain urine ☐
- Indwelling catheter ☑
- Date inserted _11/12/02_
- Size: _16 Fr._
- Intermittent catheter ☐
  - Frequency: _____

Side rails
- Constant ☐
- PRN ☐
- Nights ☐

Restraints
Date: _____
Type: _____

Specimens and tests
CBC daily
24-hour collection
Other (specify)_____

Stools

Special notes

Social services
Consulted 11/12/02

Monitoring
- Hardwire ☑
- Telemetry ☐

Pulmonary artery catheter ☑
  Pulmonary artery
  pressure _8/_
  Pulmonary artery
  wedge pressure: _8 2°_
CVP _____
Arterial line ☐
Other (specify) _ICP_ ☑

Mechanical ventilation
Type: _____
Tidal volume: _700 ml_
FiO$_2$ _50%_
Mode: _AC_
Rate: _12_

> On an obstetrics unit, you might find additional information on the Kardex cover sheet.

Delivery
Date: _____
Time: _____
Type of delivery: _____

Special procedures
- Perineal rinse ☐
- Sitz bath ☐
- Witch hazel compress ☐
- Breast binders ☐
- Ice ☐
- Abdominal binders ☐
- Other (specify)_____ ☐

Mother
Due date: _____
Gravida: _____
Para: _____
Rh: _____
Blood type: _____
Membranes ruptured: _____
Episiotomy ☐
Lacerations ☐
RhoGAM studies?
  Yes ☐
  No ☐
Rubella titer?
  Yes ☐
  No ☐

Infant
- Male ☐
- Female ☐
- Full term ☐
- Premature ☐
  - Weeks ☐
- Apgar score ☐
- Nursing ☐
- Formula ☐
- Condition (specify): _____
- Other (specify): _____

• nursing diagnoses, listed by priority
• current doctors' orders for medication, treatments, diet, I.V. therapy, diagnostic tests, procedures, and other measures
• consultations
• results of diagnostic tests and procedures
• permitted activities, functional limitations, assistance that's needed, and safety precautions.

All shapes and sizes

Kardexes come in various shapes, sizes, and types and may be computer-generated. Some facilities use different Kardexes to document specific information, such as medication information, test results, and nonnursing data.

Computerized Kardex

Typically used to record laboratory or diagnostic test results and X-ray findings, a computerized Kardex usually includes information on medical orders, referrals, consultations, specimens (for culture and sensitivity tests or for blood glucose analysis, for example), vital signs, diet, and activity restrictions. (See *Computer-generated patient care Kardex.*)

The Kardex can be all aces

The Kardex has some good points, including:
• It allows quick access to information about task-oriented interventions, such as specific patient care, medication administration, and I.V. therapy.
• The plan of care may be added to the Kardex to provide all the necessary data for patient care, although this duplicates information.

A key Kardex kriticism

The Kardex has one major drawback: It's only as useful as nurses make it. It isn't an effective charting tool if there isn't enough space for appropriate information, if it isn't updated frequently, if it isn't completed, or if it isn't read before giving patient care.

In addition, Kardexes aren't usually part of the permanent record, so be sure the information on the Kardex is also found elsewhere on the patient's chart.

How to use the Kardex

The Kardex is most effective when you tailor the information to the needs of a particular setting. For instance, an intensive care unit Kardex should include information on hardwire or telemetry monitoring and arterial pressure monitoring.

Art of the chart

Computer-generated patient care Kardex

In the computer-generated Kardex shown below, you'll find a detailed list of medical orders and other patient care data.

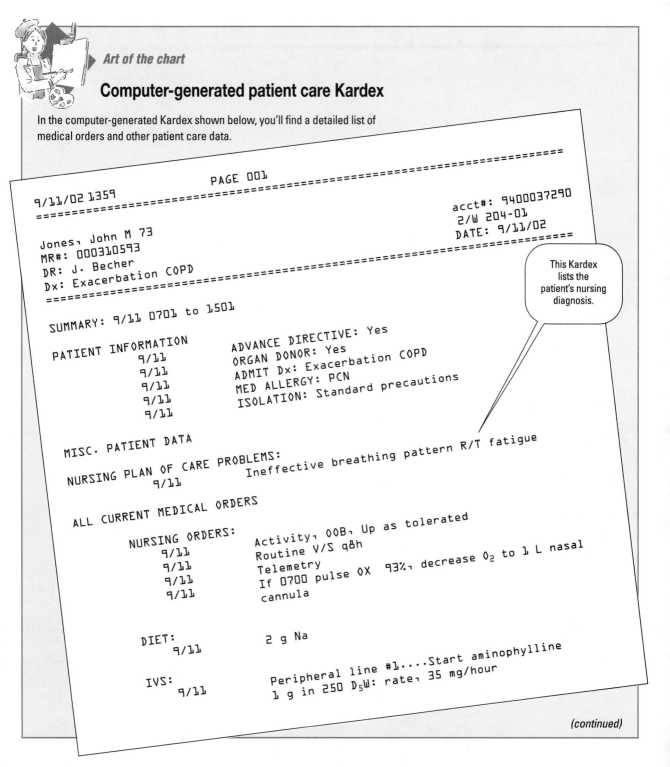

```
                                                              =================================
                              PAGE 001
                    ==========================================================
9/11/02 1359                                                  acct#: 9400037290
==========================================================   2/W 204-01
                                                             DATE: 9/11/02
Jones, John M 73                                             =================
MR#: 000310593
DR: J. Becher
Dx: Exacerbation COPD
==========================================================

SUMMARY: 9/11 0701 to 1501

  PATIENT INFORMATION          ADVANCE DIRECTIVE: Yes
            9/11               ORGAN DONOR: Yes
            9/11               ADMIT Dx: Exacerbation COPD
            9/11               MED ALLERGY: PCN
            9/11               ISOLATION: Standard precautions
            9/11


  MISC. PATIENT DATA

    NURSING PLAN OF CARE PROBLEMS:
            9/11               Ineffective breathing pattern R/T fatigue


  ALL CURRENT MEDICAL ORDERS

        NURSING ORDERS:        Activity, OOB, Up as tolerated
            9/11               Routine V/S q8h
            9/11               Telemetry
            9/11               If 0700 pulse OX  93%, decrease O2 to 1 L nasal
            9/11               cannula


        DIET:                  2 g Na
            9/11

        IVS:                   Peripheral line #1....Start aminophylline
            9/11               1 g in 250 D5W: rate, 35 mg/hour
```

This Kardex lists the patient's nursing diagnosis.

(continued)

Computer-generated patient care KARDEX (continued)

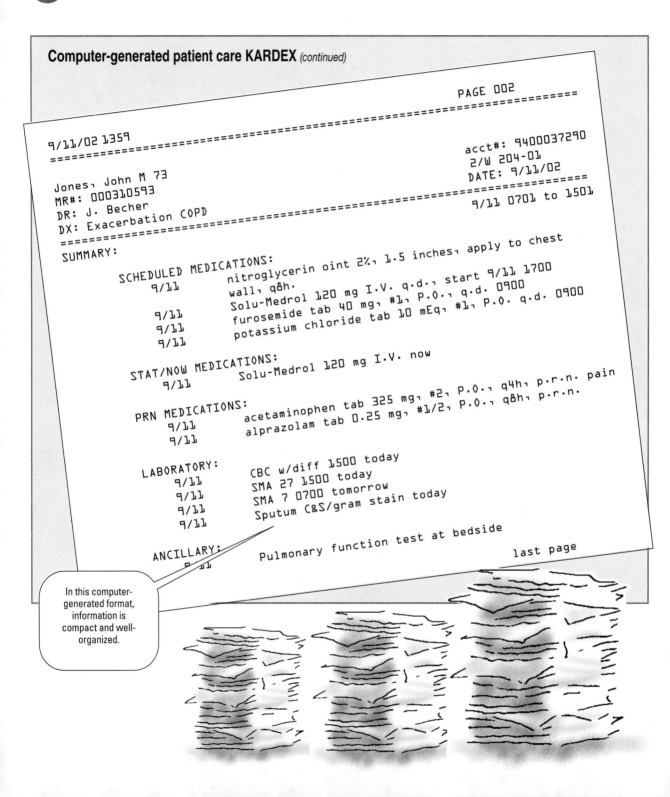

```
                                                        PAGE 002
                                                ==============================

9/11/02 1359
=====================================================================
                                                acct#: 9400037290
                                                2/W 204-01
Jones, John M 73                                DATE: 9/11/02
MR#: 000310593                                  ==============================
DR: J. Becher                                   9/11 0701 to 1501
DX: Exacerbation COPD
=====================================================================
SUMMARY:

        SCHEDULED MEDICATIONS:
        9/11            nitroglycerin oint 2%, 1.5 inches, apply to chest
                        wall, q8h.
                        Solu-Medrol 120 mg I.V. q.d., start 9/11 1700
        9/11            furosemide tab 40 mg, #1, P.O., q.d. 0900
        9/11            potassium chloride tab 10 mEq, #1, P.O. q.d. 0900
        9/11

        STAT/NOW MEDICATIONS:
        9/11            Solu-Medrol 120 mg I.V. now

        PRN MEDICATIONS:
        9/11            acetaminophen tab 325 mg, #2, P.O., q4h, p.r.n. pain
        9/11            alprazolam tab 0.25 mg, #1/2, P.O., q8h, p.r.n.

        LABORATORY:
        9/11            CBC w/diff 1500 today
        9/11            SMA 27 1500 today
        9/11            SMA 7 0700 tomorrow
        9/11            Sputum C&S/gram stain today

        ANCILLARY:
        9/11            Pulmonary function test at bedside          last page
```

In this computer-generated format, information is compact and well-organized.

A Kardex a day keeps confusion away

Use the Kardex to record information that helps nurses plan daily interventions. For example, record the time a patient prefers to bathe, his food preferences before and during chemotherapy, and which analgesics or positions are usually required to ease pain.

The medication Kardex

If your facility uses a separate medication Kardex on acute care units, you'll find this document on the medication cart or other designated place. The medication Kardex may include the medication administration record (MAR), which lists medications, doses, and frequency and route of administration. Medication administration is documented on this form, which is a permanent part of the patient's record. (See *The medication Kardex*, pages 114 and 115.)

Getting the most out of your medication Kardex

When recording information on a medication Kardex, here are some tips:
• Include the date and administration time as well as the medication dose, route, and frequency. Don't forget to initial the entry.
• Indicate when you administer a stat dose of a medication and, if appropriate, the number of doses ordered and the stop date.
• Write legibly, using only standard abbreviations. When in doubt about how to abbreviate a term, spell it out. Remember, the MAR is a legal record, so any information entered there should be legible and above question.
• After giving the first dose of a medication, sign your full name, your licensure status, and your initials in the appropriate space.
• After withholding a medication dose, document which dose wasn't given (usually by circling the time it was scheduled). Also document the reason it was omitted — for example, withholding oral medications from a patient because he has surgery scheduled that day.

How are things progressing? Need more space?

If you administer all medications according to the plan of care, you don't need to document further. However, if your MAR doesn't have space for some information, such as the parenteral administration site, the patient's response to as-needed medications, or deviations from the medication order, you'll need to record this information

Now what does this say? I can't stress enough how important it is to write legibly!

(Text continues on page 116.)

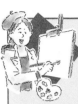

Art of the chart

The medication Kardex

One type of Kardex is the medication Kardex. It contains a permanent record of the patient's medications. The medication Kardex may also include the patient's diagnosis and information about allergies and diet. A sample form is shown here.

NURSE'S FULL SIGNATURE, STATUS AND INITIALS	INIT.		INIT.		INIT.
Roy Charles, RN	RC				
Theresa Hopkins, RN	TH				

Don't forget to sign your name.

DIAGNOSIS: Heart failure, Atrial flutter

ALLERGIES: ASA   **DIET:** Cardiac

ROUTINE/DAILY ORDERS/FINGERSTICKS/INSULIN COVERAGE	DATE: 11/25/02	DATE:	DATE:	DATE:	DATE:	DATE:	DATE:	DATE:	DATE:	DATE:

ORDER DATE INIT.	RE-NEWAL DATE INIT.	MEDICATIONS DOSE, ROUTE, FREQUENCY	TIME	SITE	INT.	SITE	INT.	SITE	INT.	SITE	INT.	SITE	INT.	SITE	INT.	SITE	INT.	SITE	INT.	SITE	INT.	SITE	INT.
11/24/02		digoxin 0.125 mg	0900	®s.c.	RC																		
RC		I.V. q.d.	HR		TH																		
11/24/02		furosemide 40 mg	0900	®s.c.	RC																		
11/24/02		I.V. q.2h	2100		TH																		
11/24/02		enalapril	0511	®s.c.	TH																		
RC		1.25 mg I.V. q.6h	1100		RC																		
			1700		RC																		
11/25/02		vancomycin 1 g I.V. q.d.	2100	®s.c.	TH																		
TH																							

Initial here to verify that the dose, route, and frequency were checked against the doctor's orders.

The medication Kardex (continued)

	PRN MEDICATION	

ALLERGIES: ASA

Addressograph

INITIAL	SIGNATURE & STATUS	INITIAL	SIGNATURE & STATUS	INITIAL	SIGNATURE & STATUS	INITIAL	SIGNATURE & STATUS
RC	Roy Charles, RN						
TH	Theresa Hopkins, RN						

YEAR 20 02   P.R.N. MEDICATIONS

ORDER DATE: 11 24	**RENEWAL** DATE: /	**DISCONTINUED** DATE: /	DATE	11/24										
MEDICATION: acetaminophen		**DOSE** 650 mg	TIME GIVEN	0930										
DIRECTION: p.r.n. mild pain		**ROUTE:** P.O.	DATA											
			INIT.	RC										
ORDER DATE: 11 24	**RENEWAL** DATE: /	**DISCONTINUED** DATE: /	DATE	11/24										
MEDICATION: MSO₄		**DOSE** 2 mg	TIME GIVEN	0930										
DIRECTION: 15 minutes prior to changing (R) heel dressing		**ROUTE:** I.V.	DATA											
			INIT.	RC										
ORDER DATE: 11 24	**RENEWAL** DATE: /	**DISCONTINUED** DATE: /	DATE	11/24										
MEDICATION: Milk of Magnesia		**DOSE** 30 ml	TIME GIVEN	2115										
DIRECTION: q6h p.r.n.		**ROUTE:** P.O.	DATA											
			INIT.	TH										
ORDER DATE: 11 25	**RENEWAL** DATE: /	**DISCONTINUED** DATE: 11 25	DATE	11/25										
MEDICATION: prochlorperazine		**DOSE** 5 mg	TIME GIVEN	1100	2230									
DIRECTION: q6h p.r.n.		**ROUTE:** I.M.	DATA	(R) glut	(L) glut									
prn nausea and vomiting			INIT.	RC	TH									
ORDER DATE: /	**RENEWAL** DATE: /	**DISCONTINUED** DATE: /	DATE											
MEDICATION:		**DOSE**	TIME GIVEN											
DIRECTION:		**ROUTE:**	DATA											
			INIT.											
ORDER DATE: /	**RENEWAL** DATE: /	**DISCONTINUED** DATE: /	DATE											
MEDICATION:		**DOSE**	TIME GIVEN											
DIRECTION:		**ROUTE:**	DATA											
			INIT.											
ORDER DATE: /	**RENEWAL** DATE: /	**DISCONTINUED** DATE: /	DATE											
MEDICATION:		**DOSE**	TIME GIVEN											
DIRECTION:		**ROUTE:**	DATA											
			INIT.											

I.M. sites must be charted.

in the progress notes. For example, consider the progress note shown below.

12/8/02	0900	Digoxin held per order of Dr. John because of
		pt's heart rate of 53. Digoxin level pending.
		———————————————— Dave Bevins, RN

Graphic form

The graphic form is used to plot the patient's vital signs. Weight, intake and output, appetite, and activity level also may be documented on the graphic form. (See *Plotting along: Using a graphic form.*)

The graphic form usually has a column of data printed on the left side of the page, times and dates written across the top, and open blocks within the side and top borders.

Advantages — in graphic terms

The graphic form has two important advantages:
• It presents information at a glance. This allows more visual comparison of data than is possible in narrative-style forms. For example, if a patient's temperature goes up or down or fluctuates over time, this can be detected much more readily on a graph than in a narrative account of the patient's temperature.
• Unlicensed personnel, such as nursing assistants and technicians, are allowed to document measurements on graphic forms, saving nurses valuable time.

Disadvantages — in graphic terms

Guess what? Graphic forms also have disadvantages:
• If data placed on the graph aren't accurate, legible, and complete, the form is useless. Every vital sign you take should be transcribed onto the form. For accuracy, double-check the graph after transcribing information.
• If you use information from the graph alone, you won't get a complete picture of the patient's clinical condition. You must combine the graph with narrative documentation.

How to use a graphic form

To avoid transcription errors, document directly onto a graphic form when information is obtained.

Art of the chart

Plotting along: Using a graphic form

Plotting information on a graphic form helps you visualize changes in your patient's temperature, blood pressure, heart rate, weight, and intake and output. Review the sample form below.

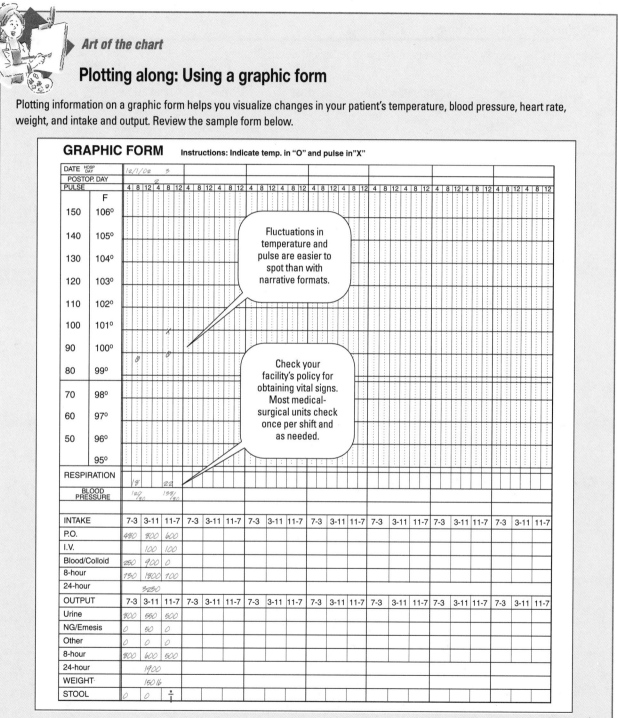

GRAPHIC FORM   Instructions: Indicate temp. in "O" and pulse in "X"

DATE HOSP DAY		12/1/02	3										
POSTOP. DAY			2										
PULSE		4 8 12	4 8 12	4 8 12	4 8 12	4 8 12	4 8 12	4 8 12	4 8 12	4 8 12	4 8 12	4 8 12	4 8 12

	F
150	106°
140	105°
130	104°
120	103°
110	102°
100	101°
90	100°
80	99°
70	98°
60	97°
50	96°
	95°

> Fluctuations in temperature and pulse are easier to spot than with narrative formats.

> Check your facility's policy for obtaining vital signs. Most medical-surgical units check once per shift and as needed.

RESPIRATION	18	22
BLOOD PRESSURE	120/80	138/80

INTAKE	7-3	3-11	11-7	7-3	3-11	11-7	7-3	3-11	11-7	7-3	3-11	11-7	7-3	3-11	11-7	7-3	3-11	11-7	7-3	3-11	11-7
P.O.	480	800	600																		
I.V.		100	100																		
Blood/Colloid	250	900	0																		
8-hour	730	1800	700																		
24-hour		3230																			
OUTPUT	7-3	3-11	11-7	7-3	3-11	11-7	7-3	3-11	11-7	7-3	3-11	11-7	7-3	3-11	11-7	7-3	3-11	11-7	7-3	3-11	11-7
Urine	800	550	500																		
NG/Emesis	0	50	0																		
Other	0	0	0																		
8-hour	800	600	500																		
24-hour		1900																			
WEIGHT		150 lb																			
STOOL	0	0	÷																		

(continued)

Plotting along: Using a graphic form (continued)

Additional space is usually provided for more frequently monitored vital signs.

DATE	TIME	BLOOD PRESSURE	PULSE	RESP.	MISCELLANEOUS
12/1/02	0800	130/80	96	20	T 99⁴ blood transfusion
	0815	134/82	102	18	T 99⁸ no s/s of reaction
	0830	128/84	91	16	T 99²

A few more charting opportunities

If a medication (an antipyretic or antihypertensive, for example) precipitates a change in a particular vital sign, document this in the progress notes as well as on the graphic form. Specify the relationship between the medication and its effect.

Make sure you also document vital signs on both the graphic form and the progress notes when a patient has an acute episode, such as chest pain or a seizure. Be sure to:
• chart legibly
• put data in the correct time line
• make the dots you plot on the graph large enough to be seen easily (connect the dots if your facility requires this).

Progress notes and flow sheets

In the acute care setting, progress notes and flow sheets are used to record the patient's status and monitor changes in his condition.

Making progress with progress notes

Progress notes are written chronologically. The standard format for nursing progress notes has a column for the date and time and a column for detailed comments about:
• the patient's problems (the nursing diagnoses)
• the patient's needs
• pertinent nursing observations
• nursing reassessments and interventions
• the patient's responses to interventions
• evaluation of expected outcomes.

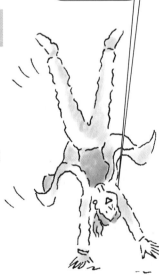

I love observing a patient's steady progress toward achieving outcomes!

All members of the health care team can document integrated progress notes, which are in chronological order based on the date. (See *A group effort: Integrated progress notes.*)

Making good progress

Progress notes are helpful for the following reasons:
- They're written chronologically and reflect the nursing diagnoses.
- They contain narrative information that doesn't easily fit into available space or format provided by other documentation forms.

Progress? More like stumbling into pitfalls...

On the other hand, progress notes have these pitfalls:

Art of the chart

A group effort: Integrated progress notes

One key advantage of integrated progress notes: Every member of the health care team can document on them. Integrated progress notes are written in chronological order and dated.

Don't skip lines between entries.

INTEGRATED PROGRESS NOTES

11/24/02 0800	Nursing note	
Pt with temp. 102°F. Doctor Weber notified. No order at this time.		P. Smith, RN
11/24/02 0830	MICU attending	
Pt continues to appear w/o change in status. Remains febrile and unresponsive. Will discuss code status		
with family. Prognosis poor.		R. Weber, MD
11/24/02 1030	Infectious disease attending	
Pt continues with fever of unknown origin. T max. 104°F. Tylenol ineffective. Cultures from 11/23 pend-		
ing. Change all central line a_____ _____ tips for culture. Continue vancomycin, gentamicin, and		
amikacin. Monitor trough leve____ ____s accordingly. Try to obtain HIV testing consent from fami-		
ly. Send fungal cultures. If ___ ___ amphotericin B. Use test dose. Consult renal for worsen-		
ing renal failure.		J. Barry, MD
11/24/02 1545	Intern progress note	
HIV consent obtained. Labs to be drawn.		J. Krimm, DO

Make sure you record the date and time.

- If they aren't well-organized, you may have to read through the entire form to find what you're looking for. To help prevent this, some facilities require you to put a heading on each note.
- You may waste time recording information on progress notes that you have already recorded on other forms.

How to write progress notes

When writing progress notes, include the following information:
- date and time of the entry
- the patient's condition
- interventions
- the patient's response to care
- details of changes in the patient's condition
- evaluation of interventions.

A solid base of nursing diagnoses

Some progress notes are designed to focus on nursing diagnoses. If your facility uses this type of note, be sure to record the nursing diagnosis that relates to your entry. (See *Nursing diagnosis–based progress notes.*)

Set your watch

Every time you write a progress note, be sure to record the exact time you gave the care or noted the observation. Don't record entries in blocks of time, such as 3:30 to 8:30. Years ago, when nurses were required to write progress notes every 2 hours, charting blocks of time was common. But today, most nurses use a flow sheet to chart how often they check on a patient. Together, flow sheets and progress notes usually provide adequate evidence of nursing care.

Change in condition? Chart it.

Be sure to document new patient problems, such as onset of seizures, and the resolution of old problems, such as no complaint of pain in 12 hours. Also, record deteriorations in the patient's condition—for example, *Pt has increasing dyspnea, causing him to remain on bed rest. ABG values show PaO$_2$ of 55. O$_2$ provided by rebreather mask as ordered.*

Document your observations of the patient's response to the plan of care. If his behaviors are similar to agreed-upon objectives, document that the goals are being met. If not, document that they aren't being met.

> **Art of the chart**

Nursing diagnosis–based progress notes

Progress notes can be written using a nursing diagnosis, as the sample below shows.

Patient identification information
Robert Burns
131 Green Ave.
Tempe, AZ
(123) 666-7777

Memorial General, Tempe, AZ

> Notes are directly related to the patient problem.

PROGRESS NOTES

Date and time	Nursing diagnosis and related problems	Notes
11/11/02 - 1100	Excess fluid volume R/T chronic renal insufficiency	Bilat. +4 pretibial and pedal edema. #16 Fr. Foley with urimeter inserted to monitor hourly output.
		Furosemide 40 mg I.V. given at 1055. HOB elevated to 45 ; O₂ 2 L. Nasal cannula in place. P. Smith, RN
11/11/02 - 1130	Excess fluid volume R/T chronic renal insufficiency	200 ml clear yellow urine in urimeter. Edema unchanged. Pt states: "It isn't as hard to catch my breath." ———————— P. Smith, RN

Don't repeat yourself

Avoid including information that's already on the flow sheet, except when there's a sudden change in the patient's condition, such as a decreased level of consciousness, a change in skin condition, or swelling at an I.V. site.

Say what you did

Sometimes, nurses document a problem but fail to describe what they did about it. Outline your interventions clearly, including such information as notification of other health team members, interventions, and the patient's response. For example, *Patient at 8 a.m. had oral temp of 102° F, Dr. Bard notified. Acetaminophen 650 mg given P.O. At 10 a.m. patient had oral temp. of 100° F.*

Avoid vague wording. Using a phrase like "appears to be" indicates uncertainty about what you're charting. Phrases like "no problems" and "had a good day" are also ambiguous. Chart specific observations instead. For example, *Pa-*

> Didn't I already document that? I have to remember not to repeat myself.

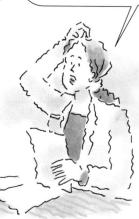

tient reports his left hip has less pain, a 2 on a scale of 1 to 10. Yesterday it was a 5.

Flow sheets

Flow sheets highlight specific patient information according to preestablished parameters of nursing care. They have spaces for recording dates, times, and specific interventions, which are set by each facility.

Charting with a nice flow

Flow sheets are used for charting data related to physical assessment of the patient and for recording routine aspects of patient care, such as activities of daily living, fluid balance, nutrition, pain, and skin integrity. They're also useful for recording specific nursing interventions.

Many facilities also document I.V. therapy and patient education on flow sheets. The style and format of flow sheets may vary to fit the needs of patients on particular units. Using flow sheets doesn't exempt you from narrative charting to describe your observations, patient teaching, patient responses, detailed interventions, and unusual circumstances. (See *Go with the flow sheets.*)

Go flow sheets!

Flow sheets have many sterling qualities:
• You can insert nursing data quickly and concisely, preferably at the time you give care or observe a change in the patient's condition.
• Because they provide an easy-to-read record of changes in the patient's condition over time, flow sheets allow all members of the health care team to compare data and assess the patient's progress.
• The concise format enables you to evaluate patient trends at a glance.
• They're less time-consuming to read because they tend to be more legible than handwritten progress notes.
• The format reinforces standards of nursing care and facilitates precise and less-fragmented nursing documentation.

Flow sheet faults

Flow sheets also have some less-than-ideal qualities:
• They may not have enough space for recording unusual events.
• Overuse of these forms can lead to incomplete documentation that obscures the patient's clinical picture.
• They may cause legal hassles if they aren't consistent with the progress notes. What's checked off on the flow sheet needs to agree with what's documented on the progress notes.

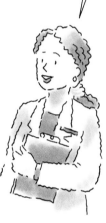

Flow sheets are easy to prepare and easy to read!

Art of the chart

Go with the flow sheets

As this sample shows, a patient care flow sheet lets you quickly document routine interventions.

Be sure to initial your entry.

PATIENT CARE FLOW SHEET

Date: 11/22/02	2300-0700	0700-1500	1500-2300
RESPIRATORY			
Breath sounds	clear 2330 AS	Crackles LLL 0800 JM	clear 1600 HM
Treatments/Results		Nebulizer 0830 JM	
Cough/Results		Mod. amt. tenacious yellow mucus 0900 JM	
O$_2$ therapy	Nasal cannula @2 L / min AS	Nasal cannula @2 L/ min JM	Nasal cannula @2 L/min HM
CARDIAC			
Chest pain			
Heart sounds	Normal S$_1$ and S$_2$ AS	Normal S$_1$ and S$_2$ JM	S$_2$ HM
Telemetry	N/A	N/A	
PAIN			
Type and location	(L) flank 0400 AS	(L) flank 1000 JM	(L) flank 1600 HM
Intervention	meperidine 0415 AS	reposition and meperidine 1010 JM	meperidine 1615 HM
Pt response	Improved from #9 to #3 in 1/2 hour AS	Improved from #8 to #2 in 1/2 hr JM	complete relief in 1 hr HM
NUTRITION			
Type		regular JM	Regular HM
Toleration %		90% JM	80% HM
Supplement		1 can Ensure JM	
ELIMINATION			
Stool appearance			
Enema	N/A	N/A	N/A
Results			
Bowel sounds	present all quadrants 2330 AS	present all quadrants 0800 JM	hyperactive all quadrants 1600 HM
Urine appearance	Clear amber 0400 AS	Clear amber 1000 JM	Dark yellow 1500 HM
Indwelling urinary catheter	N/A	N/A	N/A
Catheter irrigations			

Note the exact time.

Make sure you document your patient's response to medications.

Use the flow sheet to track changes in your patient's responses.

(continued)

Go with the flow sheets (continued)

PATIENT CARE FLOW SHEET

Date 11/22/02	2300-0700	0700-1500	1500-2300
TUBES			
Type	N/A	N/A	N/A
Irrigation			
Drainage appearance			
HYGIENE			
Self/partial/ complete		Partial 1000 JM	Partial 2100 HM
Oral care		1000 JM	2100 HM
Back care	0400 AS	1000 JM	2100 HM
Foot care		1000 JM	
Remove/reapply elastic stockings	2330 AS	1000 JM	2100 HM
ACTIVITY			
Type	bed rest AS	OOB to chair x 20 min 1000 JM	OOB to chair x 20 min 1800 HM
Toleration	Turns self AS	Tol. well JM	Tol. well
Repositioned	2330 supine AS 0400 (L) side AS	(L) side 0800 JM (R) side 1400 JM	self HM
ROM		1000 (active) JM 1400 (active) JM	1800 (active) HM 2200 (active) HM
SLEEP			
Sleeps well	0400 AS 0600 AS	N/A	N/A
Awake at intervals	2300 AS 0400 AS		
Awake most of the time			
SAFETY			
ID bracelet on	2330 AS 0200 AS	0800 JM 1200 JM 1500 JM	1600 HM 2100 HM
Call button in reach	2330 AS 0200 AS	0800 JM 1200 JM 1500 JM	1600 HM 2100 HM
Side rails up	2330 AS 0200 AS	0800 JM 1200 JM 1500 JM	1600 HM 2100 HM

Don't leave space blank. Write "none" or "N/A" or draw a line through the space.

Flow sheets encourage you to chart care promptly.

• The format may fail to reflect the patients' needs as well as the nurses' documentation needs on each unit. Flow sheets can become a liability if they aren't tailored to each unit and revised as needed.

How to use flow sheets

Ideally, flow sheets are used to document all routine assessment data and nursing interventions. Some common examples of these are:
• repositioning or turning the patient
• range-of-motion exercises
• patient education
• wound care
• medication administration.

Charting routine assessment data this way allows you to focus on changes in the patient's condition, his complex needs, and his progress toward achieving expected outcomes.

Be sure data on the flow sheet are consistent with data in your progress notes. Of course, all entries should accurately reflect the care given. Discrepancies can damage your credibility and increase your chance of liability.

Completing the picture

Sometimes, recording only the information requested isn't enough to give a complete picture of the patient's health. If this is the case, record additional information in the space provided on the flow sheet. If additional information isn't necessary, draw a line through the space to indicate this.

If your flow sheet doesn't have additional space and you need to record more information, use the progress notes.

Symbolic significance

Fill out flow sheets completely, using the specified symbols — such as check marks, "X"s, initials, circles, or the time — to indicate assessment of a parameter or performance of an intervention. When necessary, use the abbreviation "N/A" (not applicable) or another abbreviation recognized by your facility.

A ban on blanks

Don't leave blank spaces, which may imply that an intervention wasn't completed, wasn't attempted, or wasn't recognized. If you must omit something, document the reason for the omission.

Discharge summaries

Discharge summaries reflect the reassessment and evaluation components of the nursing process. To comply with JCAHO requirements, you must document your assessment of a patient's

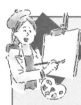

Art of the chart

Moving on: Discharge summaries

By combining the patient's discharge summary with instructions for care after discharge, you can fulfill two requirements with a single form. When using this documentation method, be sure to give one copy to the patient and keep one for the record.

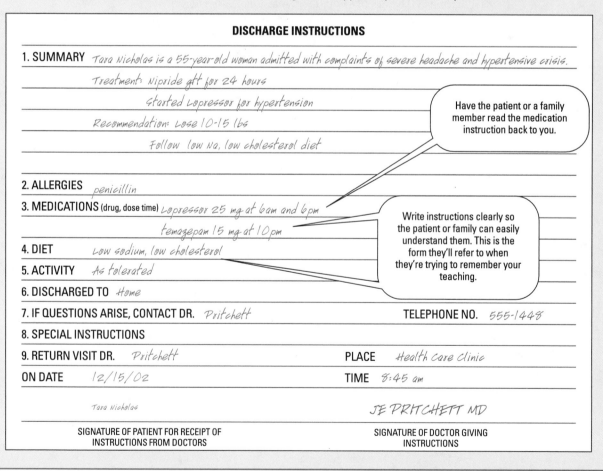

DISCHARGE INSTRUCTIONS

1. SUMMARY Tara Nicholas is a 55-year-old woman admitted with complaints of severe headache and hypertensive crisis.

Treatment: Nipride gtt for 24 hours

Started Lopressor for hypertension

Recommendation: Lose 10-15 lbs

Follow low Na, low cholesterol diet

> Have the patient or a family member read the medication instruction back to you.

2. ALLERGIES penicillin

3. MEDICATIONS (drug, dose time) Lopressor 25 mg at 6am and 6pm

temazepam 15 mg at 10pm

> Write instructions clearly so the patient or family can easily understand them. This is the form they'll refer to when they're trying to remember your teaching.

4. DIET Low sodium, low cholesterol

5. ACTIVITY As tolerated

6. DISCHARGED TO Home

7. IF QUESTIONS ARISE, CONTACT DR. Pritchett   TELEPHONE NO. 555-1448

8. SPECIAL INSTRUCTIONS

9. RETURN VISIT DR. Pritchett   PLACE Health Care Clinic

ON DATE 12/15/02   TIME 8:45 am

Tara Nicholas   JE PRITCHETT MD

SIGNATURE OF PATIENT FOR RECEIPT OF
INSTRUCTIONS FROM DOCTORS

SIGNATURE OF DOCTOR GIVING
INSTRUCTIONS

continuing care needs as well as any referrals for care and begin discharge planning early in the patient's stay.

Before we say good-bye...

To help in this kind of documentation, many facilities combine discharge summaries and patient instructions in one form. This form contains sections for recording patient assessment, patient education, detailed special instructions, and the circumstances of discharge. It uses a narrative style along with open- and closed-ended styles. (See *Moving on: Discharge summaries.*)

In sum, discharge summaries are all good

We have only good things to say about discharge summary forms:

• The combined form provides useful data about additional teaching needs and points out whether the patient has the information he needs to care for himself or to get further help.

• The form establishes compliance with JCAHO requirements and helps safeguard you from malpractice accusations.

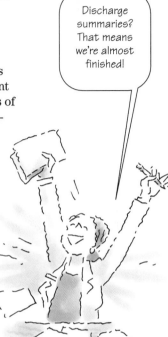

Discharge summaries? That means we're almost finished!

Art of the chart

Parting words: Narrative discharge notes

Some health care facilities use a narrative-style discharge summary, which is similar to a progress note. Here's a sample.

Date	Time	Progress notes
12/1/02	Discharge	68 y.o. black male admitted 11/28/02 with chest pain, hypertension; BP 190/100, and SOB. MI ruled
	1530	out. Chest pain relieved with sublingual nitroglycerin and O_2. Persantine thallium performed 11/30.
	(summary)	Tolerated procedure well. Has been OOB ambulating in the hallway without chest pain or SOB since 11/30.
		BP remains stable (144/86 at 1215). Drug regimen includes daily aspirin 325 mg, and captopril
		25 mg b.id. Verbalized understanding of medication times, dosages, and adverse effects. Will call
		Dr. Harris for 10 day postdischarge appointment. Discharge instruction sheet given. ——— B. McCort, RN

How to use discharge summaries

After completing your discharge summary form, give one copy to the patient and put another copy in the medical record for future reference. Be sure that the completed form outlines the patient's care, provides useful information for further teaching and evaluation, and documents that the patient has the information he needs to care for himself or to get further help.

Taking note of narrative discharge notes

Not all facilities use combined forms—some use narrative discharge notes. (See *Parting words: Narrative discharge notes*, page 127.) If your facility uses these, be sure to include the following information on the form:
• the patient's status at admission and discharge
• significant information about the patient's stay in the facility, including resolved and unresolved patient problems and referrals for continuing care
• instructions given to the patient, his family members, and other caregivers about medications, treatments, activity, diet, referrals, follow-up appointments, and any other special instructions.

Cheat sheet

Acute care documentation review

Admission database form
• Documents patient's initial assessment
• Must be completed within 24 hours of admission
• May be integrated with nursing and medical assessments
• Contains physiologic, psychosocial, and cultural information that's used throughout hospitalization

Plan of care
• Outlines the patient's nursing care
• Includes ongoing assessments, nursing diagnoses, expected outcomes, nursing interventions, and evaluation of care

Critical pathway
• Is a multidisciplinary plan of care that helps standardize care for routine conditions
• Determines the patient's daily care requirements and desired outcomes

Patient care Kardex
• Gives a quick overview of basic patient care information
• Allows quick access to information about task-oriented interventions, such as specific patient care, medication administration, and I.V. therapy
• Isn't usually a part of the permanent record, so information must also be recorded in another part of the chart

Graphic form
• Is used to plot vital signs and other standard data
• Presents information at a glance
• Saves the nurse time because unlicensed personnel are allowed to record data on it

Progress notes
• Are used to record the patient's status and monitor his condition

Acute care documentation review *(continued)*

• Reflect the nursing process in a format that's arranged chronologically, making it easy to follow
• Allow the nurse to record information that doesn't fit into other documentation forms

Flow sheets
• Are used to record the routine aspects of care as well as specific nursing interventions, allowing you to focus on changes in the patient's condition
• Highlight specific information according to preestablished parameters of nursing care
• Commonly used to document I.V. therapy and patient education

Discharge summary
• Reflects the reassessment and evaluation components of the nursing process
• Commonly combined with patient discharge instruction forms
• Provides useful data about additional teaching needs and the patient's ability to care for himself
• Establishes compliance with JCAHO requirements

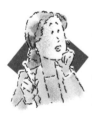

Quick quiz

1. An admission database is:
  A. a collection of computer information about your patient's psychosocial status.
  B. a form that documents the initial patient assessment data.
  C. a collection of data printed by a computer.

Answer: B. It's also known as an admission assessment form.

2. A responsibility of the staff nurse in the discharge planning process is:
  A. initiating a referral for home health services.
  B. evaluating the patient's mental status when his competence is an issue.
  C. deciding when the patient should be discharged.

Answer: A. Initiating a referral for home health services is within the nurse's scope of practice.

3.   A care track is an important part of which of the following documentation methods?
   A.   Computer-generated Kardex
   B.   Critical pathway
   C.   Flow sheet

Answer: B. The care track, or case map, defines a patient's daily care requirements and desired outcomes, consistent with the average length of stay for a specified DRG.

4.   Progress notes are organized according to what order?
   A.   Alphabetical
   B.   Numerical
   C.   Chronological

Answer: C. Progress notes chronologically record the patient's status and track changes in his condition.

5.   JCAHO asks nurses to do all of the following except:
   A.   include a patient care Kardex in the medical record.
   B.   include ongoing assessments related to illness in plans of care.
   C.   use flow sheets to document basic assessment findings and wound care, hygiene, and routine care interventions.

Answer: A. A Kardex isn't a JCAHO requirement, so some facilities have eliminated it and have incorporated the information into the patient's plan of care.

Scoring

☆☆☆   If you answered all five items correctly, amazing! You're destined to be acclaimed for accurate observation of acute care.

☆☆   If you answered three or four items correctly, wonderful! Your progress is well noted.

☆   If you answered fewer than three items correctly, don't worry. You can take the test as many times as you want and record your scores on a flow sheet.

Home health care

Just the facts

In this chapter, you'll learn:

♦ current and future trends in home health care

♦ risks and responsibilities in documenting home health care

♦ forms used for home health care documentation

♦ documenting patient teaching in home health care.

A look at home health care

The purpose of home health nursing is to restore, maintain, or promote health and function for patients and their families at home. A home health agency plans, coordinates, and supplies care based on the needs of the patient and family and the resources available to them. Think of the home health agency as a hospital without walls. Home care is one component of comprehensive health care.

An emerging health care powerhouse

Recent trends have contributed to the growth of the home health care industry, including:
• the development of a prospective payment system (PPS) for home health agencies
• the use of the Outcome and Assessment Information Set (OASIS), a tool used to help assess the patient's condition
• the increasing number of patients of advanced age
• the increased availability of sophisticated home care equipment

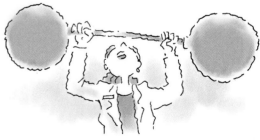

• the use of electronic claim processing and surveillance of the Health Care Financing Administration (HCFA) and fiscal intermediaries.

The Balanced Budget Act of 1997 required the development of a PPS for Medicare home health services and the implementation of this system in October 2000. Under this system, Medicare will pay home health agencies a predetermined base payment. The payment will be adjusted for the health care needs and conditions of the patient.

Quicker has equaled sicker

Managed care organizations have identified sophisticated methods of performing utilization review, causing a decrease in the average length of stay. Therefore, patients are typically sicker when they're discharged to home.

Because support services in the home and community cost less than institutional care, government and private insurance payers are expanding their coverage of home health care. In the future, the home health industry may become the primary supplier of health care in the United States.

Not your traditional patient

Traditionally, homebound Medicare recipients have constituted the major portion of the home health caseload. Agencies have expanded services to new populations, representing all age-groups and a variety of medical conditions. This has led to the emergence of home health subspecialties, such as home infusion agencies and high-tech cancer-related home care, including stem cell transplants. These agencies may be offshoots of parent organizations or stand-alone agencies. (See *The hospice alternative.*)

New documentation requirements

Although Medicare has tied reimbursement to the OASIS assessment, all patients over age 18, excluding women receiving maternal-child services, must have an OASIS evaluation. OASIS regulations require that nurses complete an assessment and agencies transmit the assessment and other data within strict time frames.

Patient assessment must be completed:
• within 5 days of the initiation of care and at 60 days and 120 days (if needed)
• when the patient is transferred to another agency
• when the patient is discharged from home care
• when there's a significant change in the patient's condition.

The hospice alternative

Many home health care agencies provide hospice care services. Hospice programs provide palliative care to terminally ill patients in both homes and hospitals.

Medicare coverage

Since 1983, patients who have met specific admission criteria can qualify for the hospice Medicare benefit instead of the traditional Medicare benefit, allowing greater freedom to choose the hospice alternative for terminal care. The patient receives noncurative medical and support service not otherwise covered by Medicare.

Medicare coverage for hospice care is available if:

• the patient is eligible for Medicare Part A, which covers skilled nursing home and hospital care; people eligible for Medicare include those who are age 65 or older, long-term disabled patients, and people with end-stage renal disease.

• the patient's doctor and the hospice medical director certify that the patient is terminally ill with a life expectancy of 6 months or less.

• the patient receives care from a Medicare-approved hospice program.

A Medicare-approved hospice program will usually provide care in the patient's home. The hospice team and the patient's doctor establish a plan of care for medical and support services for the management of a terminal illness.

A patient without coverage for hospice benefits may be eligible for free or reduced-cost care through local programs or foundations. Alternatively, a patient may pay privately for hospice services.

Understanding and acceptance of treatment

With hospice care, the patient and primary caregiver must complete documentation, indicating their understanding of hospice care. The patient and caregiver must sign an informed consent form that outlines everyone's responsibilities. The patient and primary caregiver must also sign a form indicating understanding and acceptance of the role of the primary caregiver. The form below is an example of this type of document.

REEDSVILLE HOME HEALTH AND HOSPICE
ACCEPTANCE OF PRIMARY CAREGIVER ROLE

I have been offered the opportunity to ask questions regarding the Hospice program and Hospice care of this patient. I understand that the Hospice program provides palliative, or comfort, measures and services, but not aggressive, invasive, or life-sustaining procedures.

I also understand that the Hospice concept of care is based upon the active participation of a primary care person who is not provided through the Hospice benefit, who is and will be willing to assist this patient with personal care and with activities of daily living as well as with safety precautions when Hospice personnel are not scheduled to be in the home. I accept the responsibility of being primary caregiver, and I agree to make appropriate arrangements to provide this role to this patient.

If, for any reason, I am unable to serve in this capacity at a time as deemed necessary for the safety and care of this patient, I agree to make other arrangements to fulfill the responsibilities of primary caregiver, which are acceptable to Reedsville Home Health and Hospice. I further understand that Reedsville Home Health and Hospice will assist in making the arrangements, but that I will be financially responsible for any costs associated with them.

Name of Patient: _____ Joan Powell _____

Signature of Patient: Joan Powell _____

Date: _____ 11/17/02 _____

Name of primary caregiver: _____ Joseph Powell _____

Date: _____ 11/17/02 _____

Signature of primary caregiver: _____ Joseph Powell _____

Relationship: _____ husband _____

Witness: _____ Cathy Melvin, RN _____

Date: _____ 11/17/02 _____

> When the patient and caregiver sign this form, it indicates that they understand the purpose and goals of hospice care and agree to comply with regulations for hospice eligibility.

Creating opportunities for care

Before receiving care from a home health care agency, patients with private insurance must obtain authorization from their insurance providers. In many cases, insurance limitations restrict treatment options.

In this cost-conscious environment, nurses take on an especially important role in helping patients get coverage by educating them about local, state, and federal benefit programs. When you help a patient identify a program for which he qualifies—such as veteran's benefits or Meals On Wheels—you help him get the services he needs while ensuring that your agency receives proper reimbursement.

> I'll help you find programs that augment your health coverage. That way, we both win.

Legal risks and responsibilities

Home health agencies are licensed and regulated by state governments and accredited by private agencies such as the Community Health Accreditation Program (CHAP), which is administered through the National League for Nursing (NLN) and the Joint Commission on Accreditation of Healthcare Organizations (JCAHO). In many cases, obtaining state licensure hinges on having accreditation. Home health agencies must also adhere to Medicare and Medicaid regulations administered by the HCFA and its agencies and carriers.

Meeting standards

Home health agencies are evaluated for such factors as accurate and complete documentation and adherence to standards, particularly establishing eligibility for services and quality of care. If standards aren't met, a home health agency may fail to earn licensure or accreditation, may have its current license and accreditation revoked, or may have reimbursement privileges withheld or revoked.

Risks of poor documentation

Home health agencies must maintain complete and legally sound documentation. For reimbursable services, nurses must document each instance that the specified service is provided. Nurses must also document the services the agency refuses to provide. Inadequate or incomplete documentation can have serious consequences.

Evaluating admissions

Since the inception of PPS for home health agencies, agencies have had to carefully evaluate admissions. Because of this evaluation process, not all patients who are referred for home health care qualify. If a patient has no caregiver or has a complex chronic medical condition, the cost of his care may quickly exceed the allotted reimbursement. Therefore, home health care agencies are unable to admit these patients.

Let's admit it: Admission assessment is crucial

A complete admission assessment and detailed documentation of this assessment are crucial in determining the appropriateness of each patient referred for admission.

Liability

After a nurse or home health agency is named in a lawsuit, it's too late to correct inaccurate documentation. For example, a nurse fails to record the patient's apical pulse and rhythm before administering digoxin. Later, the family sues the home health agency, alleging the staff caused the patient to go into complete heart block by failing to recognize signs of digoxin toxicity.

No record, no proof

Without a documented record, the agency is unable to prove that the patient wasn't experiencing excessive slowing of the pulse, a classic sign of digoxin toxicity.

Financial losses

Inadequate or incomplete documentation may result in refusal by third-party payers or fiscal intermediaries to cover services.

A bad business practice

Insurance companies who negotiate preferred provider contracts may refuse to do business with home health agencies that provide incomplete documentation.

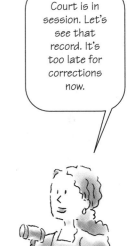

Court is in session. Let's see that record. It's too late for corrections now.

Documentation guidelines

Documentation of care and discharge planning begins when you evaluate a new patient for service. (See *Does the patient qualify?* page 136.) You may use a referral form to document the patient's needs. (See *Referral form*, pages 137 and 138.) Patients and caregivers also fill out several forms during the initial home visit. (See *Paperwork for patients*, page 136.)

Advice from the experts

Does the patient qualify?

Careful screening, which is done at the initial evaluation, is critical when determining what clinical services a patient needs. When evaluating a new patient for service, look for the following criteria.

Clinical criteria
- Skilled care needed
- Appropriately prescribed therapy that can be done in the home
- Caregiver available to assist patient

Technical criteria (patient or caregiver)
- Senses intact
- Ability to learn and follow procedures
- Ability to recognize complications and initiate emergency medical procedures

Environmental criteria
- Access to a telephone
- Access to electricity
- Access to water
- Clean living environment

Financial criteria
- Verification of insurance coverage
- Full knowledge of copayment or out-of-pocket expenses
- Agreement to comply with the conditions of participation

Be sure to begin at the beginning

When you start caring for a patient, always document activities completed during your nursing visit: assessments, interventions, the patient's response to treatment, and whether he had complications. Also, record your communications with other members of the health care team and the date of the next visit. Use your agency's flow sheets.

The information you provide gets around

The information you provide is used by third-party payers during utilization review to evaluate each claim in accordance with criteria for coverage. It may also be used by the government and oversight agencies to determine the validity of services.

Documentation details

Home care documentation should cover:
- OASIS
- evidence that the home environment is safe for the procedure or treatment or can be safely adapted; findings about the home and measures taken to ensure safe delivery of care
- rationale for treatment and patient response

Paperwork for patients

During your initial home visit, you'll ask the patient or caregiver to read and sign many forms. These required forms include:
- patient rights and responsibilities
- advance directives, including a do-not-resuscitate option
- consent for services
- medical information authorization and release
- assignment of benefits
- equipment acceptance
- patient-teaching checklist.

If an I.V. infusion is required, the forms also include:
- consent for vascular access
- infusion treatment service agreement.

Feeling validated
In addition, your agency may require the patient to cosign the Outcome and Assessment Information Set form and the nurses' notes or a time sheet to validate your visit in the home.

Art of the chart

Referral form

Also called an intake form, a referral form is used to document the patient's needs when you begin your evaluation of a new patient. Use the form shown here as a guide.

> This form provides an overview of the patient's condition, required treatment, and psychosocial and cultural concerns.

Date of referral: _11/17/02_   Bra   Chart #: _91-413_   H ✔
Info taken by: _Beth Isham, RN   North_   Admit Date: _11/18/02_
Patient's Name: _Geraldine Rush_
Address: _66 Newton St._
City: _Burlington_   State: _VT_   Zip: _05402_
Phone: _(802) 123-4561_   Date of birth: _4/3/25_
Primary caregiver name & phone number: _husband (Dennis) (802) 123-4561_
Insurance name: _Medicare_   Ins. #: _123-45-6189_
Is this a managed care policy (HMO)? _no_
Primary Dx: (Code _162.5_) _lung cancer_   Date: _12/11/02_
     (Code _811_) _pressure ulcer (coccyx)_   Date: _3/13/02_
     (Code _714.0_) _rheumatoid arthritis_   Date: _1980s_
Procedures: (Code _86.28_) _pressure ulcer_   Date: _11/1/02_
Referral source: _J. Silva, hospital SW_   Phone: _165-2813_
Doctor name & phone #: _Frank Crabbe_   Phone: _165-4321_
Doctor address: _9013 Parkway Drive, Burlington_
Hospital _University Hospital_   Admit _11/1/02_   Discharge _11/16/02_
Functional limitations: Pain management, _nonambulatory, poor fine motor skills 2° rheumatoid arthritis_
ORDERS/SERVICES: (specify amount, frequency and duration)
(SN:) _SN visits 3x/week & p.r.n. x 2 months_
(AL:) _CNA visits daily 5 days/week x 2 months_
(PT, OT,) ST: _PT & OT evaluations and visits 2-3 x/week & p.r.n. x 2 month_
(MSW) _MSW evaluation & weekly vs x 2 months_

> Check out this part of the form to determine what services the patient needs.

Spiritual Coordinator: _Rev. Carlson, St. Paul's Lutheran Church_
Counselor: _JoAnne Knowlton, MSW_
Volunteer: _Rosalie Marshall - niece will provide care on weekends_
Other services provided: _shopping, laundry, meal prep_
Goals: _wound care, pain management, terminal care @ home_
Equipment: _needs: commode, hospital bed, bedpan, Hoyer lift, side rail w/c_
Company & Phone number: _Scott Medical Equipment 165-9931_
Safety Measures _side rails ↑_   Nutritional req _diet as tolerated_

FUNCTIONAL LIMITATIONS: (Circle Applicable)			ACTIVITIES PERMITTED: (Circle Applicable)		
1 Amputation	5 Paralysis	9 Legally Blind	1. Complete bedrest	6. Partial wgt bearing	(A) Wheelchair
2 Bowel/Bladder	6 Endurance	A Dyspnea with	2. Bedrest BRP	7. Independent at home	B. Walker
3 Contracture	7 Ambulation	minimal exer	3. Up as tolerated	8. Crutches	C. No restriction
4 Hearing	8 Speech	B. Other _B. A._	4 Transfer bed/chair	9. Cane	D. Other -specify

Accessibility to bath   Y - N   Shower   Y - N   Bathroom   Y - N   Exit   Y - N
Mental status: (Circle)   Oriented   Comatose   Forgetful   Depressed   Disoriented   Lethargic   Agitated   Other

(continued)

Referral form (continued)

Allergies: _____none known_____

• Hospice appropriate meds   • Med company: _____Walker Pharmacy_____

MEDICATIONS:

_____morphine sulfate liq. 20 mg/ml 40 mg P.O. q6h p.r.n pain_____

_____Compazine 10 mg P.O. or P.R. q4-6h p.r.n n/v_____

_____Colace 200 mg P.O. q.d. p.r.n constipation_____

_____Benadryl 25-50 mg P.O. @ hs p.r.n sleeplessness_____

Living will   yes __✓__   no_____   obtained _____ Family to mail to office _____

Guardian, POA, or responsible person: _____husband_____

Address & phone number: _____same_____

Other family members: _____

ETOH _____0_____ Drug Use: _____0_____ Smoker _2 ppd x 40 years quit 2 yrs ago_

History: _other than problems associated with arthritis, was in general good health until 12/96. Dx: lung CA - husband cared for_ _@ home until 11/1/97._

Social history (place of birth, education, jobs, retirement, etc.) _Born & raised in Toronto, became U.S. citizen_ _when married in 1951. 2 yrs college - majored in music. Retired church organist._

ADMISSION NOTES: VS: T_98.4 P.O._   AP _86_   RR _18_   BP _140/72_

Lungs: _decreased breath sounds LLL._   Extremities: _cool to touch Pedal pulses present._

Wgt: _118_ Recent wgt (loss)/gain of _40 lb over 6 months_

Admission narrative: _visit made to pt/husband in hospital before discharge. Both have been told that she is failing rapidly, and_ _would like her to return home with Hospice services. Niece willing to help 2 days/week. Pt apprehensive; husband blames him_ _self for the coccygeal decubitus which developed under his care._

Psychosocial Issues _Pt has always cared for husband. Describes self as depressed that she is no longer able to do so;_ _worries who will care for him after she dies._

Environmental concerns _(need smoke detectors?)_

Are there any cultural or spiritual customs or beliefs of which we should be aware before providing Hospice services? _Pt would like Holy Communion just before death (& weekly?)_

Funeral home: _____not yet chosen_____ Contact made yes _____ no _x_

DIRECTIONS: _corner Newton / Elm   duplex, white with green trim. Door on (L) says 66. Bell broken - knock loudly._

Agency Representative Signature: _Beth Isham, RN_ _Date: _11/18/02_

Home Care Supervisor

• emergency and resource numbers given to the patient or caregiver (JCAHO requires that the patient or caregiver have 24-hour emergency telephone access to the agency or nurse)
• the patient's or caregiver's ability to perform steps in home care procedures, including the ability to perform return demonstration
• the patient's or caregiver's ability to troubleshoot equipment, including a backup plan for a power failure
• the patient's or caregiver's ability to recognize potential complications, respond appropriately, and get help when necessary.

Documenting patient teaching

Correct documentation will help justify to your agency and to third-party payers your visits to teach the patient or caregiver. Find out about the patient's and family's needs, resources, and support systems. This will help you outline the basic teaching plan.

Keeping continuity

Remember that teaching is usually an ongoing process requiring more than one visit. Until the patient becomes independent, your documentation will help other nurses continue the teaching and identify additional areas of teaching. (See *Certification of instruction*, page 140.)

Keep a list of teaching and reference materials you have supplied to the patient or caregiver. Also, document modifications made to accommodate the patient's or caregiver's literacy skills and native language.

Being there

If the patient isn't physically or mentally able to perform the skills himself and no caregiver is available, report this in your documentation. The patient most likely isn't an appropriate candidate for home care. Never leave a patient alone to perform a procedure until he can express understanding of it and perform it competently.

Setting the terms (the ones on the packages)

Be careful to call equipment by the same names used on the packages and in teaching literature. Consider providing a glossary of terms and labeling machines to match your instructions. Make sure that the patient can identify devices when speaking on the telephone. Document all teaching materials given to the patient, and keep copies of teaching materials in your records. You may want to videotape your instructions in the home if more than one caregiver will be providing care.

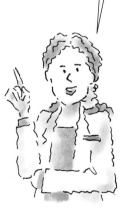

Be there for a patient until he can perform a procedure adequately on his own.

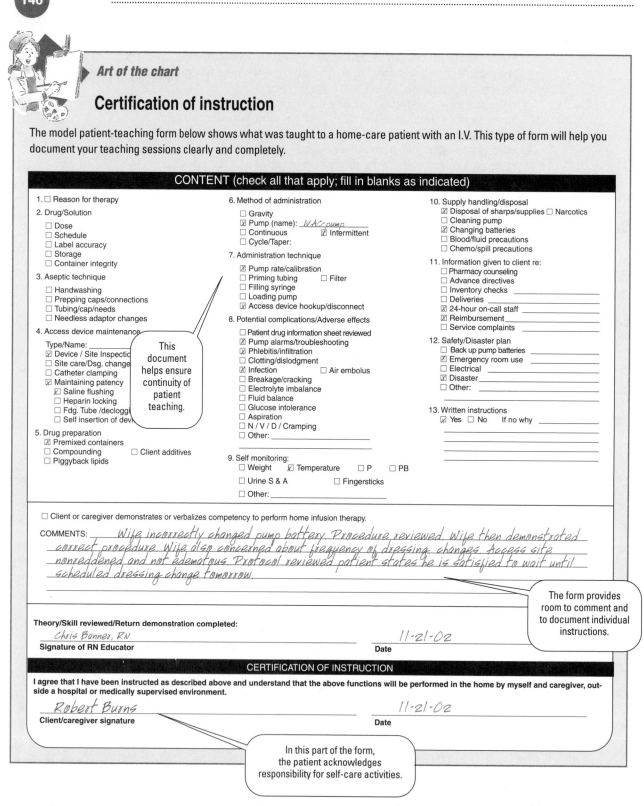

Art of the chart

Certification of instruction

The model patient-teaching form below shows what was taught to a home-care patient with an I.V. This type of form will help you document your teaching sessions clearly and completely.

CONTENT (check all that apply; fill in blanks as indicated)

1. ☐ Reason for therapy

2. Drug/Solution
   - ☐ Dose
   - ☐ Schedule
   - ☐ Label accuracy
   - ☐ Storage
   - ☐ Container integrity

3. Aseptic technique
   - ☐ Handwashing
   - ☐ Prepping caps/connections
   - ☐ Tubing/cap/needs
   - ☐ Needless adaptor changes

4. Access device maintenance
   - Type/Name:
   - ☒ Device / Site Inspection
   - ☐ Site care/Dsg. change
   - ☐ Catheter clamping
   - ☒ Maintaining patency
     - ☒ Saline flushing
     - ☐ Heparin locking
     - ☐ Fdg. Tube /declogging
     - ☐ Self insertion of device

5. Drug preparation
   - ☒ Premixed containers
   - ☐ Compounding   ☐ Client additives
   - ☐ Piggyback lipids

This document helps ensure continuity of patient teaching.

6. Method of administration
   - ☐ Gravity
   - ☒ Pump (name): _IVAC-pump_
   - ☐ Continuous   ☒ Intermittent
   - ☐ Cycle/Taper:

7. Administration technique
   - ☒ Pump rate/calibration
   - ☐ Priming tubing   ☐ Filter
   - ☐ Filling syringe
   - ☐ Loading pump
   - ☒ Access device hookup/disconnect

8. Potential complications/Adverse effects
   - ☐ Patient drug information sheet reviewed
   - ☒ Pump alarms/troubleshooting
   - ☒ Phlebitis/infiltration
   - ☐ Clotting/dislodgment
   - ☒ Infection   ☐ Air embolus
   - ☐ Breakage/cracking
   - ☐ Electrolyte imbalance
   - ☐ Fluid balance
   - ☐ Glucose intolerance
   - ☐ Aspiration
   - ☐ N / V / D / Cramping
   - ☐ Other: _____

9. Self monitoring:
   - ☐ Weight   ☒ Temperature   ☐ P   ☐ PB
   - ☐ Urine S & A   ☐ Fingersticks
   - ☐ Other: _____

10. Supply handling/disposal
    - ☒ Disposal of sharps/supplies ☐ Narcotics
    - ☐ Cleaning pump
    - ☒ Changing batteries
    - ☐ Blood/fluid precautions
    - ☐ Chemo/spill precautions

11. Information given to client re:
    - ☐ Pharmacy counseling
    - ☐ Advance directives
    - ☐ Inventory checks _____
    - ☐ Deliveries
    - ☒ 24-hour on-call staff _____
    - ☒ Reimbursement_____
    - ☐ Service complaints _____

12. Safety/Disaster plan
    - ☐ Back up pump batteries _____
    - ☒ Emergency room use _____
    - ☐ Electrical
    - ☒ Disaster_____
    - ☐ Other: _____

13. Written instructions
    - ☒ Yes ☐ No   If no why _____
    _____
    _____
    _____

☐ Client or caregiver demonstrates or verbalizes competency to perform home infusion therapy.

COMMENTS: _Wife incorrectly changed pump battery. Procedure reviewed. Wife then demonstrated correct procedure. Wife also concerned about frequency of dressing changes. Access site nonreddened and not edematous. Protocol reviewed patient states he is satisfied to wait until scheduled dressing change tomorrow._

The form provides room to comment and to document individual instructions.

Theory/Skill reviewed/Return demonstration completed:

Chris Banner, RN   _11-21-02_
Signature of RN Educator   **Date**

CERTIFICATION OF INSTRUCTION

I agree that I have been instructed as described above and understand that the above functions will be performed in the home by myself and caregiver, outside a hospital or medically supervised environment.

Robert Burns   _11-21-02_
Client/caregiver signature   **Date**

In this part of the form, the patient acknowledges responsibility for self-care activities.

Signing off

Most agencies require patients to sign a teaching documentation record indicating that they accept responsibility for learning self-care activities. This is a critical piece of documentation for the home care chart.

Home health care forms

Key forms used to document home health care include:
• agency assessment form and OASIS
• plan of care
• progress notes
• nursing and discharge summaries
• team communication
• doctor's updates to the plan of care
• communication with insurance case managers regarding authorization of care
• referrals to other service providers.

Agency assessment and OASIS forms

When a patient is referred to your home health care agency, you must complete a thorough and specific assessment and chart the information on a patient assessment form.

Assess the patient's:
• physical status
• mental and emotional status
• home environment in relation to safety and support services
• knowledge of his disease or current condition, prognosis, and treatment plan
• potential for complying with the treatment plan.

Guidelines for use

As with any setting, be thorough during home health care. A thorough patient assessment provides the information you need to plan appropriate care.

Consider the following:
• Obtain information about the patient's past and current health. Organize the interview by body system and ask open-ended questions.
• When taking a physical assessment, use a systematic approach, as is appropriate in any setting. For example, you may take a body-system or head-to-toe approach.

• When assessing the home environment, consider such factors as the presence of a caregiver, structural barriers, access to a telephone, and safety and hygiene practices.
• When assessing the patient's potential for complying with the treatment plan, consider such factors as history of psychiatric disorders, developmental status, substance abuse, comprehension, ability to read and write, and the presence of any language barriers.
• OASIS isn't a substitute for a thorough assessment; it's an addition. Some agencies have integrated their assessment forms and OASIS. (See *Using the OASIS-B1 form.*)
• OASIS guidelines specify the questions to be asked. All must be asked, even though the patient may decline to answer some. Note the ones he declines to answer on your record, and report it to your supervisor as well.

Plan of care

Professional standards dictated by CHAP in 1993 — under the guidance of NLN — require you to develop a comprehensive plan of care in cooperation with the patient and his caregivers.

Family counsel

In many aspects of care, the patient and family become the decision makers. This fact must be taken into account when developing your plan of care; adjust your interventions, patient goals, and teaching accordingly. Reimbursement must also be taken into consideration.

Don't go astray — without documenting it, at least

Legally speaking, a plan of care is the most direct evidence of your nursing judgment. If you outline a plan of care and then deviate from it, a court may decide that you strayed from a reasonable standard of care. So be sure to update your plan of care and make sure it fits the patient's needs.

Collating care

Some agencies use the home health certification form and plan of care form (required for Medicare reimbursement) as the official plan of care for Medicare patients. Most home health agencies, however, require a separate plan of care.

Agencies use a multidisciplinary, integrated plan of care for those patients receiving more than one service such as physical or occupational therapy. (See *Interdisciplinary plan of care,* page 159.)

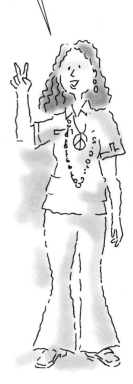

Change of plans? Just document it, man. Don't get caught out of date!

(Text continues on page 158.)

Art of the chart

Using the OASIS-B1 form

The OASIS-B1 form includes more than 80 topics, such as socioeconomic, physiologic, and functional data; service utilization information; and mental, behavioral, and emotional data.

OUTCOME AND ASSESSMENT INFORMATION SET (OASIS-B1)

START OF CARE Assessment (also used for Resumption of Care Following Inpatient Stay)	Client's Name: _____ Client Record No. _____

The Outcome and Assessment Information Set (OASIS) is the intellectual property of The Center for Health Services and Policy Research. Copyright ©2000 Used with Permission.

DEMOGRAPHIC/GENERAL INFORMATION

1. (M0010) Agency Medicare Provider Number:
_____

2. (M0012) Agency Medicaid Provider Number:
_____

> Identify the date that care is started here.

5. (M0020) Patient ID Number:
  QCB/811757

6. (M0030) Start of Care Date: _07_ / _02_ / _2002_
  month   day   year

7. (M0032) Resumption of Care Date:
  ____ / ____ / _____   ☒ NA - Not Applicable
  month   day   year

8. (M0040) Patient Name:
  Terry   _S_
  First   MI
  Elliot   _Mr._
  Last   Suffix

Patient Address:
  11 Second Street
  Street, Route, Apt. Number
  Hometown
  City

  (M0050) Patient State of Residence: _PA_
  (M0060) Patient Zip Code: _10981_ - _1234_
  Phone: (_881_) _555_ - _2937_

9. (M0063) Medicare Number:
  _134765482 A_
                including suffix
  ☐ NA - No Medicare

10. (M0064) Social Security Number:
  _111_ - _22_ - _3333_
  ☐ UK - Unknown or Not Available

11. (M0065) Medicaid Number:
  _____
  ☐ NA - No Medicaid

12. (M0066) Birth Date: _07_ / _08_ / _1926_
                        month day   year

13. (M0069) Gender:
  ☒ 1 - Male   ☐ 2 - Female

14. (M0072) Primary Referring Physician ID:
  _222222_   (UPIN#)
  ☐ UK - Unknown or Not Available
  Name _Dr. Kyle Stevens_
  Address _10 State St._
  Hometown, PA 10981
  Phone: (_881_) _555_ - _6900_
  FAX: (_881_) _555_ - _6974_

15. (M0080) Discipline of Person Completing Assessment:
  ☒ 1-RN   ☐ 2-PT   ☐ 3-SLP/ST   ☐ 4-OT

16. (M0090) Date Assessment Completed:
  _07_ / _02_ / _2002_
  month day   year

(continued)

Using the OASIS-B1 form *(continued)*

17. (M0100) This Assessment is Currently Being Completed for the Following Reason:

Start/Resumption of Care

☒ 1 - Start of care—further visits planned

☐ 2 - Start of care—no further visits planned

☐ 3 - Resumption of care (after inpatient stay)

Identify the reason for the current assessment in this section.

Follow-Up

☐ 4 - Recertification (follow-up) reassessment [Go to *M0150*]

☐ 5 - Other follow-up [Go to *M0150*]

Transfer to an Inpatient Facility

☐ 6 - Transferred to an inpatient facility—patient not discharged from agency [Go to *M0150*]

☐ 7 - Transferred to an inpatient facility—patient discharged from agency [Go to *M0150*]

Discharge from Agency—Not to an Inpatient Facility

☐ 8 - Death at home [Go to *M0150*]

☐ 9 - Discharge from agency [Go to *M0150*]

☐ 10 - Discharge from agency—no visits completed after start/resumption of care assessment [Go to *M0150*]

18. Marital status:

☐ Not Married   ☒ Married   ☐ Widowed

☐ Divorced   ☐ Separated   ☐ Unknown

19. (M0140) Race/Ethnicity (as identified by patient): (Mark all that apply.)

☐ 1 - American Indian or Alaska Native

☐ 2 - Asian

☐ 3 - Black or African-American

☐ 4 - Hispanic or Latino

☐ 5 - Native Hawaiian or Pacific Islander

☒ 6 - White

☐ UK - Unknown

This section covers patient history.

20. Emergency contact:

Name   *Susan Elliot*

Address   *11 Second St.*

Hometown, PA 10981

Phone: (*881*)   *555* - *2937*

21. (M0150) Current Payment Sources for Home Care: (Mark all that apply.)

☐ 0 - None; no charge for current services

☒ 1 - Medicare (traditional fee-for-service)

☐ 2 - Medicare (HMO/managed care)

☐ 3 - Medicaid (traditional fee-for-service)

☐ 4 - Medicaid (HMO/managed care)

☐ 5 - Workers' compensation

☐ 6 - Title programs (e.g., Title III, V, or XX)

☐ 7 - Other government (e.g., CHAMPUS, VA, etc.)

☐ 8 - Private insurance

☐ 9 - Private HMO/managed care

☐ 10 - Self-pay

☐ 11 - Other (specify) _____

☐ UK - Unknown

22. (M0160) Financial Factors limiting the ability of the patient/family to meet basic health needs: (Mark all that apply.)

☒ 0 - None

☐ 1 - Unable to afford medicine or medical supplies

☐ 2 - Unable to afford medical expenses that are not covered by insurance/Medicare (e.g., copayments)

☐ 3 - Unable to afford rent/utility bills

☐ 4 - Unable to afford food

☐ 5 - Other (specify) _____

PATIENT HISTORY

23. (M0175) From which of the following **Inpatient Facilities** was the patient discharged *during the past 14 days?* (Mark all that apply.)

☐ 1 - Hospital

☐ 2 - Rehabilitation facility

☐ 3 - Skilled nursing facility

☐ 4 - Other nursing home

☐ 5 - Other (specify) _____

☒ NA - Patient was not discharged from an inpatient facility [If NA, go to *M0200*]

24. (M0180) Inpatient Discharge Date (most recent):

____ / ____ / ____
month   day   year

☐ UK - Unknown

Using the OASIS-B1 form *(continued)*

25. (M0190) Inpatient Diagnoses and ICD code categories (three digits required; five digits optional) *for only those conditions treated during an inpatient facility stay within the last 14 days* (no surgical or V-codes):

Inpatient Facility Diagnosis　　　　　**ICD**

a.＿＿＿＿＿＿＿＿＿＿＿＿＿＿　　(＿＿＿＿ . ＿＿＿)

b.＿＿＿＿＿＿＿＿＿＿＿＿＿＿　　(＿＿＿＿ . ＿＿＿)

26. (M0200) **Medical or Treatment Regimen Change Within Past 14 Days:** Has this patient experienced a change in medical or treatment regimen (e.g., medication, treatment, or service change due to new or additional diagnosis, etc.) within the last 14 days?

☐　0 - No　　[If No, go to *M0220*]

☒　1 - Yes

27. (M0210) List the patient's **Medical Diagnoses** and ICD code categories (three digits required; five digits optional) or those conditions requiring changed medical or treatment regimen (no surgical or V-codes):

Changed Medical Regimen Diagnosis　　**ICD**

a. *open wound ℓ ankle*　　　　(*891* . *00*)

b.＿＿＿＿＿＿＿＿＿＿＿＿　　(＿＿＿＿ . ＿＿＿)

c.＿＿＿＿＿＿＿＿＿＿＿＿　　(＿＿＿＿ . ＿＿＿)

d.＿＿＿＿＿＿＿＿＿＿＿＿　　(＿＿＿＿ . ＿＿＿)

28. (M0220) **Conditions Prior to Medical or Treatment Regimen Change or Inpatient Stay Within Past 14 Days:**
If this patient experienced an inpatient facility discharge or change in medical or treatment regimen within the past 14 days, indicate any conditions which existed *prior to* the inpatient stay or change in medical or treatment regimen. **(Mark all that apply.)**

☐　1 - Urinary incontinence

☐　2 - Indwelling/suprapubic catheter

☐　3 - Intractable pain

☐　4 - Impaired decision making

☐　5 - Disruptive or socially inappropriate behavior

☐　6 - Memory loss to the extent that supervision required

☒　7 - None of the above

☐　NA - No inpatient facility discharge *and* no change in medical or treatment regimen in past 14 days

☐　UK - Unknown

29. (M0230/M0240) **Diagnoses and Severity Index:** List each medical diagnosis or problem for which the patient is receiving home care and ICD code category (three digits required; five digits optional — no surgical or V-codes) and rate them using the following severity index. (Choose one value that represents the most severe rating appropriate for each diagnosis.)

0 - Asymptomatic, no treatment needed at this time

1 - Symptoms well controlled with current therapy

2 - Symptoms controlled with difficulty, affecting daily functioning; patient needs ongoing monitoring

3 - Symptoms poorly controlled, patient needs frequent adjustment in treatment and dose monitoring

4 - Symptoms poorly controlled, history of rehospitalizations

(M0230) Primary Diagnosis　　　　　**ICD**

a. *open wound ℓ ankle*　　　(*891* . *00*)

Severity Rating ☐ 0 ☐ 1 ☒ 2 ☐ 3 ☐ 4

(M0240) Other Diagnoses　　　　　**ICD**

b. *Type 2 diabetes*　　　　(*250* . *72*)

Severity Rating ☐ 0 ☐ 1 ☒ 2 ☐ 3 ☐ 4

c. *PVD*　　　　　　　　(*443* . *89*)

Severity Rating ☐ 0 ☐ 1 ☐ 2 ☒ 3 ☐ 4

d.＿＿＿＿＿＿＿＿＿　　(＿＿＿＿ . ＿＿＿)

Severity Rating ☐ 0 ☐ 1 ☐ 2 ☐ 3 ☐ 4

e.＿＿＿＿＿＿＿＿＿　　(＿＿＿＿ . ＿＿＿)

Severity Rating ☐ 0 ☐ 1 ☐ 2 ☐ 3 ☐ 4

f.＿＿＿＿＿＿＿＿＿　　(＿＿＿＿ . ＿＿＿)

Severity Rating ☐ 0 ☐ 1 ☐ 2 ☐ 3 ☐ 4

> Be sure to include all ICD codes.

30. Patient/family knowledge and coping level regarding present illness:

Patient *Knowledgeable about disease process*

Family *Anxious to assist in care*

31. Significant past health history: ＿＿＿＿＿＿＿＿＿

PVD

Type 2 diabetes

ℝ BKA

Using the OASIS-B1 form *(continued)*

32. (M0250) Therapies the patient receives *at home*:
(**Mark all that apply.**)

☐ 1 - Intravenous or infusion therapy (excludes TPN)

☐ 2 - Parenteral nutrition (TPN or lipids)

☐ 3 - Enteral nutrition (nasogastric, gastrostomy,
jejunostomy, or any other artificial entry into the
alimentary canal)

☒ 4 - None of the above

33. (M0260) Overall Prognosis: BEST description of patient's overall prognosis
for *recovery from this episode of illness.*

☐ 0 - Poor: little or no recovery is expected and/or
further decline is imminent

☒ 1 - Good/Fair: partial to full recovery is expected

☐ UK - Unknown

34. (M0270) Rehabilitative Prognosis: BEST description of patient's prognosis for
functional status.

☒ 0 - Guarded: minimal improvement in functional
status is expected; decline is possible

☐ 1 - Good: marked improvement in functional status
is expected

☐ UK - Unknown

35. (M0280) Life Expectancy: (Physician documentation is

☐ 0 - Life expectancy is greater than 6 months

☒ 1 - Life expectancy is 6 months or fewer

36. Immunization/screening tests:

Immunizations:

Flu	☒ Yes	☐ No	Date	*10/00*
Tetanus	☒ Yes	☐ No	Date	*3/98*
Pneumonia	☒ Yes	☐ No	Date	*10/00*
Other			Date	

Screening:

Cholesterol level	☒ Yes	☐ No	Date	*11/01*
Mammogram	☐ Yes	☒ No	Date	
Colon cancer screen	☒ Yes	☐ No	Date	*11/01*
Prostate cancer screen	☒ Yes	☐ No	Date	*11/01*

Self-exam frequency:

Breast self-exam frequency _____

Testicular self-exam frequency _____

37. Allergies: *NKA*

> *Remember to list all of the patient's allergies here.*

38. (M0290) High Risk Factors characterizing this patient: (**Mark all that apply.**)

☒ 1 - Heavy smoking

☐ 2 - Obesity

☐ 3 - Alcohol dependency

☐ 4 - Drug dependency

☐ 5 - None of the above

☐ UK - Unknown

LIVING ARRANGEMENTS

39. (M0300) Current Residence:

☒ 1 - Patient's owned or rented residence (house, apartment, or mobile
home owned or rented by patient/couple/significant other)

☐ 2 - Family member's residence

☐ 3 - Boarding home or rented room

☐ 4 - Board and care or assisted living facility

☐ 5 - Other (specify) _____

40. (M0310) Structural Barriers in the patient's environment limiting independent
mobility: (**Mark all that apply.**)

☐ 0 - None

☒ 1 - Stairs inside home which *must* be used by the patient (e.g., to get to
toileting, sleeping, eating areas)

☐ 2 - Stairs inside home which are used optionally (e.g., to get to laundry
facilities)

☒ 3 - Stairs leading from inside house to outside

☐ 4 - Narrow or obstructed doorways

41. (M0320) Safety Hazards found in the patient's current place of residence:
(**Mark all that apply.**)

☒ 0 - None

☐ 1 - Inadequate floor, roof, or windows

☐ 2 - Inadequate lighting

☐ 3 - Unsafe gas/electric appliance

☐ 4 - Inadequate heating

☐ 5 - Inadequate cooling

☐ 6 - Lack of fire safety devices

☐ 7 - Unsafe floor coverings

☐ 8 - Inadequate stair railings

☐ 9 - Improperly stored hazardous materials

☐ 10 - Lead-based paint

☐ 11 - Other (specify) _____

> *Safety issues should be identified here.*

Using the OASIS-B1 form *(continued)*

42. (M0330) **Sanitation Hazards** found in the patient's current place of residence: (Mark all that apply.)

- ☒ 0 - None
- ☐ 1 - No running water
- ☐ 2 - Contaminated water
- ☐ 3 - No toileting facilities
- ☐ 4 - Outdoor toileting facilities only
- ☐ 5 - Inadequate sewage disposal
- ☐ 6 - Inadequate/improper food storage
- ☐ 7 - No food refrigeration
- ☐ 8 - No cooking facilities
- ☐ 9 - Insects/rodents present
- ☐ 10 - No scheduled trash pickup
- ☐ 11 - Cluttered/soiled living area
- ☐ 12 - Other (specify) _____

43. (M0340) **Patient Lives With:** (Mark all that apply.)

- ☐ 1 - Lives alone
- ☒ 2 - With spouse or significant other
- ☐ 3 - With other family member
- ☐ 4 - With a friend
- ☐ 5 - With paid help (other than home care agency staff)
- ☐ 6 - With other than above

Comments: _____

_____

_____

_____

44. Others living in household: _____

Name *Susan*   Age *70*   Sex *F*

Relationship *wife*   Able/willing to assist ☒ Yes ☐ No

Name_____ Age_____ Sex_____

Relationship _____ Able/willing to assist ☐ Yes ☐ No

Name_____ Age_____ Sex_____

Relationship _____ Able/willing to assist ☐ Yes ☐ No

Name_____ Age_____ Sex_____

Relationship _____ Able/willing to assist ☐ Yes ☐ No

Name_____ Age_____ Sex_____

Relationship _____ Able/willing to assist ☐ Yes ☐ No

Name_____ Age_____ Sex_____

Relationship _____ Able/willing to assist ☐ Yes ☐ No

> Caregivers and other support systems should be identified here.

SUPPORTIVE ASSISTANCE

45. Persons/Organizations providing assistance:

_____

_____

_____

_____

46. (M0350) **Assisting Person(s) Other than Home Care Agency Staff:** (Mark all that apply.)

- ☐ 1 - Relatives, friends, or neighbors living outside the home
- ☒ 2 - Person residing in the home (EXCLUDING paid help)
- ☐ 3 - Paid help
- ☐ 4 - None of the above
  [If None of the above, go to *Review of Systems*]
- ☐ UK - Unknown [If Unknown, go to *Review of Systems*]

47. (M0360) **Primary Caregiver** taking *lead* responsibility for providing or managing the patient's care, providing the most frequent assistance, etc. (other than home care agency staff):

- ☐ 0 - No one person [If No one person, go to *M0390*]
- ☒ 1 - Spouse or significant other
- ☐ 2 - Daughter or son
- ☐ 3 - Other family member
- ☐ 4 - Friend or neighbor or community or church member
- ☐ 5 - Paid help
- ☐ UK - Unknown [If Unknown, go to *M0390*]

48. (M0370) **How Often** does the patient receive assistance from the primary caregiver?

- ☒ 1 - Several times during day and night
- ☐ 2 - Several times during day
- ☐ 3 - Once daily
- ☐ 4 - Three or more times per week
- ☐ 5 - One to two times per week
- ☐ 6 - Less often than weekly
- ☐ UK - Unknown

(continued)

Using the OASIS-B1 form *(continued)*

49. (M0380) Type of Primary Caregiver Assistance:
(Mark all that apply.)

☒ 1 - ADL assistance (e.g., bathing, dressing, toileting, bowel/bladder, eating/feeding)

☒ 2 - IADL assistance (e.g., meds, meals, housekeeping, laundry, telephone, shopping, finances)

☐ 3 - Environmental support (housing, home maintenance)

☒ 4 - Psychosocial support (socialization, companionship, recreation)

☒ 5 - Advocates or facilitates patient's participation in appropriate medical care

☐ 6 - Financial agent, power of attorney, or conservator of finance

☐ 7 - Health care agent, conservator of person, or medical power of attorney

☐ UK - Unknown

Comments: _____

REVIEW OF SYSTEMS

SENSORY STATUS

(Mark S for subjective, O for objectively assessed problem. If no problem present or if not assessed, mark NA.)

Head *NA* Dizziness
       NA Headache (describe location, duration) _____

Eyes *O* Glasses *NA* Cataracts *NA* Blurred/double vision
      O PERRL ____ Other (specify) _____

50. (M0390) Vision with corrective lenses if the patient usually wears them:

☒ 0 - Normal vision: sees adequately in most situations; can see medication labels, newsprint.

☐ 1 - Partially impaired: cannot see medication labels or newsprint, but *can* see obstacles in path, and the surrounding layout; can count fingers at arm's length.

☐ 2 - Severely impaired: cannot locate objects without hearing or touching them *or* patient nonresponsive.

Ears *NA* Hearing aid *NA* Tinnitus
      ____ Other (specify) _____

This guide helps you complete all of the assessment sections.

51. (M0400) Hearing and Ability to Understand Spoken Language in patient's own language (with hearing aids if the patient usually uses them):

☒ 0 - No observable impairment. Able to hear and understand complex or detailed instructions and extended or abstract conversation.

☐ 1 - With minimal difficulty, able to hear and understand most multi-step instructions and ordinary conversation. May need occasional repetition, extra time, or louder voice.

☐ 2 - Has moderate difficulty hearing and understanding simple, one-step instructions and brief conversation; needs frequent prompting or assistance.

☐ 3 - Has severe difficulty hearing and understanding simple greetings and short comments. Requires multiple repetitions, restatements, demonstrations, additional time.

☐ 4 - *Unable* to hear and understand familiar words or common expressions consistently, *or* patient nonresponsive.

Oral ____ Gum problems ____ Chewing problems
      ____ Dentures ____ Other (specify) _____

52. (M0410) Speech and Oral (Verbal) Expression of Language (in patient's own language):

☒ 0 - Expresses complex ideas, feelings, and needs clearly, completely, and easily in all situations with no observable impairment.

☐ 1 - Minimal difficulty in expressing ideas and needs (may take extra time; makes occasional errors in word choice, grammar or speech intelligibility; needs minimal prompting or assistance).

☐ 2 - Expresses simple ideas or needs with moderate difficulty (needs prompting or assistance, errors in word choice, organization, or speech intelligibility). Speaks in phrases or short sentences.

☐ 3 - Has severe difficulty expressing basic ideas or needs and requires maximal assistance or guessing by listener. Speech limited to single words or short phrases.

☐ 4 - *Unable* to express basic needs even with maximal prompting or assistance but is not comatose or unresponsive (e.g., speech is nonsensical or unintelligible).

☐ 5 - Patient nonresponsive or unable to speak.

Nose and sinus
  NA Epistaxis ____ Other (specify) _____

Neck and throat
  NA Hoarseness *NA* Difficulty swallowing
  ____ Other (specify) _____

Using the OASIS-B1 form *(continued)*

Musculoskeletal, Neurological

N/A Hx arthritis	*N/A* Joint pain	*N/A* Syncope
N/A Gout	*N/A* Weakness	*N/A* Seizure
N/A Stiffness	*S* Leg cramps	*N/A* Tenderness
N/A Swollen joints	*S* Numbness	*N/A* Deformities
N/A Unequal grasp	*O* Temp changes	*N/A* Comatose
N/A Tremor	*N/A* Aphasia/inarticulate speech	

N/A Paralysis (describe) _____

N/A Amputation (location) _____

____ Other (specify) _____

Coordinature, gait, balance (describe) _____

Gait steady

Comments (Prosthesis, appliances) _____

Uses a walker

Patient's perceived pain level: ___*4*___ (Scale 1-10)

53. (M0420) Frequency of Pain interfering with patient's activity or movement:

☐ 0 - Patient has no pain or pain does not interfere with activity or movement

☐ 1 - Less often than daily

☒ 2 - Daily, but not constantly

☐ 3 - All of the time

54. (M0430) Intractable Pain: Is the patient experiencing pain that is *not easily relieved*, occurs at least daily, and affects the patient's sleep, appetite, physical or emotional energy, concentration, personal relationships, emotions, or ability or desire to perform physical activity?

☒ 0 - No

☐ 1 - Yes

Comments (pain management) _____

INTEGUMENTARY STATUS

O Hair changes (where) *Balding* _____

N/A Puritus _____ Other (specify) _____

Skin condition (Record type # on body area. Indicate size to right of numbered category.)

> Be sure to clearly identify the affected area on the illustration.

	Type	Size
1.	Lesions	
2.	Bruises	
3.	Masses	
4.	Scars	
5.	Stasis Ulcers	*1/2" round*
6.	Pressure Ulcers	
7.	Incisions	
8.	Other (specify)	

55. (M0440) Does this patient have a **Skin Lesion** or an **Open Wound**? This excludes "OSTOMIES."

☐ 0 - No [If No, go to *Cardio/respiratory status*]

☒ 1 - Yes

56. (M0445) Does this patient have a **Pressure Ulcer**?

☒ 0 - No [If No, go to *M0468*]

☐ 1 - Yes

(continued)

Using the OASIS-B1 form *(continued)*

57. (M0450) Current Number of Pressure Ulcers at Each Stage: (Circle one response for each stage.)

Pressure Ulcer Stages	Number of Pressure Ulcers
a) Stage 1: Nonblanchable erythema of intact skin; the heralding of skin ulceration. In darker-pigmented skin, warmth, edema, hardness, or discolored skin may be indicators.	0 1 2 3 4 or more
b) Stage 2: Partial thickness skin loss involving epidermis and/or dermis. The ulcer is superficial and presents clinically as an abrasion, blister, or shallow crater.	0 1 2 3 4 or more
c) Stage 3: Full-thickness skin loss involving damage or necrosis of subcutaneous tissue which may extend down to, but not through, underlying fascia. The ulcer presents clinically as a deep crater with or without undermining of adjacent tissue.	0 1 2 3 4 or more
d) Stage 4: Full-thickness skin loss with extensive destruction, tissue necrosis, or damage to muscle, bone, or supporting structures (e.g., tendon, joint capsule, etc.)	0 1 2 3 4 or more

e) In addition to the above, is there at least one pressure ulcer that cannot be observed due to the presence of eschar or a nonremovable dressing, including casts?

☐ 0 - No
☐ 1 - Yes

58. (M0460) Stage of Most Problematic (Observable) Pressure Ulcer:

☐ 1 - Stage 1
☐ 2 - Stage 2
☐ 3 - Stage 3
☐ 4 - Stage 4
☐ NA - No observable pressure ulcer

59. (M0464) Status of Most Problematic (Observable) Pressure Ulcer:

☐ 1 - Fully granulating
☐ 2 - Early/partial granulation
☐ 3 - Not healing
☐ NA - No observable pressure ulcer

60. (M0468) Does this patient have a Stasis Ulcer?

☐ 0 - No [If No, go to *M0482*]
☒ 1 - Yes

61. (M0470) Current Number of Observable Stasis Ulcer(s):

☐ 0 - Zero
☒ 1 - One
☐ 2 - Two
☐ 3 - Three
☐ 4 - Four or more

> This detailed scale helps you evaluate pressure ulcers.

62. (M0474) Does this patient have at least one Stasis Ulcer that Cannot be Observed due to the presence of a nonremovable dressing?

☒ 0 - No
☐ 1 - Yes

63. (M0476) Status of Most Problematic (Observable) Stasis Ulcer:

☐ 1 - Fully granulating
☒ 2 - Early/partial granulation
☐ 3 - Not healing
☐ NA - No observable stasis ulcer

64. (M0482) Does this patient have a Surgical Wound?

☒ 0 - No [If No, go to *Cardio/Respiratory Status*]
☐ 1 - Yes

65. (M0484) Current Number of (Observable) Surgical Wounds: (If a wound is partially closed but has *more* than one opening, consider each opening as a separate wound.)

☐ 0 - Zero
☐ 1 - One
☐ 2 - Two
☐ 3 - Three
☐ 4 - Four or more

66. (M0486) Does this patient have at least one Surgical Wound that Cannot be Observed due to the presence of a nonremovable dressing?

☐ 0 - No
☐ 1 - Yes

67. (M0488) Status of Most Problematic (Observable) Surgical Wound:

☐ 1 - Fully granulating
☐ 2 - Early/partial granulation
☐ 3 - Not healing
☐ NA - No observable surgical wound

Using the OASIS-B1 form *(continued)*

CARDIO/RESPIRATORY STATUS

Temperature *99*   Respirations *18*

Blood pressure
Lying *132/80*   Sitting *130/78*   Standing *130/76*

Pulse
Apical rate *72*   Radial rate *72*
Rhythm *Regular*   Quality _____

Cardiovascular

NA Palpitations   *NA* Chest pains
S Claudication   *NA* Murmurs
S Fatigues easily   *O* Edema
NA BP problems   *NA* Cyanosis
NA Dyspnea on exertion   *NA* Varicosities
NA Paroxysmal nocturnal dyspnea
NA Orthopnea (# of pillows)
NA Cardiac problems (specify) _____
NA Pacemaker _____
          (Date of last battery change)
Other (specify) _____
Comments _____
_____
_____
_____

Respiratory

History of
NA Asthma   *NA* Pleurisy
NA TB   *NA* Pneumonia
S Bronchitis   *NA* Emphysema
Other (specify) _____
Present condition
S Cough (describe) *Dry*
O Breath sounds (describe) *Clear*
NA Sputum (character and amount) _____
Other (specify) _____

68. (M0490) When is the patient dyspneic or noticeably **Short of Breath**?

- ☒ 0 - Never, patient is not short of breath
- ☐ 1 - When walking more than 20 feet, climbing stairs
- ☐ 2 - With moderate exertion (e.g., while dressing, using commode or bed-pan, walking distances less than 20 feet)
- ☐ 3 - With minimal exertion (e.g., while eating, talking, or performing other ADLs) or with agitation
- ☐ 4 - At rest (during day or night)

69. (M0500) Respiratory Treatments utilized at home:
(Mark all that apply.)

- ☐ 1 - Oxygen (intermittent or continuous)
- ☐ 2 - Ventilator (continually or at night)
- ☐ 3 - Continuous positive airway pressure
- ☐ None of the above
- _____ ts _____

Use this section to record information on the patient's cardiovascular and respiratory status.

ELIMINATION STATUS

Genitourinary Tract

NA Frequency   *NA* Prostate disorder
NA Pain   *NA* Dysmenorrhea
NA Hematuria   *NA* Lesions
NA Vaginal discharge/bleeding   *NA* Hx hysterectomy
S Nocturia   *NA* Gravida/Para
NA Urgency   *NA* Contraception
NA Date last PAP _____
Other (specify) _____

70. (M0510) Has this patient been treated for a **Urinary Tract Infection** in the past 14 days?

- ☒ 0 - No
- ☐ 1 - Yes
- ☐ NA - Patient on prophylactic treatment
- ☐ UK - Unknown

71. (M0520) Urinary Incontinence or Urinary Catheter Presence:

- ☒ 0 - No incontinence or catheter (includes anuria or ostomy for urinary drainage) [If No, go to *M0540*]
- ☐ 1 - Patient is incontinent
- ☐ 2 - Patient requires a urinary catheter (i.e., external, indwelling, intermittent, suprapubic) [Go to *M0540*]

Incontinence problems should be identified in this section.

Using the OASIS-B1 form *(continued)*

72. (M0530) When does Urinary Incontinence occur?

☐ 0 - Timed-voiding defers incontinence

☐ 1 - During the night only

☐ 2 - During the day and night

Comments (e.g., appliances and care, bladder programs, catheter type, frequency of irrigation and change) _____

_____

_____

_____

_____

Gastrointestinal Tract

NA Indigestion   *NA* Rectal bleeding

NA Nausea/vomiting   *NA* Hemorrhoids

NA Ulcers   *NA* Gallbladder problems

NA Pain   *NA* Jaundice

NA Diarrhea/constipation *NA* Tenderness

NA Hernias (where) _____

Other (specify) _____

73. (M0540) Bowel Incontinence Frequency:

☒ 0 - Very rarely or never has bowel incontinence

☐ 1 - Less than once weekly

☐ 2 - One to three times weekly

☐ 3 - Four to six times weekly

☐ 4 - On a daily basis

☐ 5 - More often than once daily

☐ NA - Patient has ostomy for bowel elimination

☐ UK - Unknown

74. (M0550) Ostomy for Bowel Elimination: Does this patient have an ostomy for bowel elimination that (within the last 14 days):

a) was related to an inpatient facility stay, *or*

b) necessitated a change in medical or treatment regimen?

☒ 0 - Patient does *not* have an ostomy for bowel elimination.

☐ 1 - Patient's ostomy was *not* related to an inpatient stay and did *not* necessitate change in medical or treatment regimen.

☐ 2 - The ostomy *was* related to an inpatient stay or *did* necessitate change in medical or treatment regimen.

Comments (bowel function, stool color, bowel program, GI series, abd. girth) ___

_____

> This section identifies the patient's level of cognitive functioning.

Nutritional status

NA Weight lose/gain last 3 mos. (Give amount _____)

NA Over/under weight   *NA* Change in appetite

Diet *20% protein 30% fat* _____

Other (specify) _____

Meals prepared by *Wife* _____

Comments _____

> This section covers diet and nutritional status.

Breasts (For both male and female)

NA Lumps   *NA* Tenderness

NA Discharge   *NA* Pain

Other (specify) _____

Comments _____

_____

_____

NEURO/EMOTIONAL/BEHAVIORAL STATUS

NA Hx of previous psych. illness

Other (specify) _____

75. (M0560) Cognitive Functioning: (Patient's current level of alertness, orientation, comprehension, concentration, and immediate memory for simple commands.)

☐ 0 - Alert/oriented, able to focus and shift attention, comprehends and recalls task directions independently.

☒ 1 - Requires prompting (cueing, repetition, reminders) only under stressful or unfamiliar conditions.

☐ 2 - Requires assistance and some direction in specific situations (e.g., on all tasks involving shifting of attention), or consistently requires low stimulus environment due to distractibility.

☐ 3 - Requires considerable assistance in routine situations. Is not alert and oriented or is unable to shift attention and recall directions more than half the time.

☐ 4 - Totally dependent due to disturbances such as constant disorientation, coma, persistent vegetative state, or delirium.

Using the OASIS-B1 form *(continued)*

76. **(M0570) When Confused (Reported or Observed):**
- ☒ 0 - Never
- ☐ 1 - In new or complex situations only
- ☐ 2 - On awakening or at night only
- ☐ 3 - During the day and evening, but not constantly
- ☐ 4 - Constantly
- ☐ NA - Patient nonresponsive

77. **(M0580) When Anxious (Reported or Observed):**
- ☐ 0 - None of the time
- ☐ 1 - Less often than daily
- ☒ 2 - Daily, but not constantly
- ☐ 3 - All of the time
- ☐ NA - Patient nonresponsive

78. **(M0590) Depressive Feelings Reported or Observed in Patient:**
    (Mark all that apply.)
- ☐ 1 - Depressed mood (e.g., feeling sad, tearful)
- ☐ 2 - Sense of failure or self-reproach
- ☒ 3 - Hopelessness
- ☐ 4 - Recurrent thoughts of death
- ☐ 5 - Thoughts of suicide
- ☐ 6 - None of the above feelings observed or reported

79. **(M0600) Patient Behaviors (Reported or Observed): (Mark all that apply.)**
- ☐ 1 - Indecisiveness, lack of concentration
- ☐ 2 - Diminished interest in most activities
- ☐ 3 - Sleep disturbances
- ☐ 4 - Recent change in appetite or weight
- ☐ 5 - Agitation
- ☐ 6 - A suicide attempt
- ☒ 7 - None of the above behaviors observed or reported

> Behavioral problems should be identified in this section.

80. **(M0610) Behaviors Demonstrated *at Least Once a Week* (Reported or Observed): (Mark all that apply.)**
- ☐ 1 - Memory deficit: failure to recognize familiar persons/places, inability to recall events of past 24 hours, significant memory loss so that supervision is required
- ☐ 2 - Impaired decision making: failure to perform usual ADLs or IADLs, inability to appropriately stop activities, jeopardizes safety through actions
- ☐ 3 - Verbal disruption: yelling, threatening, excessive profanity, sexual references, etc.

- ☐ 4 - Physical aggression: aggressive or combative to self and others (e.g., hits self, throws objects, punches, dangerous maneuvers with wheelchair or other objects)
- ☐ 5 - Disruptive, infantile, or socially inappropriate behavior (**excludes** verbal actions)
- ☐ 6 - Delusional, hallucinatory, or paranoid behavior
- ☒ 7 - None of the above behaviors demonstrated

81. **(M0620) Frequency of Behavior Problems (Reported or Observed)** (e.g., wandering episodes, self-abuse, verbal disruption, physical aggression, etc.):
- ☒ 0 - Never
- ☐ 1 - Less than once a month
- ☐ 2 - Once a month
- ☐ 3 - Several times each month
- ☐ 4 - Several times a week
- ☐ 5 - At least daily

82. **(M0630) Is this patient receiving Psychiatric Nursing Services** at home provided by a qualified psychiatric nurse?
- ☒ 0 - No
- ☐ 1 - Yes
- Comments _____
  _____
  _____

Endocrine and hematopoietic

S	Diabetes	N/A	Polydipsia
N/A	Polyuria	N/A	Thyroid problem
N/A	Excessive bleeding or bruising		
S	Intolerance to heat and cold		

Fractionals
Usual results _____
Frequency checked_____
Other (specify) _____
Comments _____

(continued)

Using the OASIS-B1 form *(continued)*

ADL/IADLs

For M0640-M0800, complete the "Current" column for all patients. For these same items, complete the "Prior" column only at start of care and at resumption of care; mark the level that corresponds to the patient's condition 14 days prior to start of care date (M0030) or resumption of care date (M0032). In all cases, record what the patient is *able to do.*

83. (M0640) Grooming: Ability to tend to personal hygiene needs (i.e., washing face and hands, hair care, shaving or makeup, teeth or denture care, fingernail care).

Prior Current

- ☒ ☐ 0 - Able to groom self unaided, with or without the use of assistive devices or adapted methods.
- ☐ ☒ 1 - Grooming utensils must be placed within reach before able to complete grooming activities.
- ☐ ☐ 2 - Someone must assist the patient to groom self.
- ☐ ☐ 3 - Patient depends entirely upon someone else for grooming needs.
- ☐ UK - Unknown

84. (M0650) Ability to Dress *Upper* Body (with or without dressing aids) including undergarments, pullovers, front-opening shirts and blouses, managing zippers, buttons, and snaps:

Prior Current

- ☒ ☐ 0 - Able to get clothes out of closets and drawers, put them on and remove them from the upper body without assistance.
- ☐ ☒ 1 - Able to dress upper body without assistance if clothing is laid out or handed to the patient.
- ☐ ☐ 2 - Someone must help the patient put on upper body clothing.
- ☐ ☐ 3 - Patient depends entirely upon another person to dress the upper body.
- ☐ UK - Unknown

85. (M0660) Ability to Dress *Lower* Body (with or without dressing aids) including undergarments, slacks, socks or nylons, shoes:

Prior Current

- ☒ ☐ 0 - Able to obtain, put on, and remove clothing and shoes without assistance.
- ☐ ☐ 1 - Able to dress lower body without assistance if clothing and shoes are laid out or handed to the patient.
- ☐ ☒ 2 - Someone must help the patient put on undergarments, slacks, socks or nylons, and shoes.
- ☐ ☐ 3 - Patient depends entirely upon another person to dress lower body.
- ☐ UK - Unknown

86. (M0670) Bathing: Ability to wash entire body. *Excludes* grooming (washing face and hands only).

Prior Current

- ☐ ☐ 0 - Able to bathe self in *shower or tub* independently.
- ☒ ☐ 1 - With the use of devices, is able to bathe self in shower or tub independently.
- ☐ ☐ 2 - Able to bathe in shower or tub with the assistance of another person:
  (a) for intermittent supervision or encouragement or reminders,

> In this section, you should rate and compare the patient's prior ability to perform activities of daily living with his current ability.

OR

- ☐ ☒ b, *but* requires pres-...th for assistance or
- ☐ ☐ 4 - *Unable* to use the shower or tub and is bathed in *bed or bedside chair.*
- ☐ ☐ 5 - Unable to effectively participate in bathing and is totally bathed by another person.
- ☐ UK - Unknown

87. (M0680) Toileting: Ability to get to and from the toilet or bedside commode.

Prior Current

- ☒ ☒ 0 - Able to get to and from the toilet independently with or without a device.
- ☐ ☐ 1 - When reminded, assisted, or supervised by another person, able to get to and from the toilet.
- ☐ ☐ 2 - *Unable* to get to and from the toilet but is able to use a bedside commode (with or without assistance).
- ☐ ☐ 3 - *Unable* to get to and from the toilet or bedside commode but is able to use a bedpan/urinal independently.
- ☐ ☐ 4 - Is totally dependent in toileting.
- ☐ UK - Unknown

Using the OASIS-B1 form *(continued)*

88. (M0690) Transferring: Ability to move from bed to chair, on and off toilet or commode, into and out of tub or shower, and ability to turn and position self in bed if patient is bedfast.

Prior Current

- ☐ ☐ 0 - Able to independently transfer.
- ☒ ☒ 1 - Transfers with minimal human assistance or with use of an assistive device.
- ☐ ☐ 2 - *Unable* to transfer self but is able to bear weight and pivot during the transfer process.
- ☐ ☐ 3 - Unable to transfer self and is *unable* to bear weight or pivot when transferred by another person.
- ☐ ☐ 4 - Bedfast, unable to transfer but is able to turn and position self in bed.
- ☐ ☐ 5 - Bedfast, unable to transfer and is *unable* to turn and position self.
- ☐ UK - Unknown

89. (M0700) Ambulation/Locomotion: Ability to *SAFELY* walk, once in a standing position, or use a wheelchair, once in a seated position, on a variety of surfaces.

Prior Current

- ☒ ☐ 0 - Able to independently walk on even and uneven surfaces and climb stairs with or without railings (i.e., needs no human assistance or assistive device).
- ☐ ☒ 1 - Requires use of a device (e.g., cane, walker) to walk alone or requires human supervision or assistance to negotiate stairs or steps or uneven surfaces.
- ☐ ☐ 2 - Able to walk only with the supervision or assistance of another person at all times.
- ☐ ☐ 3 - Chairfast, *unable* to ambulate but is able to wheel self independently.
- ☐ ☐ 4 - Chairfast, unable to ambulate and is *unable* to wheel self.
- ☐ ☐ 5 - Bedfast, unable to ambulate or be up in a chair.
- ☐ UK - Unknown

> Evaluate the patient's ambulation status in this section.

90. (M0710) Feeding or Eating: Ability to feed self meals and snacks. **Note: This refers only to the process of** *eating, chewing,* **and** *swallowing, not preparing the food to be eaten.*

Prior Current

- ☒ ☒ 0 - Able to independently feed self.
- ☐ ☐ 1 - Able to feed self independently but requires:
  - (a) meal set-up; *OR*
  - (b) intermittent assistance or supervision from another person; *OR*
  - (c) a liquid, pureed or ground meat diet.
- ☐ ☐ 2 - *Unable* to feed self and must be assisted or supervised throughout the meal/snack.
- ☐ ☐ 3 - Able to take in nutrients orally *and* receives supplemental nutrients through a nasogastric tube or gastrostomy.
- ☐ ☐ 4 - *Unable* to take in nutrients orally and is fed nutrients through a nasogastric tube or gastrostomy.
- ☐ ☐ 5 - Unable to take in nutrients orally or by tube feeding.
- ☐ UK - Unknown

91. (M0720) Planning and Preparing Light Meals (e.g., cereal, sandwich) or reheat delivered meals:

Prior Current

- ☒ ☐ 0 - (a) Able to independently plan and prepare all light meals for self or reheat delivered meals; OR
  - (b) Is physically, cognitively, and mentally able to prepare light meals on a regular basis but has not routinely performed light meal preparation in the past (i.e., prior to this home care admission).
- ☐ ☒ 1 - *Unable* to prepare light meals on a regular basis due to physical, cognitive, or mental limitations.
- ☐ ☐ 2 - Unable to prepare any light meals or reheat any delivered meals.
- ☐ UK - Unknown

92. (M0730) Transportation: Physical and mental ability to *safely* use a car, taxi, or public transportation (bus, train, subway).

Prior Current

- ☐ ☐ 0 - Able to independently drive a regular or adapted car; OR uses a regular or handicap-accessible public bus.
- ☒ ☒ 1 - Able to ride in a car only when driven by another person; OR able to use a bus or handicap van only when assisted or accompanied by another person.
- ☐ ☐ 2 - Unable to ride in a car, taxi, bus, or van, and requires transportation by ambulance.
- ☐ UK - Unknown

(continued)

Using the OASIS-B1 form *(continued)*

93. (M0740) Laundry: Ability to do own laundry — to carry laundry to and from washing machine, to use washer and dryer, to wash small items by hand.

Prior   Current

☐   ☐   0 - (a) Able to independently take care of all laundry tasks; *OR*
(b) Physically, cognitively, and mentally able to do laundry and access facilities, but has not routinely performed laundry tasks in the past (i.e., prior to this home care admission).

☒   ☐   1 - Able to do only light laundry, such as minor hand wash or light washer loads. Due to physical, cognitive, or mental limitations, needs assistance with heavy laundry such as carrying large loads of laundry.

☐   ☒   2 - *Unable* to do any laundry due to physical limitation or needs continual supervision and assistance due to cognitive or mental limitation.

☐   UK - Unknown

94. (M0750) Housekeeping: Ability to safely and effectively perform light housekeeping and heavier cleaning tasks.

Prior   Current

☐   ☐   0 - (a) Able to independently p
(b) Physically, cognitively, a
housekeeping tasks but
housekeeping tasks in the past (i.e., prior to this home car
admission).

☐   ☐   1 - Able to perform only *light* housekeeping (e.g., dusting, wiping kitchen counters) tasks independently.

☐   ☐   2 - Able to perform housekeeping tasks with intermittent assistance or supervision from another person.

☐   ☐   3 - *Unable* to consistently perform any housekeeping tasks unless assisted by another person throughout the process.

☒   ☒   4 - Unable to effectively participate in any housekeeping tasks.

☐   UK - Unknown

95. (M0760) Shopping: Ability to plan for, select, and purchase items in a store and to carry them home or arrange delivery.

Prior   Current

☐   ☐   0 - (a) Able to plan for shopping needs and independently perform shopping tasks, including carrying packages; *OR*
(b) Physically, cognitively, and mentally able to take care of shopping, but has not done shopping in the past (i.e., prior to this home care admission).

☐   ☐   1 - Able to go shopping, but needs some assistance:
(a) By self is able to do only light shopping and carry small packages, but needs someone to do occasional major shopping; *OR*
(b) *Unable* to go shopping alone, but can go with someone to assist.

☒   ☒   2 - *Unable* to go shopping, but is able to identify items needed, place orders, and arrange home delivery.

☐   ☐   3 - Needs someone to do all shopping and errands.

☐   UK - Unknown

96. (M0770) Ability to Use Telephone: Ability to answer the phone, dial numbers, and *effectively* use the telephone to communicate.

Prior   Current

☒   ☒   0 - Able to dial numbers and answer calls appropriately and as desired.

☐   ☐   1 - Able to use a specially adapted telephone (i.e., large numbers on the dial, teletype phone for the deaf) and call essential numbers.

☐   ☐   2 - Able to answer the telephone and carry on a normal conversation but has difficulty with placing calls.

☐   ☐   3 - Able to answer the telephone only some of the time or is able to carry on only a limited conversation.

☐   ☐   4 - *Unable* to answer the telephone at all but can listen if assisted with equipment.

☐   ☐   5 - Totally unable to use the telephone.

☐   ☐   NA - Patient does not have a telephone.

☐   UK - Unknown

MEDICATIONS

97. (M0780) Management of Oral Medications: *Patient's ability* to prepare and take all prescribed oral medications reliably and safely, including administration of the correct dosage at the appropriate times/intervals. *Excludes injectable and I.V. medications.* (NOTE: This refers to ability, not compliance or willingness.)

Prior   Current

☒   ☒   0 - Able to independently take the correct oral medication(s) and proper dosage(s) at the correct times.

☐   ☐   1 - Able to take medication(s) at the correct times if:
(a) individual dosages are prepared in advance by another person; *OR*
(b) given daily reminders; *OR*
(c) someone develops a drug diary or chart.

☐   ☐   2 - *Unable* to take medication unless administered by someone else.

☐   ☐   NA - No oral medications prescribed.

☐   UK - Unknown

Record your patient's ability to manage his medications in this section.

Using the OASIS-B1 form *(continued)*

98. (M0790) Management of Inhalant/Mist Medications:
Patient's ability to prepare and take all prescribed inhalant/mist medications (nebulizers, metered dose devices) reliably and safely, including administration of the correct dosage at the appropriate times/intervals. *Excludes* all other forms of medication (oral tablets, injectable and I.V. medications).

Prior   Current

☐   ☐   0 - Able to independently take the correct medication and proper dosage at the correct times.

☐   ☐   1 - Able to take medication at the correct times if:
    (a) individual dosages are prepared in advance by another person, *OR*
    (b) given daily reminders.

☐   ☐   2 - *Unable* to take medication unless administered by someone else.

☒   ☒   NA - No inhalant/mist medications prescribed.

☐   UK - Unknown

99. (M0800) Management of Injectable Medications: *Patient's ability* to prepare and take all prescribed injectable medications reliably and safely, including administration of correct dosage at the appropriate times/intervals. *Excludes* I.V. medications.

Prior   Current

☒   ☒   0 - Able to independently take the correct medication and proper dosage at the correct times.

☐   ☐   1 - Able to take injectable medication at correct times if:
    (a) individual syringes are prepared in advance by another person, OR
    (b) given daily reminders.

☐   ☐   2 - Unable to take injectable medications unless administered by someone else.

☐   ☐   NA - No injectable medications prescribed.

☐   UK - Unknown

EQUIPMENT MANAGEMENT

100. (M0810) Patient Management of Equipment (includes *ONLY* oxygen, I.V./infusion therapy, enteral/parenteral nutrition equipment or supplies):
Patient's ability to set up, monitor and change equipment reliably, and safely add appropriate fluids or medication, clean/store/dispose of equipment or supplies using proper technique. (NOTE: This refers to ability, not compliance or willingness.)

☐   0 - Patient manages all tasks related to equipment completely independently.

☐   1 - If someone else sets up equipment (i.e., fills portable oxygen tank, provides patient with prepared solutions), patient is able to manage all other aspects of equipment.

☐   2 - Patient requires considerable assistance from another person to manage equipment, but independently completes portions of the task.

☐   3 - Patient is only able to monitor equipment (e.g., liter flow, fluid in bag) and must call someone else to manage the equipment.

☐   4 - Patient is completely dependent on someone else to manage all equipment.

☒   NA - No equipment of this type used in care [If NA, go to *M0825*]

101. (M0820) Caregiver Management of Equipment (includes *ONLY* oxygen, I.V./infusion equipment, enteral/parenteral nutrition, ventilator therapy equipment or supplies): *Caregiver's ability* to set up, monitor, and change equipment reliably and safely, add appropriate fluids or medication, clean/store/dispose of equipment or supplies using proper technique. (NOTE: This refers to ability, not compliance or willingness.)

☐   0 - Caregiver manages all tasks related to equipment completely independently.

☐   1 - If someone else sets up equipment, caregiver is able to manage all other aspects.

☐   2 - Caregiver requires considerable assistance from another person to manage equipment, but independently completes significant portions of task.

☐   3 - Caregiver is only able to complete small portions of task (e.g., administer nebulizer treatment, clean/store/dispose of equipment or supplies).

☐   4 - Caregiver is completely dependent on someone else to manage all equipment.

> Record your patient's ability to safely set up, monitor, and change his equipment in this section.

es the care plan of the Medicare payment period
ill define a case mix group indicate a need for
…onal, or speech therapy) that meets the threshold
for a Medicare high-therapy case mix group?

☐   0 - No

☐   1 - Yes

☐   NA - Not applicable

Using the OASIS-B1 form (continued)

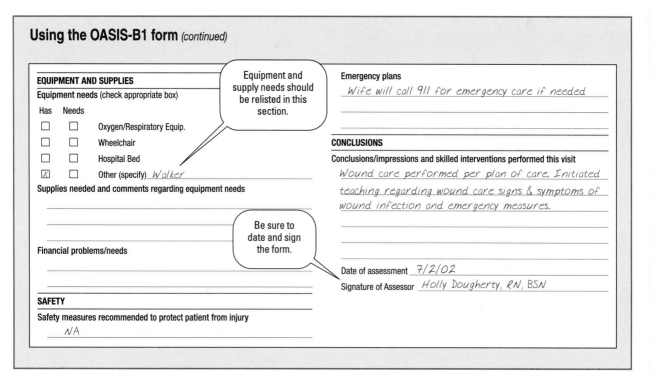

EQUIPMENT AND SUPPLIES

Equipment needs (check appropriate box)

Has   Needs

☐   ☐   Oxygen/Respiratory Equip.

☐   ☐   Wheelchair

☐   ☐   Hospital Bed

☒   ☐   Other (specify) _Walker_

Supplies needed and comments regarding equipment needs

Equipment and supply needs should be relisted in this section.

Financial problems/needs

Be sure to date and sign the form.

SAFETY

Safety measures recommended to protect patient from injury

_NA_

Emergency plans

Wife will call 911 for emergency care if needed

CONCLUSIONS

Conclusions/impressions and skilled interventions performed this visit

Wound care performed per plan of care. Initiated teaching regarding wound care signs & symptoms of wound infection and emergency measures.

Date of assessment _7/2/02_

Signature of Assessor _Holly Dougherty, RN, BSN_

Guidelines for use

To document most effectively on your plan of care, follow these suggestions:

• Keep a copy of the plan of care in the patient's home for easy reference by him and his family.

• Make sure the plan is comprehensive by including more than the patient's physiologic problems. Also chart about the home environment, the resources needed, and the attitudes of the patient, family, and caregiver.

• Document physical changes that need to be made in the patient's home for him to receive proper care. Help the family find the resources to implement them.

• Describe the primary caregiver, including whether he lives with the patient, their relationship, his age and physical ability, and his willingness to help the patient. The patient's well-being may depend on this person's abilities.

• Show in your documentation how you made the most of the patient's strengths and resources. Strengths include support systems, good health habits and coping behaviors, a safe and healthful environment, and financial security. Resources include the doctor, pharmacy, and medical equipment supplier.

Art of the chart

Interdisciplinary plan of care

The plan of care is individualized for each patient. An example of this form is shown below.

> Note that this plan of care is focused on patient problems.

Patient name: _Mary Long_

Primary nurse: _N. Smith, RN_

Init. cert. period:_____

Recert. period #1:_____

Init. cert. period:_____

PROBLEM		APPROACH	INITIAL CERT	RECERT #1	RECERT #2
Atrial fibrillation (10/1/02)	Maintain optimal cardiac output	1. Meds as ordered 2. Monitor vs. inc. apical rhythm and rate 3. observe for chest pain, dyspnea, palpitations, anxiety, etc.	GOAL MET? Y N INIT:_____	GOAL MET? Y N INIT:_____	GOAL MET? Y N INIT:_____
Heart Failure (12/1/02)	1. Maintain fluid and electrolyte balance 2. Promote optimal gas exchange.	1. Meds as ordered 2. Nebulizer as ordered 3. Draw labs as ordered 4. I & O daily 5. Monitor edema 6. ✔ for SOB, dyspnea, congestion (lung sounds) 7. amb. as tol 8. semi Fowler's when sitting	GOAL MET? Y N INIT:_____	GOAL MET? Y N INIT:_____	GOAL MET? Y N INIT:_____
Gastrostomy tube insertion (12/3/02)	1. Maintain optimal nutritional status 2. Prevent skin breakdown	1. Magnacal 80 ml/hr 2. Follow G-tube protocol, including site care & oral hygiene 3. Weekly weights 4. I&O daily 5. ✔ for N/V, diarrhea	GOAL MET? Y N INIT:_____	GOAL MET? Y N INIT:_____	GOAL MET? Y N INIT:_____

> Set realistic goals.

> Interventions are coded to allow for rapid documentation.

Intervention Codes

(please circle all that apply)

A1. Skilled observation
A2. Foley insertion
A3. Bladder installation
A4. Irrigation care (wd. dsg.)
A5. Irrigation decub. care - meds.
A6. Venipuncture
A7. Restorative nursing
A8. Postcataract care
A9. Bowel/Bladder training

A10. Chest physical (incl. postural drainage)
A11. Administer vit. B_{12}
A12. Prepare/Administer insulin
A13. Administer other
A14. Administer I.V.
A15. Teach ostomy care
A16. Teach nasogastric feeding
A17. Reposition nasogastric feeding tube
A18. Teach gastrostomy

A19. Teach parenteral nutrition
A20. Teach care of trach
A21. Administer care of trach
A22. Teach inhalation Rx
A23. Administer inhalation Rx
A24. Teach administration of injections
A25. Teach diabetic care
A26. Disimpaction/enema
A27. Other
    Foot care (diabetic)
    Teach diet

Teach disease process
Teach use of 0_2
Instruct re: Medication child
A28. Wound care/dsg - closed
A29. Decubitus care - simple
A30. Teach care of indwelling catheter
A31. Management and evaluation of patient care plan
A32. Teaching and training (other)

• Continuously identify progress toward goals. If the patient isn't able to make progress, discharge may be considered.
• If the patient is homebound, make sure this is documented at every visit and state the reason why. Medicare requires a patient receiving skilled home care to be homebound; however, some commercial insurers don't.
• Make sure that documentation reflects consistent adherence by all caregivers to the plan of care. Have caregivers demonstrate the procedures they use for the care they provide, and document their skill level.
• Keep the record updated, noting changes in the patient's condition or plan of care, and document that you reported these changes to the doctor. Medicare, Medicaid, and certain other third-party payers won't reimburse for skilled services not reported to the doctor.
• Interdisciplinary care must be documented on an ongoing basis. Collaboration on patient care problems and changes to the plan of care are described in detail on the patient's chart.

Progress notes

The home care progress note, like notes in the acute care setting, is a place to document both the patient's condition and significant events that occur while he's under your care. The progress note is written in chronological order based on each home visit. (See *Progress note.*)

Work in progress

Every time you visit a patient, you must write a progress note. These notes document:
• changes in the patient's condition
• skilled nursing interventions you performed related to the plan of care
• the patient's responses to the interventions
• events or incidents in the home that might affect the treatment plan
• patient's vital signs
• what you taught the patient and caregiver, including written instructional materials and brochures
• communication with other team members since the previous visit
• discharge plans
• time you arrived in the home and time you left the home.

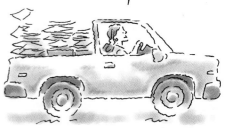

With each visit, you should add a new progress note to your records.

Art of the chart

Progress note

Use this sample progress note as a guide when charting in home care settings.

Date	Problem no.	Problem title — subjective, objective, assessment, plan
11/14/02	#2	A: L foot stasis ulcer showing no improvement in size or amount of drainage since 11/1/02
		P: Dr. Miller notified. Wound culture ordered and done. Will send specimen to lab. —————— M. A. Ford, RN

Guidelines for use

The guidelines here will help you chart safely and efficiently on progress notes:

• Chart all events in chronological order.

• Avoid addendums.

• Provide a heading for each entry because many members of the health care team use the progress notes.

• Use flow sheets and checklists to record vital signs, intake and output measurements, and nutritional data. Encourage the patient or caregiver to fill out these forms when appropriate. This gets them involved and increases their feeling of control.

• To help prevent the patient from feeling neglected, limit the time you spend charting in the home. When possible, take time to complete your charting while the patient sleeps or is otherwise occupied.

• Involve the patient in his own care and documentation by making statements like, "Here's what I've written about how your wound is healing. Is there anything else you want me to put in the notes?"

• If the patient has a medical emergency while you're there, accompany him to the hospital or emergency unit and stay until another caregiver takes over. Notify your supervisor, who will arrange coverage for your other patients, if necessary. Record all assessments and interventions performed until you're relieved. Note the date and time of transfer and the name of the caregiver who assumes responsibility.

• If documentation materials were completed and left in the patient's home, collect them at least once a week and take them to your home health care agency. This keeps volumes of paper from piling up or becoming misplaced and also makes the records available for review by the agency supervisor.

Nursing and discharge summaries

As a home health nurse, you must submit a regular patient progress report to the attending doctor and the reimburser to confirm the need for continuing services. You must also complete a summary of the patient's progress and a discharge summary.

Summing it all up

When writing a summary of the patient's progress, include:
• current problems, treatments, interventions, and instructions
• home care provided by other health care professionals, such as a physical therapist or speech pathologist
• the reason for a change in services
• patient outcomes and responses—physical and emotional—to the services provided
• discharge plan.

Guidelines for use

You'll prepare a discharge summary to get the doctor's approval to discharge a patient, to notify third-party payers that services have been terminated, and to officially close the case. The discharge summary also serves as a brief history for quick review if the patient is readmitted at a later date.

When writing these summaries, record:
• the time frame covered
• the services provided and the names and titles of assigned staff
• the third-party payer and whether the patient is eligible for future payment (he may have exhausted his annual benefits)
• the clinical and psychosocial condition of the patient at discharge
• recommendations for further care
• caregiver involvement in care
• interruptions in home care such as readmissions to the hospital
• referrals to community agencies
• OASIS discharge information
• the patient's response to and comprehension of patient-teaching efforts
• the outcomes attained.

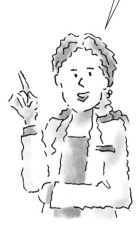

In your summary of the patient's progress, document physical and emotional responses to care.

Art of the chart

Home health certification and plan of care

The form below is the official form for authorizing Medicare coverage for home care (also known as form 485). It includes space for assessing functional abilities and documenting plan of care information.

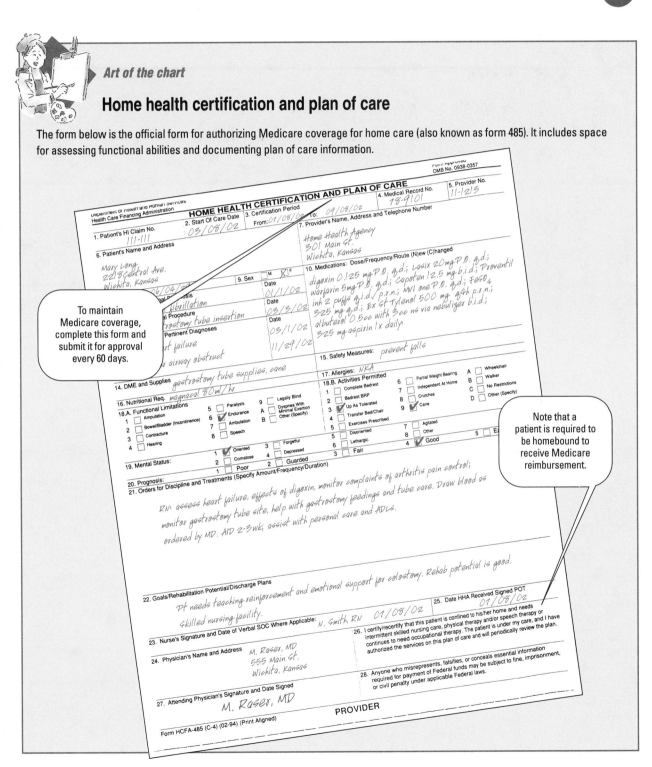

To maintain Medicare coverage, complete this form and submit it for approval every 60 days.

Note that a patient is required to be homebound to receive Medicare reimbursement.

Art of the chart

Medical update and patient information

To continue providing reimbursable skilled nursing care to a patient at home, Medicare requires you to complete the Medical Update and Patient Information form (also known as form 486).

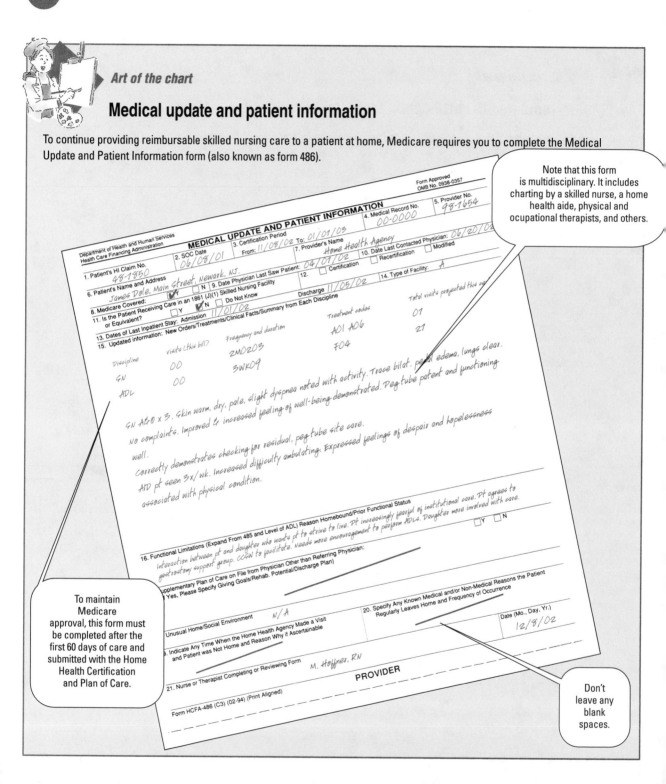

Note that this form is multidisciplinary. It includes charting by a skilled nurse, a home health aide, physical and occupational therapists, and others.

To maintain Medicare approval, this form must be completed after the first 60 days of care and submitted with the Home Health Certification and Plan of Care.

Don't leave any blank spaces.

Medicare-mandated forms

HCFA, the federal watchdog agency that oversees Medicare and Medicaid programs, requires home health agencies that receive Medicare funding to standardize their record keeping and documentation methods. Home health agencies must maintain the following forms for each qualified Medicare recipient:

• OASIS

• home health certification and plan of care (see *Home health care certification and plan of care*, page 163)

• health update and patient information (see *Medical update and patient information*)

• notice of nondiscrimination.

Art of the chart

Doctor's telephone orders

Home health nurses rely heavily on the use of telephone orders. The agency must follow guidelines established by the Health Care Financing Administration for taking and documenting these orders. Below is an example of a form used by one agency to fulfill documentation requirements. The order must be signed by the doctor within 48 hours.

Facility name	Address		
Suburban Home Health Agency	123 Main Street		
Last name	**First name**	**Attending doctor**	**Admission no.**
Smith	Kevin	Baker	141-111-471
Date ordered	**Date discontinued**	**ORDERS**	
12/18/02	12/21/02	Tylenol 650 mg P.O. q6h p.r.n. Temp 7 101° F	
Signature of nurse receiving order	**Time**	**Signature of doctor**	**Date**
Mary Reo, RN	1820		

Doctor calls

In addition, home care nurses must document a doctor's telephone orders. (See *Doctor's telephone orders*, page 165.)

Fill out and sign, please...

Medicare, via the fiscal intermediary, won't pay unless the required forms are properly completed, signed, and submitted. Forms are usually filled out by the nurse assigned to the patient, although some agencies have an admission team and a care team.

Future developments

Several major trends are emerging as the home health care industry continues to evolve:
• More private insurers require preauthorization for home health care services, which increases the paperwork burden for nurses.
• Fewer visits per episode of care are allowed. More focused reimbursement will dramatically alter the amount of home care patients will receive.
• The depth and breadth of federal regulations have placed increasing demands on care providers, and agencies will need to computerize record keeping.

One predicted outcome: More reliance on outcomes

Increased reliance on disease-specific management programs will eventually lead to the use of critical pathways that incorporate patient outcomes in home health care. Both HCFA and JCAHO are focused on outcomes. State departments of health services surveyors also have access to data. In addition, an agency's data is compared with data from similar agencies.

Blazing new trails with computers — Yee-ha!

Increasingly, home health care nurses are using laptop computers or handheld devices equipped with software designed to speed clinical documentation. Many of these programs are designed to help nurses develop a plan of care, formulate goals, monitor patient progress, update medications, and generate visit notes.

This technology expedites the exchange of data between care providers and third-party payers. Nurses inexperienced in using computers should be aware that documentation may take longer until they adjust to the new equipment.

Private insurers may mean more paperwork.

Keeping it confidential

New technology raises new concerns about confidentiality. For example, e-mail and faxes can easily end up in the wrong hands. When using either to transmit information about a patient, consider blacking out identifying data. Arrange for the recipient of a fax to wait at the other end for the fax to print.

Confidentiality when transmitting OASIS data on patients who aren't Medicare recipients continues to be a source of concern. Legislators and lawmakers will ultimately reconcile the parameters of government access to non-Medicare patients' clinical data.

In many cases, a home health agency will supply its nurses with laptop computers to streamline documentation. Laptop computers shouldn't be used by anyone other than agency personnel. You may be tempted to allow a computer-savvy spouse, friend, or child to add programs or manipulate data with all good intentions, but this is no more appropriate than it would be to let them read a patient's record. Finally, access to computer files should be protected by a password to prevent unauthorized individuals from entering files.

Cheat sheet

Home health documentation review

• For each visit, covers assessment, interventions, the patient's treatment and response to treatment, any complications, and communication with other team members
• Is used by third-party payers to evaluate claims
• Should include OASIS, evidence of a safe home environment, the rationale for the treatment, the patient's response to treatment, emergency and resource numbers given to the patient, and the patient's or caregiver's ability to perform steps in home care procedures, troubleshoot equipment problems, and recognize and handle potential complications
• Includes any patient teaching that has occurred, including a list of the teaching and reference materials provided, and the patient's response

• Is used to evaluate home health agencies for such factors as accurate, complete documentation and adherence to standards
• May consist of these forms and data: agency assessment form and OASIS, plan of care, progress notes, nursing and discharge summaries, team communication, doctor's updates to the plan of care, communication with insurance case managers regarding authorization of care, and referrals to other service providers

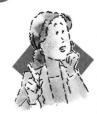

Quick quiz

1. Which of the following agencies requires standardized record keeping and documentation for Medicare recipients?

    A.   JCAHO
    B.   HCFA
    C   CHAP

Answer: B. The HCFA requires that documentation and record keeping be standardized for Medicare reimbursement.

2. OASIS is a tool now used in home health care to assess a patient's condition. It's required to be done on all patients except:

    A.   Medicare patients.
    B.   non-Medicare patients over age 18.
    C.   women receiving maternal-child services.

Answer: C. All patients over age 18, except those receiving maternal-child services, are required to have an OASIS evaluation.

3. Changes in the patient's condition should be documented in which of the following nursing records?

    A.   Progress notes
    B.   Plan of care
    C.   Both

Answer: C. Significant events that occur during your care of the patient are documented in both the progress notes and the plan of care. Any changes in the patient's condition must be integrated throughout the chart.

Scoring

☆☆☆ If you answered all three items correctly, turn off your laptop and hop into a hammock! Rest assured that you're home-free with documentation.

☆☆ If you answered two items correctly, good for you! You meet all certification and utilization review requirements, which allows you to go on to the next chapter.

☆ If you answered only one item correctly, keep at it! You'll always come across new opportunities to use your charting know-how. Just turn to the next chapter and see.

Long-term care and rehabilitation

Just the facts

In this chapter, you'll learn:

♦ about agencies that regulate documentation in long-term care settings

♦ specific forms required in long-term care settings and how to complete them

♦ guidelines for correct documentation.

A look at charting in long-term care

A long-term care facility provides continuing care for chronically ill or disabled patients. The purpose of care is to promote the highest level of functioning possible for the patient. Long-term care is an increasingly important form of health care delivery, especially because the elderly segment of the population is rapidly growing. (See *Elder power*, page 170.)

Maintaining accurate, complete documentation in long-term care is vital. Consider the following points:

• Long-term care facilities are highly regulated by state and federal agencies and therefore must live up to high standards of documentation.

• Information in your records may be used to defend you and your facility in court.

• Your employer views documentation records as evidence of standardized, high-quality nursing care.

• Good record keeping ensures certification, licensure, reimbursement, and accreditation.

Elder power

The number of persons age 65 or older numbered 34.5 million—or 12.7% of the U.S. population—in 1999. Specifically, in 1999, the 65 through 74 age-group numbered 18.2 million, the 75 through 84 age-group was 12.1 million, and the 85 and older age-group totaled 4.2 million. The older population will continue to increase, especially between the years 2010 and 2030 when the baby-boomer generation reaches age 65.

Chances are you're caring for many elderly patients right now. Studies show that people age 65 and older require health care services more often than any other age-group. Most older persons have at least one chronic condition, and many have multiple conditions. That's why we need to focus increasingly on the needs of elderly patients in long-term nursing care (as well as in subacute and home care) and in inpatient and outpatient rehabilitative and psychiatric care.

There's strength in numbers!

Documentation distinctions

Two key differences exist between documenting in long-term care settings and other settings:

Patients stay at long-term care facilities for weeks or months, so documentation isn't done as often. This takes the emphasis off charting and puts it on helping the patient relearn basic skills.

Some of the government forms used in long-term facilities are long and involved. So, even though charting isn't emphasized, it can still be extensive.

Categories of care

Long-term care facilities usually offer two levels of care: skilled and intermediate. The level of care administered to your patient should be your primary consideration when documenting.

Care may be complex...

In a skilled care facility, patient care involves specialized nursing skills, such as I.V. therapy, parenteral nutrition, respiratory care, and mechanical ventilation.

...or not so complex

An intermediate care facility deals with patients who have chronic illnesses and need less complex care. For example, they may simply need assistance with activities of daily living (ADLs), such as bathing and dressing.

Patients at both levels may need short- or long-term care and may move from one level to another according to their progress or decline. Living arrangements, geography, family and community support networks, and other factors determine the patient's length of stay.

Regulatory agencies

Documentation in long-term care facilities is regulated by both federal and state agencies. Documentation is influenced by:
• federal programs, such as Medicare and Medicaid
• government agencies such as the Health Care Financing Administration (HCFA)
• laws such as the Omnibus Budget Reconciliation Act (OBRA) of 1987
• state regulations for each facility
• accrediting agencies such as the Joint Commission on Accreditation of Healthcare Organizations (JCAHO).

Most elderly patients entering long-term care facilities pay for the services privately. When their funds become exhausted, they apply to Medicaid for coverage. If the patient requires services and is unable to pay initially, he can apply to receive Medicaid.

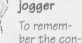

Memory jogger

To remember the conditions that affect length of stay, think of the word **FOCUS.**

• **F**unctional skills (and disabilities)
• **O**ther diseases
• **C**hronicity
• **U**rgency of needs
• **S**upport systems

Medicare

Few of the services provided in long-term care facilities are eligible for Medicare reimbursement. However, Medicare does provide reimbursement for patients requiring skilled care, such as chemotherapy or tube feeding. For these patients, Medicare requires certain minimum daily documentation to prove that a service was needed. If the patient's status changes, you must supply a revised plan of care within 7 days.

Making reimbursement a reality

Be sure to document changes in status because a patient who isn't improving or expected to improve according to his plan of care is ineligible for coverage. You must also document the need for new or continuing skilled services you provide. Medicare also requires documentation of your evaluations for expected outcomes.

According to Medicare guidelines, charting must clearly show that a patient needed care by a professional or technical staff member. To verify the need for skilled rehabilitative care, you must describe a reasonable expectation of improvement or

Medicare does cover some skilled services in long-term care, but daily documentation is required.

services needed to establish a maintenance program. The amount, duration, and frequency of services must be reasonable and necessary.

Medicaid

Most patients who receive skilled care in long-term care facilities either pay for it themselves or are on Medicaid. To ensure Medicaid reimbursement for these patients, document patient care once a day.

Reimbursement for intermediate care

To secure payment for patients receiving intermediate care, medications and treatments are documented daily. Document other types of care weekly, unless the patient's status changes and he requires a change in services. In this case, chart the change and document his status more frequently. Also, perform a monthly reevaluation for these patients and an evaluation of expected outcomes for all Medicaid patients.

> For skilled care, Medicaid requires daily documentation of patient care.

> For intermediate care, Medicaid requires daily documentation of medications and treatments.

HCFA

A branch of the Department of Health and Human Services, HCFA regulates compliance with federal Medicare and Medicaid standards. HCFA regulations are usually enforced at the state level.

To comply with HCFA regulations, staff members at a long-term care facility must complete a lengthy form called the Minimum Data Set (MDS) for Resident Assessment and Care Screening, review the patient's status every 3 months, and perform a comprehensive reassessment annually.

OBRA

In 1987, Congress enacted OBRA, which imposed dozens of new requirements on long-term care facilities and home health agencies to protect the rights of patients receiving long-term care. OBRA requires that a comprehensive assessment be performed within 4 days of a patient's admission to a long-term care facility and then be charted on the MDS form. The assessment and care screening process must be reviewed every 3 months and repeated annually—more often if the patient's condition changes.

In addition, a comprehensive nursing assessment and a formulated plan of care must be completed. The comprehensive plan of care must be completed within 7 days of the completion of the MDS. This date may vary depending on whether it's a Medicare Prospective Payment System (PPS) or an intermediate assessment.

JCAHO

JCAHO accredits long-term care facilities using standards developed in conjunction with health care experts. Standard performance is documented in assessments, progress notes, plans of care, and discharge plans. The ORYX initiative, begun in 1997, is another part of the accreditation process. It focuses on outcomes and other performance measurement data. The purpose of the initiative is to support quality improvements, not just in long-term care but in all health care organizations.

Forms used in long-term care

Many forms are used in both acute care and home health care settings as well as in long-term care; others are used only in long-term care. Forms discussed in this chapter include:
- MDS
- Resident Assessment Protocol (RAP)
- Preadmission Screening and Annual Resident Review (PASARR)
- initial nursing assessment form
- nursing summaries
- ADL checklists or flow sheets
- plans of care
- discharge and transfer forms.

In addition, many long-term care facilities have their own strict and comprehensive protocols. Typical protocols are those for

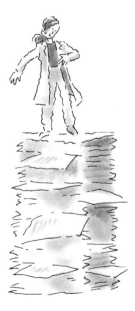

bowel and bladder monitoring, physical and chemical restraints, safety, and infection control. Charting requirements when using these protocols vary, so check your facility's policies.

MDS

Mandated by OBRA, the MDS is a federal regulatory form that must be filled out for every patient admitted to a long-term care facility. (See *Minimum Data Set form.*)

The MDS form proves compliance with quality improvement and reimbursement requirements, standardizes information, and helps health care team members and agencies communicate. Doctors, nurses, social workers, and other staff members complete and sign different sections of the form.

The requirements for completion of the MDS vary with the type of admission. For skilled care residents under PPS, Medicare requires completion at these times:
- 5-day assessment
- 14-day assessment
- 30-day assessment
- 60-day assessment
- 90-day assessment
- Readmission or return assessment.

For intermediate care residents, the MDS is completed at these times:
- admission assessment—required by day 14
- annual assessment
- significant change in status assessment
- quarterly review assessment—performed every 3 months.

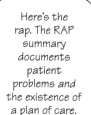

Here's the rap. The RAP summary documents patient problems and the existence of a plan of care.

RAP

Once an MDS form is completed, coded, computed, and processed, the patient's primary problems can be identified. These problems provide the basis for the patient's plan of care. Another federally mandated form, the RAP summary lists identified problem areas and documents the existence of a corresponding plan of care. For example, if the patient has a stage 2 pressure ulcer documented in the MDS, the RAP summary indicates the need for a plan of care to treat the pressure ulcer.

PASARR

For a patient to qualify for Medicare or Medicaid reimbursement, his mental status must also be documented. Federal regulations

(Text continues on page 184.)

Art of the chart

Minimum Data Set form

Patients in long-term care facilities that receive federal funds must have their health status evaluated at admission, and a plan of care must be devised. The patient's health status and plan of care are revised every 7 days.

Numeric Identifier_____

MINIMUM DATA SET (MDS) — *VERSION 2.0*
FOR NURSING HOME RESIDENT ASSESSMENT AND CARE SCREENING

BASIC ASSESSMENT TRACKING FORM

SECTION AA. IDENTIFICATION INFORMATION

1.	RESIDENT NAME	Amy J. Gaston			
		a. (First)	b. (Middle Initial)	c. (Last)	d. (Jr/Sr)
2.	GENDER	1. Male	2. Female		2
3.	BIRTHDATE	1 2 - 3 0 - 1 9 3 2			
		Month	Day	Year	
4.	RACE/ ETHNICITY	1. American Indian/Alaskan Native 4. Hispanic			
		2. Asian/Pacific Islander 5. White, not of			5
		3. Black, not of Hispanic origin Hispanic origin			
5.	SOCIAL SECURITY AND MEDICARE NUMBERS [C in 1st box if non med. no.]	a. Social Security Number			
		0 4 1 - 2 4 - 0 0 0 0			
		b. Medicare number (or comparable railroad insurance number)			
6.	FACILITY PROVIDER NO.	a. State No.			
		b. Federal No.			
7.	MEDICAID NO. ["+" if pending, "N" if not a Medicaid recipient]				

8. REASONS FOR ASSESS-MENT [Note—Other codes do not apply to this form]

a. Primary reason for assessment
1. Admission assessment (required by day 14)
2. Annual assessment
3. Significant change in status assessment
4. Significant correction of prior full assessment
5. Quarterly review assessment
10. Significant correction of prior quarterly assessment
0. NONE OF ABOVE

b. Codes for assessments required for Medicare PPS or the State
1. Medicare 5 day assessment
2. Medicare 30 day assessment
3. Medicare 60 day assessment
4. Medicare 90 day assessment
5. Medicare readmission/return assessment
6. Other state required assessment
7. Medicare 14 day assessment
8. Other Medicare required assessment

9. Signatures of Persons who Completed a Portion of the Accompanying Assessment or Tracking Form

I certify that the accompanying information accurately reflects resident assessment or tracking information for this resident and that I collected or coordinated collection of this information on the dates specified. To the best of my knowledge, this information was collected in accordance with applicable Medicare and Medicaid requirements. I understand that this information is used as a basis for ensuring that residents receive appropriate and quality care, and as a basis for payment from federal funds. I further understand that payment of such federal funds and continued partici-pation in the government-funded health care programs is conditioned on the accuracy and truthful-ness of this information, and that I may be personally subject to or may subject my organization to substantial criminal, civil, and/or administrative penalties for submitting false information. I also certify that I am authorized to submit this information by this facility on its behalf.

	Signature and Title	Sections	Date
a.	Christine Saslo, RN, MSN		12/7/02
b.	Susan Rowe, MSN		
c.	James Shaw, RN, BSN		
d.			
e.			
f.			
g.			
h.			
i.			
j.			
k.			
l.			

GENERAL INSTRUCTIONS

Complete this information for submission with all full and quarterly assessments (Admission, Annual, Significant Change, State or Medicare required assessments, or Quarterly Reviews, etc.)

○ = Key items for computerized resident tracking

☐ = When box blank, must enter number or letter   a. = When letter in box, check if condition applies

MDS 2.0 September, 2000

Place the patient's name on each assessment.

(continued)

Minimum Data Set form *(continued)*

> **The patient's name goes at the top of each page.**

Resident ___Amy J. Gaston___   Numeric Identifier _____

MINIMUM DATA SET (MDS) — *VERSION 2.0*
FOR NURSING HOME RESIDENT ASSESSMENT AND CARE SCREENING
BACKGROUND (FACE SHEET) INFORMATION AT ADMISSION

SECTION AB. DEMOGRAPHIC INFORMATION

1.	DATE OF ENTRY	Date the stay began. Note — Does not include readmission if record was closed at time of temporary discharge to hospital, etc. In such cases, use prior admission date

`1 2 - 0 3 - 2 0 0 2`
Month Day Year

2.	ADMITTED FROM (AT ENTRY)	1. Private home/apt. with no home health services 2. Private home/apt. with home health services 3. Board and care/assisted living/group home 4. Nursing home 5. Acute care hospital 6. Psychiatric hospital, MR/DD facility 7. Rehabilitation hospital 8. Other	`1`
3.	LIVED ALONE (PRIOR TO ENTRY)	0. No 1. Yes 2. In other facility	`0`
4.	ZIP CODE OF PRIOR PRIMARY RESIDENCE	`1 9 0 0 0`	
5.	RESIDENTIAL HISTORY 5 YEARS PRIOR TO ENTRY	*(Check all settings resident lived in during 5 years prior to date of entry given in item AB1 above)* Prior stay at this nursing home — a. Stay in other nursing home — b. Other residential facility—board and care home, assisted living, group home — c. MH/psychiatric setting — d. MR/DD setting — e. NONE OF ABOVE — f. ✓	
6.	LIFETIME OCCUPATION(S) [Put "/" between two occupations]	`T E A C H E R`	
7.	EDUCATION (Highest Level Completed)	1. No schooling 5. Technical or trade school 2. 8th grade/less 6. Some college 3. 9-11 grades 7. Bachelor's degree 4. High school 8. Graduate degree	`8`
8.	LANGUAGE	*(Code for correct response)* a. Primary Language 0. English 1. Spanish 2. French 3. Other b. If other, specify	`0`
9.	MENTAL HEALTH HISTORY	Does resident's RECORD indicate any history of mental retardation, mental illness, or developmental disability problem? 0. No 1. Yes	`0`
10.	CONDITIONS RELATED TO MR/DD STATUS	*(Check all conditions that are related to MR/DD status that were manifested before age 22, and are likely to continue indefinitely)* Not applicable—no MR/DD (Skip to AB11) — a. ✓ MR/DD with organic condition — b. Down's syndrome — c. Autism — d. Epilepsy — e. Other organic condition related to MR/DD — MR/DD with no organic condition — f.	
11.	DATE BACKGROUND INFORMATION COMPLETED	`1 2 - 0 7 - 2 0 0 2` Month Day Year	

SECTION AC. CUSTOMARY ROUTINE

1.	CUSTOMARY ROUTINE	*(Check all that apply. If all information UNKNOWN, check last box only)*

(In year prior to DATE OF ENTRY to this nursing home, or year last in community if now being admitted from another nursing home)

CYCLE OF DAILY EVENTS

Stays up late at night (e.g., after 9 pm)	a.
Naps regularly during day (at least 1 hour)	b. ✓
Goes out 1+ days a week	c.
Stays busy with hobbies, reading, or fixed daily routine	d. ✓
Spends most of time alone or watching TV	e.
Moves independently indoors (with appliances, if used)	f.
Use of tobacco products at least daily	g.
NONE OF ABOVE	h.

EATING PATTERNS

Distinct food preferences	i.
Eats between meals all or most days	j. ✓
Use of alcoholic beverage(s) at least weekly	k.
NONE OF ABOVE	l.

ADL PATTERNS

In bedclothes much of day	m.
Wakens to toilet all or most nights	n. ✓
Has irregular bowel movement pattern	o.
Showers for bathing	p.
Bathing in PM	q. ✓
NONE OF ABOVE	r.

INVOLVEMENT PATTERNS

Daily contact with relatives/close friends	s. ✓
Usually attends church, temple, synagogue (etc.)	t.
Finds strength in faith	u. ✓
Daily animal companion/presence	v.
Involved in group activities	w.
NONE OF ABOVE	x.
UNKNOWN—Resident/family unable to provide information	y.

> **Use check marks to identify relevant information.**

SECTION AD. FACE SHEET SIGNATURES

SIGNATURES OF PERSONS COMPLETING FACE SHEET:

Christine Saslo, RN, MSN

a. Signature of RN Assessment Coordinator	Date

James Shaw, RN, BSN 12/07/02

I certify that the accompanying information accurately reflects resident assessment or tracking information for this resident and that I collected or coordinated collection of this information on the dates specified. To the best of my knowledge, this information was collected in accordance with applicable Medicare and Medicaid requirements. I understand that this information is used as a basis for ensuring that residents receive appropriate and quality care, and as a basis for payment from federal funds. I further understand that payment of such federal funds and continued participation in the government-funded health care programs is conditioned on the accuracy and truthfulness of this information, and that I may be personally subject to or may subject my organization to substantial criminal, civil, and/or administrative penalties for submitting false information. I also certify that I am authorized to submit this information by this facility on its behalf.

Signature and Title	Sections	Date
b. *Susan Rowe, MSN*		*12/07/02*
c.		
d.		
e.		
f.		
g.		

☐ = When box blank, must enter number or letter   a. = When letter in box, check if condition applies

MDS 2.0 September, 2000

Minimum Data Set form *(continued)*

Resident __Amy J. Gaston__   Numeric Identifier_____

MINIMUM DATA SET (MDS) — *VERSION 2.0*
FOR NURSING HOME RESIDENT ASSESSMENT AND CARE SCREENING
FULL ASSESSMENT FORM
(Status in last 7 days, unless other time frame indicated)

SECTION A. IDENTIFICATION AND BACKGROUND INFORMATION

1.	RESIDENT NAME	Amy	J.	Gaston	
		a. (First)	b. (Middle Initial)	c. (Last)	d. (Jr/Sr)

2. ROOM NUMBER: 402

3. ASSESSMENT REFERENCE DATE
a. Last day of MDS observation period: 12 - 07 - 2002 (Month - Day - Year)
b. Original (0) or corrected copy of form (enter number of correction)

4a. DATE OF REENTRY — Date of reentry from most recent temporary discharge to a hospital in last 90 days (or since last assessment or admission if less than 90 days): [ ][ ] - [ ][ ] - [ ][ ][ ][ ] (Month Day Year)

5. MARITAL STATUS
1. Never married   3. Widowed   5. Divorced
2. Married   4. Separated — **3**

6. MEDICAL RECORD NO.: M M 0 0 0 9 9 2 2 6 8 1

7. CURRENT PAYMENT SOURCES FOR N.H. STAY (Billing Office to indicate; check all that apply in last 30 days)
- Medicaid per diem — a.
- Medicare per diem — b. **X** (Self or family pays for full per diem)
- Medicare ancillary part A — c.
- Medicare ancillary part B — d.
- CHAMPUS per diem — e.
- VA per diem — f.
- Self or family pays for full per diem — g. **X**
- Medicaid resident liability or Medicare co-payment — h.
- Private insurance per diem (including co-payment) — i.
- Other per diem — j.

8. REASONS FOR ASSESSMENT
[Note—If this is a discharge or reentry assessment, only a limited subset of MDS items need be completed]
a. Primary reason for assessment — **1**
1. Admission assessment (required by day 14)
2. Annual assessment
3. Significant change in status assessment
4. Significant correction of prior full assessment
5. Quarterly review assessment
6. Discharged—return not anticipated
7. Discharged—return anticipated
8. Discharged prior to completing initial assessment
9. Reentry
10. Significant correction of prior quarterly assessment
0. NONE OF ABOVE
b. Codes for assessments required for Medicare PPS or the State
1. Medicare 5 day assessment
2. Medicare 30 day assessment
3. Medicare 60 day assessment
4. Medicare 90 day assessment
5. Medicare readmission/return assessment
6. Other state required assessment
7. Medicare 14 day assessment
8. Other Medicare required assessment

9. RESPONSIBILITY/ LEGAL GUARDIAN (Check all that apply)
- Legal guardian — a.
- Other legal oversight — b.
- Durable power of attorney/health care — c. **X**
- Durable power attorney/financial — d.
- Family member responsible — e.
- Patient responsible for self — f.
- NONE OF ABOVE — g.

10. ADVANCED DIRECTIVES (For those items with supporting documentation in the medical record, check all that apply)
- Living will — a. **X**
- Do not resuscitate — b.
- Do not hospitalize — c.
- Organ donation — d.
- Autopsy request — e.
- Feeding restrictions — f.
- Medication restrictions — g.
- Other treatment restrictions — h.
- NONE OF ABOVE — i.

SECTION B. COGNITIVE PATTERNS

1. COMATOSE (Persistent vegetative state/no discernible consciousness)
0. No   1. Yes   (If yes, skip to Section G) — **0**

2. MEMORY (Recall of what was learned or known)
a. Short-term memory OK—seems/appears to recall after 5 minutes
0. Memory OK   1. Memory problem — **1**
b. Long-term memory OK—seems/appears to recall long past
0. Memory OK   1. Memory problem — **1**

This section is for your assessment of the patient's mental status.

3. MEMORY/ RECALL ABILITY (Check all that resident was normally able to recall during last 7 days)
- Current season — a.
- Location of own room — b.
- Staff names/faces — c.
- That he/she is in a nursing home — d.
- NONE OF ABOVE are recalled — e. **X**

4. COGNITIVE SKILLS FOR DAILY DECISION-MAKING (Made decisions regarding tasks of daily life)
0. INDEPENDENT—decisions consistent/reasonable
1. MODIFIED INDEPENDENCE—some difficulty in new situations only
2. MODERATELY IMPAIRED—decisions poor; cues/supervision required
3. SEVERELY IMPAIRED—never/rarely made decisions — **2**

5. INDICATORS OF DELIRIUM— PERIODIC DISORDERED THINKING/ AWARENESS (Code for behavior in the last 7 days.) [Note: Accurate assessment requires conversations with staff and family who have direct knowledge of resident's behavior over this time].
0. Behavior not present
1. Behavior present, not of recent onset
2. Behavior present, over last 7 days appears different from resident's usual functioning (e.g., new onset or worsening)
a. EASILY DISTRACTED—(e.g., difficulty paying attention; gets sidetracked) — **1**
b. PERIODS OF ALTERED PERCEPTION OR AWARENESS OF SURROUNDINGS—(e.g., moves lips or talks to someone not present; believes he/she is somewhere else; confuses night and day) — **0**
c. EPISODES OF DISORGANIZED SPEECH—(e.g., speech is incoherent, nonsensical, irrelevant, or rambling from subject to subject; loses train of thought) — **0**
d. PERIODS OF RESTLESSNESS—(e.g., fidgeting or picking at skin, clothing, napkins, etc; frequent position changes; repetitive physical movements or calling out) — **0**
e. PERIODS OF LETHARGY—(e.g., sluggishness; staring into space; difficult to arouse; little body movement) — **0**
f. MENTAL FUNCTION VARIES OVER THE COURSE OF THE DAY—(e.g., sometimes better, sometimes worse; behaviors sometimes present, sometimes not) — **0**

6. CHANGE IN COGNITIVE STATUS — Resident's cognitive status, skills, or abilities have changed as compared to status of 90 days ago (or since last assessment if less than 90 days)
0. No change   1. Improved   2. Deteriorated — **0**

SECTION C. COMMUNICATION/HEARING PATTERNS

1. HEARING (With hearing appliance, if used)
0. HEARS ADEQUATELY—normal talk, TV, phone
1. MINIMAL DIFFICULTY when not in quiet setting
2. HEARS IN SPECIAL SITUATIONS ONLY—speaker has to adjust tonal quality and speak distinctly
3. HIGHLY IMPAIRED/absence of useful hearing — **1**

2. COMMUNICATION DEVICES/ TECHNIQUES (Check all that apply during last 7 days)
- Hearing aid, present and used — a.
- Hearing aid, present and not used regularly — b.
- Other receptive comm. techniques used (e.g., lip reading) — c.
- NONE OF ABOVE — d. **X**

3. MODES OF EXPRESSION (Check all used by resident to make needs known)
- Speech — a. **X**
- Writing messages to express or clarify needs — b.
- American sign language or Braille — c.
- Signs/gestures/sounds — d.
- Communication board — e.
- Other — f.
- NONE OF ABOVE — g.

4. MAKING SELF UNDERSTOOD (Expressing information content—however able)
0. UNDERSTOOD
1. USUALLY UNDERSTOOD—difficulty finding words or finishing thoughts
2. SOMETIMES UNDERSTOOD—ability is limited to making concrete requests
3. RARELY/NEVER UNDERSTOOD — **1**

5. SPEECH CLARITY (Code for speech in the last 7 days)
0. CLEAR SPEECH—distinct, intelligible words
1. UNCLEAR SPEECH—slurred, mumbled words
2. NO SPEECH—absence of spoken words — **0**

6. ABILITY TO UNDERSTAND OTHERS (Understanding verbal information content—however able)
0. UNDERSTANDS
1. USUALLY UNDERSTANDS—may miss some part/intent of message
2. SOMETIMES UNDERSTANDS—responds adequately to simple, direct communication
3. RARELY/NEVER UNDERSTANDS — **2**

7. CHANGE IN COMMUNICATION/ HEARING — Resident's ability to express, understand, or hear information has changed as compared to status of 90 days ago (or since last assessment if less than 90 days)
0. No change   1. Improved   2. Deteriorated — **0**

[ ] = When box blank, must enter number or letter   [a.] = When letter in box, check if condition applies

MDS 2.0 September, 2000

(continued)

Minimum Data Set form *(continued)*

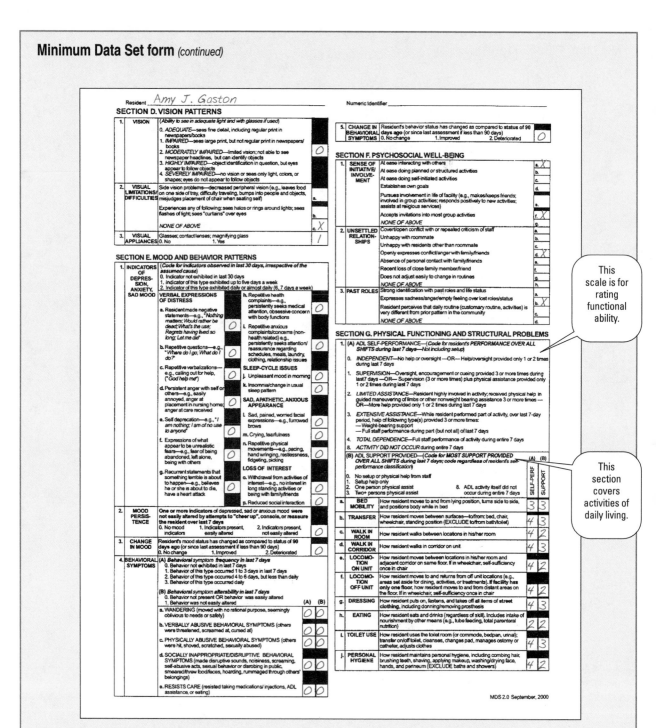

MDS 2.0 September, 2000

Minimum Data Set form *(continued)*

Resident **Amy J. Gaston**

Numeric Identifier _____

2. BATHING — How resident takes full-body bath/shower, sponge bath, and transfers in/out of tub/shower (EXCLUDE washing of back and hair.) Code for most dependent in self-performance and support.
(A) BATHING SELF-PERFORMANCE codes appear below

		(A)	(B)
0.	Independent—No help provided	4	3
1.	Supervision—Oversight help only		
2.	Physical help limited to transfer only		
3.	Physical help in part of bathing activity		
4.	Total dependence		
8.	Activity itself did not occur during entire 7 days		

(Bathing support codes are as defined in Item 1, code B above)

3. TEST FOR BALANCE *(see training manual)* — *(Code for ability during test in the last 7 days)*
0. Maintained position as required in test
1. Unsteady, but able to rebalance self without physical support
2. Partial physical support during test; or stands (sits) but does not follow directions for test
3. Not able to attempt test without physical help

a. Balance while standing	3
b. Balance while sitting—position, trunk control	3

4. FUNCTIONAL LIMITATION IN RANGE OF MOTION *(see training manual)* — *(Code for limitations during last 7 days that interfered with daily functions or placed resident at risk of injury)*

(A) RANGE OF MOTION
0. No limitation
1. Limitation on one side
2. Limitation on both sides

(B) VOLUNTARY MOVEMENT
0. No loss
1. Partial loss
2. Full loss

	(A)	(B)
a. Neck		
b. Arm—Including shoulder or elbow		
c. Hand—Including wrist or fingers		
d. Leg—Including hip or knee		
e. Foot—Including ankle or toes		
f. Other limitation or loss	0	0

5. MODES OF LOCOMOTION — *(Check all that apply during last 7 days)*

Cane/walker/crutch	a.	Wheelchair primary mode of locomotion	d. X
Wheeled self	b.	NONE OF ABOVE	e.
Other person wheeled	c.		

6. MODES OF TRANSFER — *(Check all that apply during last 7 days)*

Bedfast all or most of time	a. X	Lifted mechanically	d.
Bed rails used for bed mobility or transfer	b.	Transfer aid (e.g., slide board, trapeze, cane, walker, brace)	e.
Lifted manually	c.	NONE OF ABOVE	f.

7. TASK SEGMENTATION — Some or all of ADL activities were broken into subtasks during last 7 days so that resident could perform them
0. No   1. Yes → 0

8. ADL FUNCTIONAL REHABILITATION POTENTIAL

Resident believes he/she is capable of increased independence in at least some ADLs	a.
Direct care staff believe resident is capable of increased independence in at least some ADLs	b.
Resident able to perform tasks/activity but is very slow	c.
Difference in ADL Self-Performance or ADL Support, comparing mornings to evenings	d.
NONE OF ABOVE	e. 0

9. CHANGE IN ADL FUNCTION — Resident's ADL self-performance status has changed as compared to status of 90 days ago (or since last assessment if less than 90 days)
0. No change   1. Improved   2. Deteriorated → 0

SECTION H. CONTINENCE IN LAST 14 DAYS

1. CONTINENCE SELF-CONTROL CATEGORIES
(Code for resident's PERFORMANCE OVER ALL SHIFTS)

0. CONTINENT—Complete control [includes use of indwelling urinary catheter or ostomy device that does not leak urine or stool]

1. USUALLY CONTINENT—BLADDER, incontinent episodes once a week or less; BOWEL, less than weekly

2. OCCASIONALLY INCONTINENT—BLADDER, 2 or more times a week but not daily; BOWEL, once a week

3. FREQUENTLY INCONTINENT—BLADDER, tended to be incontinent daily, but some control present (e.g., on day shift); BOWEL, 2-3 times a week

4. INCONTINENT—Had inadequate control BLADDER, multiple daily episodes; BOWEL, all (or almost all) of the time

a.	BOWEL CONTINENCE	Control of bowel movement, with appliance or bowel continence programs, if employed	2
b.	BLADDER CONTINENCE	Control of urinary bladder function (if dribbles, volume insufficient to soak through underpants), with appliances (e.g., foley) or continence programs, if employed	2

2. BOWEL ELIMINATION PATTERN

Bowel elimination pattern regular—at least one movement every three days	a. X	Diarrhea	c.
		Fecal impaction	d.
Constipation	b.	NONE OF ABOVE	e.

MDS 2.0 September, 2000

3. APPLIANCES AND PROGRAMS

Any scheduled toileting plan	a.	Did not use toilet room/commode/urinal	f.
Bladder retraining program	b.	Pads/briefs used	g. X
External (condom) catheter	c.	Enemas/irrigation	h.
Indwelling catheter	d.	Ostomy present	i.
Intermittent catheter	e.	NONE OF ABOVE	

4. CHANGE IN URINARY CONTINENCE — Resident's urinary continence has changed as compared to status of 90 days ago (or since last assessment if less than 90 days)
0. No change   1. Improved   2. Deteriorated → 0

SECTION I. DISEASE DIAGNOSES

Check only those diseases that have a relationship to current ADL status, cognitive status, mood and behavior status, medical treatments, nursing monitoring, or risk of death. (Do not list inactive diagnoses.)

1. DISEASES *(If none apply, CHECK the NONE OF ABOVE box)*

ENDOCRINE/METABOLIC/NUTRITIONAL		Hemiplegia/Hemiparesis	v.
		Multiple sclerosis	w.
Diabetes mellitus	a.	Paraplegia	x.
Hyperthyroidism	b.	Parkinson's disease	y.
Hypothyroidism	c. X	Quadriplegia	z.
HEART/CIRCULATION		Seizure disorder	aa.
Arteriosclerotic heart disease (ASHD)	d.	Transient ischemic attack (TIA)	bb.
Cardiac dysrhythmias	e.	Traumatic brain injury	cc.
Congestive heart failure	f.	PSYCHIATRIC/MOOD	
Deep vein thrombosis	g.	Anxiety disorder	dd.
Hypertension	h.	Depression	ee.
Hypotension	i.	Manic depression (bipolar disease)	ff.
Peripheral vascular disease	j. X	Schizophrenia	gg.
Other cardiovascular disease	k.	PULMONARY	
MUSCULOSKELETAL		Asthma	hh.
Arthritis	l.	Emphysema/COPD	ii.
Hip fracture	m.	SENSORY	
Missing limb (e.g., amputation)	n.	Cataracts	jj.
Osteoporosis	o.	Diabetic retinopathy	kk.
Pathological bone fracture	p.	Glaucoma	ll.
NEUROLOGICAL		Macular degeneration	mm.
Alzheimer's disease	q.	OTHER	
Aphasia	r.	Allergies	nn.
Cerebral palsy	s.	Anemia	oo.
Cerebrovascular accident (stroke)	t.	Cancer	pp.
Dementia other than Alzheimer's disease	u. X	Renal failure	qq.
		NONE OF ABOVE	rr.

2. INFECTIONS *(If none apply, CHECK the NONE OF ABOVE box)*

Antibiotic resistant infection (e.g., Methicillin resistant staph)	a.	Septicemia	g.
		Sexually transmitted diseases	h.
Clostridium difficile (c. diff.)	b.	Tuberculosis	i.
Conjunctivitis	c. X	Urinary tract infection in last 30 days	j.
HIV infection	d.	Viral hepatitis	k.
Pneumonia	e.	Wound infection	l.
Respiratory infection	f.	NONE OF ABOVE	m.

3. OTHER CURRENT OR MORE DETAILED DIAGNOSES AND ICD-9 CODES

a.	*Hypertension*	402.11
b.		
c.		
d.		
e.		

List other diseases here.

Identify other health problems here.

SECTION J. HEALTH CONDITIONS

1. PROBLEM CONDITIONS *(Check all problems present in last 7 days unless other time frame is indicated)*

INDICATORS OF FLUID STATUS		Dizziness/Vertigo	f.
		Edema	g.
Weight gain or loss of 3 or more pounds within a 7 day period	a.	Fever	h.
		Hallucinations	i.
Inability to lie flat due to shortness of breath	b.	Internal bleeding	j.
		Recurrent lung aspirations in last 90 days	k.
Dehydrated; output exceeds input	c.	Shortness of breath	l.
		Syncope (fainting)	m.
Insufficient fluid; did NOT consume all/almost all liquids provided during last 3 days	d.	Unsteady gait	n.
		Vomiting	o.
OTHER		NONE OF ABOVE	p. X
Delusions	e.		

(continued)

Minimum Data Set form *(continued)*

> A detailed scale helps you assess pressure ulcers.

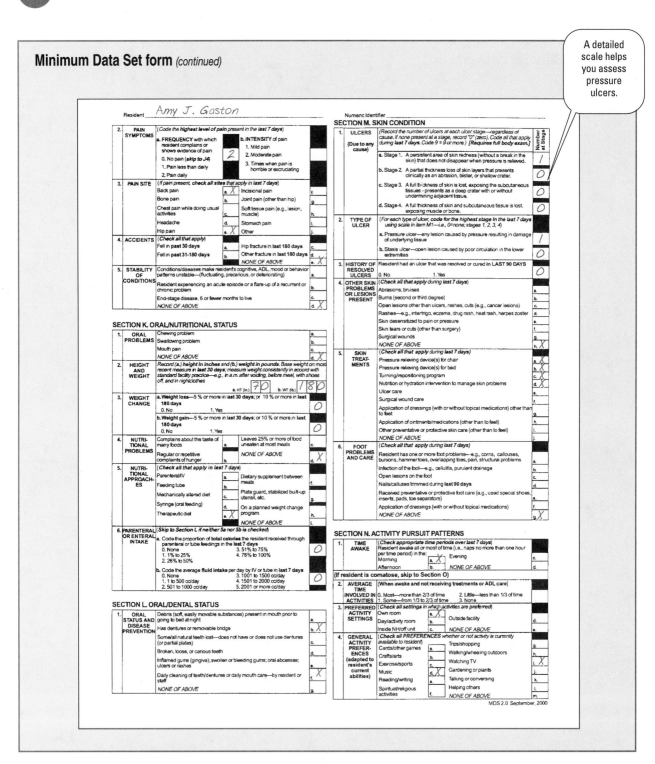

Resident: **Amy J. Gaston**

Numeric Identifier: _____

2.	PAIN SYMPTOMS	*(Code the highest level of pain present in the last 7 days)*
		a. FREQUENCY with which resident complains or shows evidence of pain — 0. No pain *(skip to J4)*; 1. Pain less than daily; 2. Pain daily → **2**	**b. INTENSITY** of pain — 1. Mild pain; 2. Moderate pain; 3. Times when pain is horrible or excruciating

3.	PAIN SITE	*(If pain present, check all sites that apply in last 7 days)*		
		Back pain	a.	Incisional pain — f.
		Bone pain		Joint pain (other than hip) — g.
		Chest pain while doing usual activities		Soft tissue pain (e.g., lesion, muscle) — h.
		Headache	d.	Stomach pain — i.
		Hip pain	e.	Other — j.

4.	ACCIDENTS	*(Check all that apply)*		
		Fell in past 30 days	a.	Hip fracture in last 180 days — c.
		Fell in past 31-180 days	b.	Other fracture in last 180 days — d.
				NONE OF ABOVE — e. X

5.	STABILITY OF CONDITIONS	Conditions/diseases make resident's cognitive, ADL, mood or behavior patterns unstable—(fluctuating, precarious, or deteriorating) — a.
		Resident experiencing an acute episode or a flare-up of a recurrent or chronic problem — b.
		End-stage disease, 6 or fewer months to live — c.
		NONE OF ABOVE — d.

SECTION K. ORAL/NUTRITIONAL STATUS

1.	ORAL PROBLEMS	Chewing problem — a.
		Swallowing problem — b.
		Mouth pain — c.
		NONE OF ABOVE — d.

2.	HEIGHT AND WEIGHT	Record (a.) height in inches and (b.) weight in pounds. Base weight on most recent measure in last 30 days; measure weight consistently in accord with standard facility practice—e.g., in a.m. after voiding, before meal, with shoes off, and in nightclothes. **a. HT (in.) 70** **b. WT (lb.) 180**

3.	WEIGHT CHANGE	a. Weight loss—5 % or more in last 30 days; or 10 % or more in last 180 days. 0. No 1. Yes → **0**
		b. Weight gain—5 % or more in last 30 days; or 10 % or more in last 180 days. 0. No 1. Yes → **0**

4.	NUTRITIONAL PROBLEMS	Complains about the taste of many foods — a.	Leaves 25% or more of food uneaten at most meals — c.
		Regular or repetitive complaints of hunger — b.	NONE OF ABOVE — d. X

5.	NUTRITIONAL APPROACHES	*(Check all that apply in last 7 days)*	
		Parenteral/IV — a.	Dietary supplement between meals — f.
		Feeding tube — b.	Plate guard, stabilized built-up utensil, etc. — g.
		Mechanically altered diet — c.	On a planned weight change program — h.
		Syringe (oral feeding) — d.	
		Therapeutic diet — e. X	NONE OF ABOVE — i.

6.	PARENTERAL OR ENTERAL INTAKE	*(Skip to Section L if neither 5a nor 5b is checked)*
		a. Code the proportion of total calories the resident received through parenteral or tube feedings in the last 7 days — 0. None; 1. 1% to 25%; 2. 26% to 50%; 3. 51% to 75%; 4. 76% to 100% → **0**
		b. Code the average fluid intake per day by IV or tube in last 7 days — 0. None; 1. 1 to 500 cc/day; 2. 501 to 1000 cc/day; 3. 1001 to 1500 cc/day; 4. 1501 to 2000 cc/day; 5. 2001 or more cc/day → **0**

SECTION L. ORAL/DENTAL STATUS

1.	ORAL STATUS AND DISEASE PREVENTION	Debris (soft, easily movable substances) present in mouth prior to going to bed at night — a.
		Has dentures or removable bridge — b. X
		Some/all natural teeth lost—does not have or does not use dentures (or partial plates) — c.
		Broken, loose, or carious teeth — d.
		Inflamed gums (gingiva); swollen or bleeding gums; oral abscesses; ulcers or rashes — e.
		Daily cleaning of teeth/dentures or daily mouth care—by resident or staff — f.
		NONE OF ABOVE — g.

SECTION M. SKIN CONDITION

1.	ULCERS (Due to any cause)	*(Record the number of ulcers at each ulcer stage—regardless of cause. If none present at a stage, record "0" (zero). Code all that apply during last 7 days. Code 9 = 9 or more.) [Requires full body exam.]*	Number at Stage
		a. Stage 1. A persistent area of skin redness (without a break in the skin) that does not disappear when pressure is relieved.	1
		b. Stage 2. A partial thickness loss of skin layers that presents clinically as an abrasion, blister, or shallow crater.	0
		c. Stage 3. A full thickness of skin is lost, exposing the subcutaneous tissues - presents as a deep crater with or without undermining adjacent tissue.	0
		d. Stage 4. A full thickness of skin and subcutaneous tissue is lost, exposing muscle or bone.	0

2.	TYPE OF ULCER	*(For each type of ulcer, code for the highest stage in the last 7 days using scale in item M1—i.e., 0=none; stages 1, 2, 3, 4)*	
		a. Pressure ulcer—any lesion caused by pressure resulting in damage of underlying tissue	1
		b. Stasis ulcer—open lesion caused by poor circulation in the lower extremities	

3.	HISTORY OF RESOLVED ULCERS	Resident had an ulcer that was resolved or cured in LAST 90 DAYS. 0. No 1. Yes → **0**

4.	OTHER SKIN PROBLEMS OR LESIONS PRESENT	*(Check all that apply during last 7 days)*	
		Abrasions, bruises	a.
		Burns (second or third degree)	b.
		Open lesions other than ulcers, rashes, cuts (e.g., cancer lesions)	c.
		Rashes—e.g., intertrigo, eczema, drug rash, heat rash, herpes zoster	d.
		Skin desensitized to pain or pressure	e.
		Skin tears or cuts (other than surgery)	f.
		Surgical wounds	g.
		NONE OF ABOVE	h. X

5.	SKIN TREATMENTS	*(Check all that apply during last 7 days)*	
		Pressure relieving device(s) for chair	a.
		Pressure relieving device(s) for bed	b.
		Turning/repositioning program	c.
		Nutrition or hydration intervention to manage skin problems	d.
		Ulcer care	e.
		Surgical wound care	f.
		Application of dressings (with or without topical medications) other than to feet	g.
		Application of ointments/medications (other than to feet)	h.
		Other preventative or protective skin care (other than to feet)	i.
		NONE OF ABOVE	j.

6.	FOOT PROBLEMS AND CARE	*(Check all that apply during last 7 days)*	
		Resident has one or more foot problems—e.g., corns, callouses, bunions, hammer toes, overlapping toes, pain, structural problems	a.
		Infection of the foot—e.g., cellulitis, purulent drainage	b.
		Open lesions on the foot	c.
		Nails/calluses trimmed during last 90 days	d.
		Received preventative or protective foot care (e.g., used special shoes, inserts, pads, toe separators)	e.
		Application of dressings (with or without topical medications)	f.
		NONE OF ABOVE	g. X

SECTION N. ACTIVITY PURSUIT PATTERNS

1.	TIME AWAKE	*(Check appropriate time periods over last 7 days)* Resident awake all or most of time (i.e., naps no more than one hour per time period) in the:	
		Morning — a. X	Evening — c.
		Afternoon — b.	NONE OF ABOVE — d.

(If resident is comatose, skip to Section O)

2.	AVERAGE TIME INVOLVED IN ACTIVITIES	*(When awake and not receiving treatments or ADL care)* 0. Most—more than 2/3 of time; 1. Some—from 1/3 to 2/3 of time; 2. Little—less than 1/3 of time; 3. None

3.	PREFERRED ACTIVITY SETTINGS	*(Check all settings in which activities are preferred)*	
		Own room — a. X	Outside facility — d.
		Day/activity room — b.	NONE OF ABOVE — e.
		Inside NH/off unit — c.	

4.	GENERAL ACTIVITY PREFERENCES (adapted to resident's current abilities)	*(Check all PREFERENCES whether or not activity is currently available to resident)*	
		Cards/other games — a.	Trips/shopping — g.
		Crafts/arts — b.	Walking/wheeling outdoors — h.
		Exercise/sports — c.	Watching TV — i. X
		Music — d. X	Gardening or plants — j.
		Reading/writing — e.	Talking or conversing — k.
		Spiritual/religious activities — f.	Helping others — l.
			NONE OF ABOVE — m.

MDS 2.0 September, 2000

Minimum Data Set form *(continued)*

Resident ___Amy J. Gaston___   Numeric Identifier _____

5.	PREFERS CHANGE IN DAILY ROUTINE	Code for resident preferences in daily routines 0. No change 1. Slight change 2. Major change a. Type of activities in which resident is currently involved b. Extent of resident involvement in activities	

SECTION O. MEDICATIONS

1.	NUMBER OF MEDICA-TIONS	(Record the number of different medications used in the *last 7 days*; enter "0" if none used)	4
2.	NEW MEDICA-TIONS	(Resident currently receiving medications that were initiated during the *last 90 days*) 0. No 1. Yes	0
3.	INJECTIONS	(Record the number of DAYS injections of any type received during the *last 7 days*; enter "0" if none used)	0
4.	DAYS RECEIVED THE FOLLOWING MEDICATION	(Record the number of DAYS during last 7 days; enter "0" if not used. Note—enter "1" for long-acting meds used less than weekly) a. Antipsychotic d. Hypnotic b. Antianxiety c. Antidepressant e. Diuretic	X

SECTION P. SPECIAL TREATMENTS AND PROCEDURES

1.	SPECIAL TREAT-MENTS, PROCE-DURES, AND PROGRAMS	a. SPECIAL CARE—Check treatments or programs received during the *last 14 days*	

TREATMENTS		PROGRAMS	
Chemotherapy	a.	Ventilator or respirator	l.
Dialysis	b.	Alcohol/drug treatment program	m.
IV medication	c.	Alzheimer's/dementia special care unit	n. X
Intake/output	d.	Hospice care	o.
Monitoring acute medical condition	e.	Pediatric unit	p.
Ostomy care	f.	Respite care	q.
Oxygen therapy	g.	Training in skills required to return to the community (e.g., taking medications, house work, shopping, transportation, ADLs)	r.
Radiation	h.		
Suctioning	i.		
Tracheostomy care	j.		
Transfusions	k.	NONE OF ABOVE	s.

b. THERAPIES - Record the number of days and total minutes each of the following therapies was administered (for at least 15 minutes a day) in the *last 7 calendar days* (Enter 0 if none or less than 15 min. daily) [Note—count only post admission therapies]

(A) = # of days administered for 15 minutes or more (B) = total # of minutes provided in last 7 days	DAYS (A)	MIN (B)
a. Speech - language pathology and audiology services	0	
b. Occupational therapy	0	
c. Physical therapy	1	
d. Respiratory therapy	0	
e. Psychological therapy (by any licensed mental health professional)	0	

2.	INTERVEN-TION PROGRAMS FOR MOOD, BEHAVIOR, COGNITIVE LOSS	(Check all interventions or strategies used in last 7 days—no matter where received)	
		Special behavior symptom evaluation program	a. X
		Evaluation by a licensed mental health specialist in **last 90 days**	b.
		Group therapy	c.
		Resident-specific deliberate changes in the environment to address mood/behavior patterns—e.g., providing bureau in which to rummage	d. X
		Reorientation—e.g., cueing	e.
		NONE OF ABOVE	f.

3.	NURSING REHABILITA-TION/ RESTOR-ATIVE CARE	Record the NUMBER OF DAYS each of the following rehabilitation or restorative techniques or practices was provided to the resident for more than or equal to 15 minutes per day in the last 7 days (Enter 0 if none or less than 15 min. daily)	
		a. Range of motion (passive)	/	f. Walking	
		b. Range of motion (active)		g. Dressing or grooming	
		c. Splint or brace assistance		h. Eating or swallowing	
		TRAINING AND SKILL PRACTICE IN:		i. Amputation/prosthesis care	
		d. Bed mobility		j. Communication	
		e. Transfer		k. Other	

4.	DEVICES AND RESTRAINTS	(Use the following codes for *last 7 days:*) 0. Not used 1. Used less than daily 2. Used daily	
		Bed rails	
		a. — Full bed rails on all open sides of bed	0
		b. — Other types of side rails used (e.g., half rail, one side)	0
		c. Trunk restraint	0
		d. Limb restraint	0
		e. Chair prevents rising	0
5.	HOSPITAL STAY(S)	Record number of times resident was admitted to hospital with an overnight stay in **last 90 days** (or since last assessment if less than 90 days). *(Enter 0 if no hospital admissions)*	0
6.	EMERGENCY ROOM (ER) VISIT(S)	Record number of times resident visited ER without an overnight stay in **last 90 days** (or since last assessment if less than 90 days). *(Enter 0 if no ER visits)*	0
7.	PHYSICIAN VISITS	In the LAST 14 DAYS (or since admission if less than 14 days in facility) how many days has the physician (or authorized assistant or practitioner) examined the resident? *(Enter 0 if none)*	1
8.	PHYSICIAN ORDERS	In the LAST 14 DAYS (or since admission if less than 14 days in facility) how many days has the physician (or authorized assistant or practitioner) changed the resident's orders? *Do not include order renewals without change. (Enter 0 if none)*	0
9.	ABNORMAL LAB VALUES	Has the resident had any abnormal lab values during the **last 90 days** (or since admission)? 0. No 1. Yes	0

SECTION Q. DISCHARGE POTENTIAL AND OVERALL STATUS

1.	DISCHARGE POTENTIAL	a. Resident expresses/indicates preference to return to the community 0. No 1. Yes	0
		b. Resident has a support person who is positive towards discharge 0. No 1. Yes	0
		c. Stay projected to be of a short duration— discharge projected within **90 days** (do not include expected discharge due to death) 0. No 2. Within 31-90 days 1. Within 30 days 3. Discharge status uncertain	0
2.	OVERALL CHANGE IN CARE NEEDS	Resident's overall self sufficiency has changed significantly as compared to status of 90 days ago (or since last assessment if less than 90 days) 0. No change 1. Improved—receives fewer supports, needs less restrictive level of care 2. Deteriorated—receives more support	2

SECTION R. ASSESSMENT INFORMATION

1.	PARTICIPA-TION IN ASSESS-MENT	a. Resident: 0. No 1. Yes	1
		b. Family: 0. No 1. Yes 2. No family	1
		c. Significant other: 0. No 1. Yes 2. None	0

2. SIGNATURE OF PERSON COORDINATING THE ASSESSMENT:

a. Signature of RN Assessment Coordinator (sign on above line)

Christine Saslo, RN, MSN

b. Date RN Assessment Coordinator signed as complete	1 2	0 7	2 0 0 2
	Month	Day	Year

> This section covers special treatments and procedures that may affect patient care.

MDS 2.0 September, 2000

(continued)

Minimum Data Set form *(continued)*

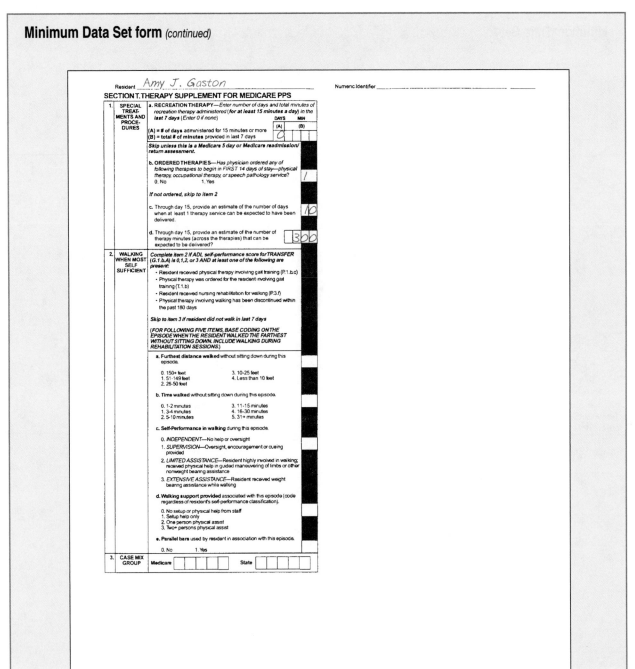

Resident **Amy J. Gaston**   Numeric Identifier _____

SECTION T. THERAPY SUPPLEMENT FOR MEDICARE PPS

1.	SPECIAL TREATMENTS AND PROCEDURES	

a. RECREATION THERAPY—*Enter number of days and total minutes of recreation therapy administered (**for at least 15 minutes a day**) in the last 7 days (Enter 0 if none)*

	DAYS (A)	MIN (B)
(A) = # of days administered for 15 minutes or more (B) = total # of minutes provided in last 7 days	0	

Skip unless this is a Medicare 5 day or Medicare readmission/ return assessment.

b. ORDERED THERAPIES—*Has physician ordered any of following therapies to begin in FIRST 14 days of stay—physical therapy, occupational therapy, or speech pathology service?*
0. No   1. Yes   **1**

If not ordered, skip to item 2

c. Through day 15, provide an estimate of the number of days when at least 1 therapy service can be expected to have been delivered.   **10**

d. Through day 15, provide an estimate of the number of therapy minutes (across the therapies) that can be expected to be delivered?   **300**

2.	WALKING WHEN MOST SELF SUFFICIENT	

Complete item 2 if ADL self-performance score for TRANSFER (G.1.b.A) is 0,1,2, or 3 AND at least one of the following are present:
- Resident received physical therapy involving gait training (P.1.b.c)
- Physical therapy was ordered for the resident involving gait training (T.1.b)
- Resident received nursing rehabilitation for walking (P.3.f)
- Physical therapy involving walking has been discontinued within the past 180 days

Skip to item 3 if resident did not walk in last 7 days

(FOR FOLLOWING FIVE ITEMS, BASE CODING ON THE EPISODE WHEN THE RESIDENT WALKED THE FARTHEST WITHOUT SITTING DOWN. INCLUDE WALKING DURING REHABILITATION SESSIONS.)

a. Furthest distance walked without sitting down during this episode.

0. 150+ feet   3. 10-25 feet
1. 51-149 feet   4. Less than 10 feet
2. 26-50 feet

b. Time walked without sitting down during this episode.

0. 1-2 minutes   3. 11-15 minutes
1. 3-4 minutes   4. 16-30 minutes
2. 5-10 minutes   5. 31+ minutes

c. Self-Performance in walking during this episode.

0. *INDEPENDENT*—No help or oversight
1. *SUPERVISION*—Oversight, encouragement or cueing provided
2. *LIMITED ASSISTANCE*—Resident highly involved in walking; received physical help in guided maneuvering of limbs or other nonweight bearing assistance
3. *EXTENSIVE ASSISTANCE*—Resident received weight bearing assistance while walking

d. Walking support provided associated with this episode (code regardless of resident's self-performance classification).

0. No setup or physical help from staff
1. Setup help only
2. One person physical assist
3. Two+ persons physical assist

e. Parallel bars used by resident in association with this episode.

0. No   1. Yes

3.	CASE MIX GROUP	Medicare ☐☐☐☐☐ State ☐☐☐☐☐

MDS 2.0 September, 2000

Minimum Data Set form *(continued)*

SECTION V. RESIDENT ASSESSMENT PROTOCOL SUMMARY   Numeric Identifier _____

Resident's Name: *Amy J. Gaston*	Medical Record No.: *MM0009922681*

1. Check if RAP is triggered.

2. For each triggered RAP, use the RAP guidelines to identify areas needing further assessment. Document relevant assessment information regarding the resident's status.

   • Describe:
     — Nature of the condition (may include presence or lack of objective data and subjective complaints).
     — Complications and risk factors that affect your decision to proceed to care planning.
     — Factors that must be considered in developing individualized care plan interventions.
     — Need for referrals/further evaluation by appropriate health professionals.

   • Documentation should support your decision-making regarding whether to proceed with a care plan for a triggered RAP and the type(s) of care plan interventions that are appropriate for a particular resident.

   • Documentation may appear anywhere in the clinical record (e.g., progress notes, consults, flowsheets, etc.).

3. Indicate under the Location of RAP Assessment Documentation column where information related to the RAP assessment can be found.

4. For each triggered RAP, indicate whether a new care plan, care plan revision, or continuation of current care plan is necessary to address the problem(s) identified in your assessment. The Care Planning Decision column must be completed within 7 days of completing the RAI (MDS and RAPs).

A. RAP PROBLEM AREA	(a) Check if triggered	Location and Date of RAP Assessment Documentation	(b) Care Planning Decision—check if addressed in care plan
1. DELIRIUM			
2. COGNITIVE LOSS	X	*progress notes*	X
3. VISUAL FUNCTION			
4. COMMUNICATION	X	*progress notes*	X
5. ADL FUNCTIONAL/ REHABILITATION POTENTIAL			
6. URINARY INCONTINENCE AND INDWELLING CATHETER			
7. PSYCHOSOCIAL WELL-BEING			
8. MOOD STATE			
9. BEHAVIORAL SYMPTOMS			
10. ACTIVITIES			
11. FALLS			
12. NUTRITIONAL STATUS			
13. FEEDING TUBES			
14. DEHYDRATION/FLUID MAINTENANCE			
15. DENTAL CARE			
16. PRESSURE ULCERS	X	*progress notes*	X
17. PSYCHOTROPIC DRUG USE			
18. PHYSICAL RESTRAINTS			

B. *James Shaw, RN, BSN*
1. Signature of RN Coordinator for RAP Assessment Process   2. |1|2|–|0|7|–|2|0|0|2| Month Day Year

Christine Saslo, RN, MSN
3. Signature of Person Completing Care Planning Decision   4. |1|2|–|0|7|–|2|0|0|2| Month Day Year

MDS 2.0 September, 2000

> The RAP summary lists identified problem areas and documents the existence of a corresponding plan of care.

require that a long-term care facility performs a complete mental status assessment and documents it on a PASARR form. (See *PASARR identification form.*)

Initial nursing assessment

This required form is similar to the initial assessment form used in other settings. When documenting your initial assessment in a long-term care setting, place special emphasis on the patient's:

- activity level
- hearing and vision
- bowel and bladder control
- ability to communicate
- safety
- need for adaptive devices to assist dexterity and mobility
- family relationships
- transition from home or hospital to the long-term care facility.

Nursing summaries

Care and status updates must be completed regularly in long-term care facilities. Usually, you must complete a standard nursing care summary at least once every 2 to 4 weeks for patients with specific problems, such as pressure ulcers, who are receiving skilled care. A summary addressing the specific problems must be done weekly. For patients receiving intermediate care, a standard nursing care summary is usually required every 4 weeks.

Summing it up

The nursing summary describes:

- patient's ability to perform ADLs
- nutrition and hydration
- safety measures, such as bed rails, restraints, or adaptive devices
- medications and other treatments
- problems the patient has adjusting to the long-term care facility.

In addition, you must complete a nursing assessment summary at least monthly to comply with Medicare and Medicaid standards.

ADL checklists and flow sheets

ADL checklists and flow sheets are forms that are usually completed by a nursing assistant or a restorative nurse on each shift; then you review and sign them. These forms tell the health care team members about the patient's abilities, degree of indepen-

(Text continues on page 188.)

Art of the chart

PASARR identification form

Before a patient covered by Medicare or Medicaid enters a long-term care facility, he must undergo an evaluation of mental status, using the Preadmission Screening and Annual Resident Review (PASARR). This form is shown here.

SECTION A. IDENTIFYING INFORMATION FOR APPLICANT/RESIDENT

Last name Perrone **First Name** Joseph **MI** R

Sex M M = Male F = Female **Date of birth** 081083 **Social security number** 012345678 **Medicaid Recipient?** N Y = Yes N = No P = Pending

SECTION B: REASON FOR SCREENING

Enter code /

Preadmission Screening Codes
1-Nursing Facility Applicant
2-PASSPORT waiver Applicant

Annual RESIDENT REVIEW CODES
3-Expired Time Limit for Convalescent Stay
4-Expired Time for Emergency Admission
5-Expired Time Limit for Respite Admission
6-Significant Change in Condition
7-No Previous PASARR Records
8-ODMH Use Only
9-Other

SECTION C: DEMENTIA QUESTIONS

Yes	No	
	✓	(1) Does the individual have a documented PRIMARY diagnosis of dementia, Alzheimer's disease, or some other organic mental disorder as defined in *DSM-IV-TR*? If YES, the individual does not have indications of serious MI, go to Section E. If NO, go to the next question.
	✓	(2) Does the individual have a SECONDARY diagnosis of dementia, Alzheimer's disease, or some other organic mental disorder as defined in *DSM-IV-TR*? If YES, go to the next question. If NO, go to Section D.
	✓	(3) Does the individual have a PRIMARY diagnosis of one of the mental disorders listen in Question D (1) below? If YES, go to Section D. If NO, and the individual does not have indications of serious MI, go to Section E.

SECTION D: INDICATIONS OF SERIOUS MENTAL ILLNESS

Yes No

(1) Does the individual have a diagnosis of any of the mental disorders listed below? Check all that apply.

a. [ ] Schizophrenic Disorder
b. [ ] Mood Disorder
c. [ ] Delusional (Paranoid) Disorder
d. [ ] Panic or Other Severe Anxiety Disorder

e. [ ] Somatoform Disorder
f. [ ] Personality Disorder
g. [ ] Other Psychotic Disorder
h. [ ] Another Mental Disorder Other Than MR That May Lead to a Chronic Disability
   Describe:_____

Yes No

(2) Within the past 2 years, DUE TO THE MENTAL DISORDER, has the individual:

(a) Utilized intensive psychiatric services more than once? Indicate the number of times the individual utilized each service over the last 2 years (e.g., 0,1, 2, 7 times).

a. [ ] Ongoing case management from a MH agency? ("1" if continuously receiving over the last 2 years.)
b. [ ] Emergency mental health services?
c. [ ] Number of admissions to inpatient hospital settings for psychiatric reasons?
d. [ ] Number of admissions to partial hospitalization treatment programs for psychiatric reasons?
e. [ ] Number of admissions to Residential Care Facilities (RCFs) providing MH services or operated by an MH agency?
f. [ ] TOTAL SCORE: If total score equals 2 or more, answer YES to Question D(2). Regardless of score, answer Question D(2)(b).

OR

Yes No

(b) Had a disruption to his/her usual living arrangement (e.g., arrest, eviction, inter- or intra-facility transfer, locked seclusion)? If YES, answer YES to Question D(2).

> If the patient is diagnosed as having a serious mental disorder, document the diagnosis here.

(continued)

PASARR identification form *(continued)*

SECTION D: INDICATIONS OF SERIOUS MENTAL ILLNESS *(continued)*

Yes | No

(3) Within the past 6 months, DUE TO THE MENTAL DISORDER, has the individual experienced one or more of the following functional limitations on a continuing or intermittent basis? Check all that apply.

a. Maintaining Personal Hygiene
b. Dressing Self
c. Walking or Getting Around
d. Maintaining Adequate Diet
e. Preparing or Obtaining Own Meals
f. Maintaining Prescribed Medication Regimen
g. Performing Household Chores
h. Going Shopping
i. Using Available Transportation
j. Managing Available Funds
k. Securing Necessary Support Services
l. Verbalizing Needs

Yes | No

(4) Within the past 2 years, has the individual received SSI or SSDI due to a mental impairment?

Yes | No

(5) Does the individual have indications of serious mental illness?
The individual has indications of serious mental illness if the individual received:
- *Yes to AT LEAST 2 of Questions D(1), D(2), or D(3); OR*
- *Yes to Question D(4).*

SECTION E: INDICATIONS OF MR OR RELATED CONDITION

Yes | No [✓]

(1) Does the individual have a diagnosis of mental retardation (mild, moderate, severe, or profound as described in the *American Association of Mental Retardation's Manual on Classification in Mental Retardation,* 1989)?

Yes | No [✓]

(2) Does the individual have a severe, chronic disability that is attributable to a condition other than mental illness but is closely related to MR because this condition results in impairment of general intellectual functioning or adaptive behavior similar to that of a person with MR and requires treatment or services similar to those required for persons with MR? If YES, specify:_____

If NO, go to question E(6).

Yes | No

(3) Did the disability manifest symptoms before the individual's 22nd birthday?

Yes | No

(4) Is the disability likely to continue indefinitely?

Yes | No

(5) Did the disability result in functional limitations, prior to age 22, in 3 or more of the following major life activities? Check all that apply:

a. Self Care
b. Mobility
c. Economic Self Sufficiency
d. Understanding and Use of Language
e. Self Direction
f. Learning
g. Capacity for Independen

> Fill out this section if your patient has mental retardation or a related condition.

Yes | No [✓]

(6) Does the person currently receive services from the County Board of MR/DD?

Yes | No [✓]

(7) Does the person have indications of MR or a related condition?
The individual has indications of MR or a related condition if the individual received:
- *Yes to Question E(1); OR*
- *Yes to all of the following in this Section; Questions 2, 3, 4 AND 5; OR*
- *Yes to Question E(6).*

SECTION F: SUBMITTER INFORMATION/CERTIFICATION

In order to process the screen, the submitter must provide his/her name and address and sign below. If the individual has indications of serious MI (YES to D[5]) and/or MR or a related condition (YES to E[7]), submitters must also complete Section G (next page). If the individual has indications of neither, submitters do not have to complete Section G. The NF may not admit or retain individuals with indications of serious MI and/or MR or a related condition without further review by ODMH and/or ODMR/DD (OAC Rules 5101:3-3-151 and 5101:3-3-152).

Last name: Brown

First Name: Lisa

PASARR identification form *(continued)*

Street address
4 5 6 Main street

City
Springhouse

State
PA

Zip
1 9 4 7 7

Telephone Number
(2 1 4) 999-9900

I understand that this screening information may be relied upon in the payment of claims that will be from Federal and State funds, and that any willful falsification, or concealment of a material fact, may be prosecuted under Federal and State laws. I certify that to the best of my knowledge the foregoing information is true, accurate, and complete.

Signature *Lisa Brown*

Title *RN*

Date
06-10-02
Month   Day   Year

Employer *Sunnyside Care Facility*

PASARR IDENTIFICATION SCREEN

SECTION G: MAILING ADDRESSES

Complete this section ONLY if the individual has indications of serious MI, MR, or a related condition.

(1) What address should be used for mailing results of the PASARR evaluation to the applicant/resident?

In care of

Street address

City

State

Zip

Telephone Number
(   )

(2) Please provide the following information about the individual's attending physician:

Last name

First Name

Street address

City

State

Zip

Telephone Number
(   )

(3) If the individual has a legal representative, please provide the following information about the representative:

Last name

First Name

Street address

City

State

Zip

Telephone Number
(   )

(continued)

PASARR identification form (continued)

(4) If the individual is an applicant to or resident of an NF, please provide the name and address of the NF:

Name of NF

Street address

| City | State | Zip | First 4 letters of county |

(5) If the individual is being discharged from a hospital, and the submitter is not employed by the discharging hospital, please provide the name of a contact person and the name and address of the discharging hospital:

Last name   **First Name**

Discharging hospital

Street address

| City | State | Zip | Telephone Number ( ) |

---

dence, and special needs so they can determine the type of assistance he requires.

The following tools are examples of checklists and flow sheets that can be used to assess ADLs:

- Katz index
- Lawton scale
- Barthel index and scale.

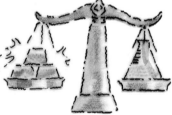

Katz index

The Katz index ranks the patient's ability in six areas:

- bathing
- dressing
- toileting
- moving from wheelchair to bed and returning
- continence
- feeding.

It describes his functional level at a specific time and rates his performance of each function on three levels: performing without help, needing some help, or having complete disability. (See *Rating ability to perform basic tasks*, page 190.)

Lawton scale

The Lawton scale of instrumental activities evaluates the patient's ability to perform complex personal care activities necessary for independent living. Activities include:
- using the telephone
- cooking
- shopping
- doing laundry
- managing finances
- taking medications
- preparing meals.

Activities are rated on a three-point scale, ranging from without help (3), to needing some help (2), to complete disability (1). (See *Rating ability to perform complex tasks*, page 191.)

Barthel index and scale

The Barthel index and scale is used to evaluate:
- feeding
- moving from wheelchair to bed and returning
- performing personal hygiene
- getting on and off the toilet
- bathing
- walking on a level surface or propelling a wheelchair
- going up and down stairs
- dressing and undressing
- maintaining bowel continence
- controlling the bladder.

Each item is scored according to the amount of assistance needed. Over time, results reveal improvement or decline. Another scale, the Barthel self-care rating scale, evaluates function in more detail. (See *Getting better or worse?* pages 192 and 193.)

Plans of care

Standards for plans of care are developed by individual long-term care facilities. When a patient is admitted to a facility, an interim plan of care is used until there's an interdisciplinary care conference regarding the patient. The interim plan of care should be in place within 24 hours of admission. After this, a full plan of care is developed for the patient. The interdisciplinary plan of care should be completed within 7 days of the completion of the MDS.

(Text continues on page 194.)

Art of the chart

Rating ability to perform basic tasks

The Katz index, shown below, is used to assess six basic ADLs.

> Resident's name and the date

Evaluation Form   Name _Henry Dancer_   Date _12/4/02_

For each area of functioning listed below, check the description that applies. (The word "assistance" means supervision, direction, or personal assistance.)

Bathing: Sponge bath, tub bath, or shower.
- ☐ Receives no assistance; gets into and out of tub, if tub is usual means of bathing.
- ☑ Receives assistance in bathing only one part of the body, such as the back or leg.
- ○ Receives assistance in bathing more than one part of the body, or can't bathe.

Dressing: Gets outer garments and underwear from closets and drawers and uses fasteners, including suspenders, if worn.
- ☐ Gets clothes and gets completely dressed without assistance.
- ☐ Gets clothes and gets dressed without assistance except for tying shoes.
- ☑ Receives assistance in getting clothes or in getting dressed, or stays partly or completely undressed.

Toileting: Goes to the room termed "toilet" for bowel movement ~~...~~ ans self afterward, and arranges clothes.
- ☐ Goes to toilet room, cleans self, and arranges clothes without assistance. May use object for support, such as cane, walker, or wheelchair and may manage night bedpan or commode, emptying it in the morning.
- ☑ R~~...~~ in going to toilet room or ~~...~~ arranging clothes after elimina~~...~~ t bedpan or commode.
- ○ Doesn't go to toilet room for the elimination process.

> The focus of this chart is on basic activities

Transfer
- ☐ Moves into and out of bed and chair without assistance. May use object, such as cane or walker for support.
- ☑ Moves into or out of bed or chair with assistance.
- ○ Doesn't get out of bed.

Continence
- ☑ Controls urination and bowel movement completely by self.
- ○ Has occasional accidents.
- ○ Supervision helps keep control of urination or bowel movement, or catheter is used, or is incontinent.

Feeding
- ☐ Feeds self without assistance.
- ☑ Feeds self except for assistance in cutting meat or buttering bread.
- ○ Receives assistance in feeding or is fed partly or completely through tubes or by I.V. fluids.

Evaluator: _Germaine Fried, RN_

Index   ☐ **Indicates independence**   ○ **Indicates dependence**

A: Independent in all six functions.
B: Independent in all but one of these functions.
C: Independent in all but bathing and one additional function.
D: Independent in all but bathing, dressing and one additional function.
E: Independent in all but bathing, dressing, toileting, and one additional function.

F: Independent in all but bathing, dressing, toileting, transferring, and one additional function.
G: Dependent in all six functions.
Other: Dependent in at least two functions but not classifiable as C, D, E, or F.

Adapted with permission from Katz, S. et al. "Studies of Illness in the Aged: The Index of ADL-A Standardized Measure of Biological and Psychosocial Function," *JAMA* 185:914-19, ©1996, American Medical Association.

Art of the chart

Rating ability to perform complex tasks

The Lawton scale of instrumental activities (shown below) provides information about a patient's ability to perform more sophisticated tasks than basic activities of daily living.

Name _John Shapiro_   Rated by _James Mott, RN_   Date _Dec. 12, 2002_

1. Can you use the telephone?
   without help .... (3) *(Your name)*
   with some help 2
   completely unable 1

2. Can you get to places beyond walking distance?
   without help 3
   with some help .... (2)
   not without special arrangements 1

3. Can you go shopping for groceries?
   without help 3
   with some help .... (2)
   completely unable 1

4. Can you prepare your own meals?
   without help .... (3)
   with some help 2
   completely unable 1

5. Can you do your own housework?
   without help .... (3)
   with some help 2
   completely unable 1

6. Can you do your own handyman work?
   without help 3
   with some help .... (2)
   completely unable 1

Patient's name

Questions may need to be modified for individual patients.

7. Can you do your own laundry?
   without help .... *(Date)* .... (3)
   with some help 2
   completely unable 1

8a. Do you take or use any medications?
   Yes (If yes, answer question 8b.) .... (1)
   No (If no, answer question 8c.) 2

8b. Do you take your own medication?
   without help (in the right doses at the right times) .... (3)
   with some help (if someone prepares it for you or reminds you to take it) 2
   completely unable 1

8c. If you had to take medication, could you do it?
   without help (in the right doses at the right time) 3
   with some help (if someone prepared it for you or reminded you to take it) 2
   completely unable 1

9. Can you manage your own money?
   without help .... (3)
   with some help 2
   completely unable 1

Activities are rated on a three-point scale.

The first answer in each case — except for 8a — indicates independence; the second indicates capability with assistance; and the third, dependence. In this version the maximum score is 29, although scores have meaning only for a particular patient, such as when declining scores over time reveal deterioration.

Adapted with permission from Lawton, M.P., and Brody, E.M. "Assessment of Older People: Self-Maintaining and Instrumental Activities of Daily Living," *The Journal of Gerontology* 9(3):179-86, Autumn 1969.

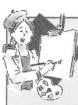

Art of the chart

Getting better or worse?

The Barthel index and scale (shown below) is used to assess the patient's ability to perform 10 activities of daily living, document findings for other health care team members, and reveal improvement or decline.

Date *December 14, 2002*
Patient's name *Jack Boyd*
Evaluator *Kate Roth, RN*

Action	With help	Independent
Feeding (if food needs to be cut up = help)	5	⑩
Moving from wheelchair to bed and return (includes sitting up in bed)	5 to ⑩	15
Personal toilet (wash face, comb hair, shave, clean teeth)	0	⑤
Getting on and off toilet (handling clothes, wipe, flush)	⑤	10
Bathing self	0	⑤
Walking on level surface (or, if unable to walk, propelling wheelchair)	0	⑤ or 15
Ascending and descending stairs	⑤	10
Dressing (includes tying shoes, fastening fasteners)	⑤	10
Controlling bowels	⑤	⑩
Controlling bladder	⑤	10

> Reading the definitions of the numbers will enable you to interpret the scale.

Definition and Discussion of Scoring

A person scoring 100 is continent, feeds himself, dresse[...]d and chairs, bathes himself, walks at least a block, and can ascend and descend stairs. This doesn't [...] alone; he may not be able to cook, keep house, or meet the public, but he's able to get along without att[...]

Feeding

10 = Independent. The person can feed hi[...]en a meal [...] en someone puts the food within his reach. He must be able to put on an assistive device if needed, cut up the food, use salt and pepper, spread butter, and so forth. Also, he must accomplish these tasks in a reasonable time.

5 = The person needs some help with cutting up food and other tasks, as listed above.

Moving from wheelchair to bed and return

15 = The person operates independently in all phases of this activity. He can safely approach the bed in his wheelchair, lock brakes, lift footrests, move safely from bed, lie down, come to a sitting position on the side of the bed, change the position of the wheelchair, if necessary, to transfer back into it safely, and return to the wheelchair.

10 = Either the person needs some minimal help in some step of this activity, or needs to be reminded or supervised for safety in one or more parts of this activity.

5 = The person can come to a sitting position without the help of a second person but needs to be lifted out of bed, or needs a great deal of help with transfers.

Handling personal toilet

5 = The person can wash his hands and face, comb hair, clean teeth, and shave. He may use any kind of razor but he must be able to get it from the drawer or cabinet and plug it in or put in a blade without help. A female must put on her own makeup, if any, but need not braid or style her hair.

(continued)

Getting better or worse? *(continued)*

Getting on and off toilet

10 = The person is able to get on and off the toilet, unfasten and refasten clothes, prevent soiling of clothes, and use toilet paper without help. He may use a wall bar or other stable object for support, if needed. If he needs to use a bed pan instead of toilet, he must be able to place it on a chair, use it competently, and empty and clean it.

5 = The person needs help to overcome imbalance, handle clothes, or use toilet paper.

Bathing self

5 = The person may use a bath tub or shower or give himself a complete sponge bath. Regardless of method, he must be able to complete all the steps involved without another person's presence.

Walking on a level surface

15 = The person can walk at least 50 yards without help or supervision. He may wear braces or prostheses and use crutches, canes, or a walkerette, but not a rolling walker. He must be able to lock and unlock braces, if used, get the necessary mechanical aids into position for use, stand up and sit down, and dispose of the aids when he sits. (Putting on, fastening, and taking off braces is scored under Dressing).

5 = If the person can't ambulate but can propel a wheelchair independently, he must be able to go around corners, turn around, maneuver the chair to table, bed, toilet, and other locations. He must be able to push a chair at least 150' (45 m). Don't score this item if the person receives a score for walking.

0 = unable to walk

Ascending and descending stairs

10 = The person can go up and down a flight of stairs safely without help or supervision. He may and should use handrails, canes, or crutches when needed, and he must be able to carry canes or crutches as he ascends or descends.

5 = The person needs help with or supervision of any one of the above items.

Dressing and undressing

10 = The person can put on, fasten, and remove all clothing (including any prescribed corset or braces) and tie shoe laces (unless he requires adaptations for this). Such special clothing as suspenders, loafers, and dresses that open down the front may be used when necessary.

5 = The person needs help in putting on, fastening, or removing any clothing. He must do at least half the work himself and must accomplish the task in a reasonable time. Women need not be scored on use of a brassiere or girdle unless these are prescribed garments.

Controlling bowels

10 = The person can control his bowels without accidents. He can use a suppository or take an enema when necessary (as in spinal cord injury patients who have had bowel training).

5 = The person needs help in using a suppository or taking an enema or has occasional accidents.

Controlling bladder

10 = The person can control his bladder day and night. Spinal cord injury patients who wear an external device and leg bag must put them on independently, clean and empty the bag, and stay dry, day and night.

5 = The person has occasional accidents, can't wait for the bed pan or get to the toilet in time, or needs help with an external device.

The total score is less significant or meaningful than the individual items, because these indicate where the deficiencies lie. Any applicant to a long-term care facility who scores 100 should be evaluated carefully before admission to see whether admission is indicated. Discharged patients with scores of 100 shouldn't require further physical therapy but may be evaluated to see whether any environmental adjustments are needed.

This scale clearly explains how to rate the patient.

Adapted with permission from Mahoney, F.I. and Barthel, D.W. "Functional Evaluation: The Barthel Index," *Maryland State Medical Journal* 14:62, 1965.

A documented review of the plan must be completed every 3 months or when the patient's status changes.

In long-term care settings, plans of care usually evolve from an interdisciplinary approach to care, with contributions by the patient, members of his family, and other health care providers.

As always, base your plan of care on the patient's health problems, nursing diagnoses, and expected treatment outcomes. Include measurable patient outcomes with reasonable time frames and specific interventions to achieve them.

Discharge and transfer forms

When the facility discharges a patient to home or to a hospital, you must document the reason for discharge, the patient's destination, his mode of transportation, and the person or staff member accompanying him, if appropriate.

Other important data to include in this document are a list of prescribed medications, skin assessment findings, overall condition, the disposition of personal belongings, and teaching topics that you covered (such as diet, medications, skin care, and other areas).

Guidelines drawn up by JCAHO emphasize the need to assess and summarize the patient's condition at transfer time. (See *Transfer and personal belongings form.*)

Documentation guidelines

In long-term care facilities, consider the following points when updating your records:
• When writing nursing summaries, address specific patient problems noted in the plan of care.
• When writing progress notes, confirm that the patient's progress is being evaluated and reevaluated in relation to the goals or outcomes in the plan of care. If goals aren't met, address this. Also, describe and document additional actions.
• Record transfers and discharges according to facility protocol.
• Document changes in the patient's condition and report them to the doctor and the family within 24 hours.
• Document follow-up interventions or other measures taken in response to a change in the patient's condition.

Art of the chart

Transfer and personal belongings form

Patients in long-term care facilities may be admitted to the hospital, discharged to home, or transferred to other facilities. The forms below are used during this process.

1. PATIENT'S LAST NAME _Clark_	FIRST NAME _Robert_	MI _T_	2. SEX _Male_	3. SOCIAL SECURITY NUMBER _144-44-4444_

4. PATIENT'S ADDRESS (Street, City, State, Zip Code) _1 Wise street Springhouse, PA 19411_	5. DATE OF BIRTH _2-8-28_	6. RELIGION _unknown_

7. DATE OF THIS TRANSFER _12/29/02_	8. FACILITY NAME AND ADDRESS TRANSFERRING TO _Seniors Care Facility 22 Elderly Way Phila., PA_	9. PHYSICIAN IN CHARGE AT TIME OF TRANSFER _Dr. Nicholas_ Will this physician care for patient after admission to new facility? ☐ YES ☒ NO

10. DATES OF STAY AT FACILITY

TRANSFERRING FROM

ADMISSION _11/14/02_   DISCHARGE _12/29/02_

11. PAYMENT SOURCE FOR CHARGES TO PATIENT

A. ☒ SELF OR FAMILY
B. ☐ PRIVATE INSURANCE
C. ☐ BLUE CROSS BLUE SHIELD
D. ☐ EMPLOYER OR UNION
E. ☐ PUBLIC AGENCY (Give name)
F. ☐ OTHER (Explain)

12-A. NAME AND ADDRESS OF FACILITY TRANSFERRING FROM _Community Hospital 3000 Medical Way, Phila., PA_	12-B. NAMES AND ADDRESSES OF ALL HOSPITALS AND EXTENDED CARE FACILITIES FROM WHICH PATIENT WAS DISCHARGED IN PAST 60 DAYS.

13. CLINIC APPOINTMENT DATE TIME CLINIC APPOINTMENT CARD ATTACHED	14. DATE OF LAST PHYSICAL EXAMINATION _12/26/02_

15. RELATIVE OR GUARDIAN: Name _Katherine Clark_   Address _1 Wise Street Springhouse, PA 19411_   Phone number _1-215-999-9000_

16. DIAGNOSES AT TIME OF TRANSFER
(a) Primary ⓡ CVA
(b) Secondary IDDM

EMPLOYMENT RELATED:
☐ YES
☒ NO

VITALS AT TIME OF TRANSFER
T _98⁶_   P _68_   R _20_   B/P _140/82_

ADVANCE DIRECTIVES   ☐ YES ☒ NO ☐ COPY ATTACHED
CODE STATUS _Full code_

CHECK ALL THAT APPLY
Disabilities
☐ Amputation
☑ Paralysis _(L) side_
☐ Contracture
☐ Pressure Ulcer
Impairments
☐ Mental

☑ Speech
☑ Hearing
☑ Vision
☐ Sensation
Incontinence
☑ Bladder
☑ Bowel
☑ Saliva

Activity Tolerance Limitations
☐ None
☑ Moderate
☐ Severe
Patient knows diagnosis?
☑ Yes
☐ No

Potential for Rehabilitation
☐ Good
☑ Fair
☐ Poor
IMPORTANT MEDICAL INFORMATION
(State allergies if any)
PCN

DIET, DRUGS, AND OTHER THERAPY at time of discharge
-Mechanical soft diet (2,000 cal)
-Megace 4 tabs Q6h
-Lasix 40 mg P.O. b.i.d.
-Aspirin 81mg P.O. q.d.
-Humulin 70/30 20 units q.a.m. & h.s.
-Sliding scale coverage: BG <40 7400
-Call Dr. Nicholas, BG 200-250:2u | 301-350:4u ⟩ Humulin R
       251-300:3u | 351-400:5u
(Physician, please sign below)

SUGGESTIONS FOR ACTIVE CARE
BED
Position in good body alignment and change position every _2_ hrs.
Avoid _flat supine_ position
Prone position _2_ time/day as tolerated.
SITTING
_4_ hr _3_ times/day

Signature of Physician or Nurse _John Brown, RN_

WEIGHT BEARING
☐ Full
☑ Partial
☐ None
on _____ Leg

EXERCISES
Range of motion _3_ times/day.
to _(L) extremities_ by
☐ patient ☐ nurse ☐ family
Stand _3_ min. _2_ times/day.

LOCOMOTION
Walk _unable_ times/day.

SOCIAL ACTIVITIES
Encourage (☑ Group ☐ Individual) activities (☑ within ☐ outside) home.
☐ Transportation: ☑ Ambulance
☐ Car ☐ Car for handicapped
☐ Bus

Date _12 / 29 / 02_

(continued)

Transfer and personal belongings form *(continued)*

Any articles of clothing or other belongings left at the hospital will be held for 30 days after discharge. Items remaining after this period will be disposed of by the hospital.

		COMMENTS
Date: *12/29/02*		
Initials: *CR*		
VALUABLES DESCRIBE		
Wallet:	✔	*1 brown leather wallet*
Money (Amount): *$25.00*	✔	*1-$20.00 bill* *5 $1 bills*
Watch:		
Jewelry:		
Glasses/Contacts: *Glasses*	✔	*Wire rim-gold*
Hearing Aids:		
Dentures:	✔	
Partial		
Complete	✔	*Container labeled*
Keys		
ARTICLE DESCRIBE		
Ambulatory Aids:		
Cane, Walker, Etc.		
Bedclothes	✔	*1 pair plaid pajamas*
Belt		
Dress		
Outer Wear		
Pants		
Pocketbook		
Shirt		
Shoes		
Sweater		
Undergarments		
Other		

All belongings were sent home with patient's family: YES   (NO)

Patient's Signature ——— *Bob Park* ———

Witnessed by Hospital Personnel *Mary Jones, RN*

- Keep a record of visits from family or friends and of phone calls about the patient. State or federal regulators may fine your facility if these aren't charted.
- If an incident occurs, such as a fall or a treatment error, fill out an incident report and write follow-up notes for at least 48 hours after the incident (or follow your facility's policy).
- During the patient's first week of residence, keep detailed records on each shift.
- Flag a new patient by putting a red dot on the chart, bed, or door or by using a similar system so that all staff members are aware of the new resident and become familiar with him. (Remember, however, to be sensitive to each patient's need for confidentiality and dignity.)
- Keep reimbursement in mind when documenting. For a facility to qualify for payment, its records must clearly reflect the level of care given to the patient.
- Make sure that your records accurately reflect skilled services the patient receives.
- Always record a doctor's verbal and telephone orders and have the doctor countersign them within 48 hours.
- Document visits by the doctor to the patient. Generally accepted standards require one visit after admission, another after the first 30 days, and at least one every 60 days thereafter. However, the resident's condition ultimately guides the frequency of doctor's visits.

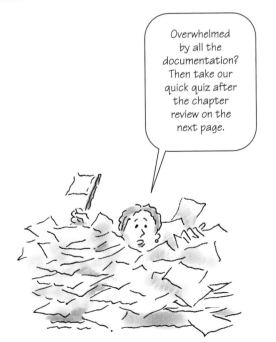

Overwhelmed by all the documentation? Then take our quick quiz after the chapter review on the next page.

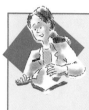

Cheat sheet

Long-term care and rehabilitation documentation review

The basics
- It isn't done as often in long-term care and rehabilitation facilities.
- It can be extensive because of the long government forms involved.
- It's influenced by federal programs, government agencies, laws, state regulations, and accrediting agencies.

Types of forms
- MDS—is a multidisciplinary form that's mandated by OBRA and must be completed for every long-term care patient
- RAP—includes the patient's primary problems and documents the corresponding plan of care
- PASARR—documents complete assessment of the patient's mental status
- Initial assessment form—is similar to the initial assessment form used in other settings but places greater emphasis on activity, hearing and vision, bowel and bladder control, communication, safety, assistive devices, family rela-

tionships, and transition
- Nursing summary—must be completed once a month and describes the patient's ability to performs ADLs, his nutrition and hydration status, safety measures, treatments, and problems adjusting to the long-term care facility
- ADL checklists and flow sheets—indicate the patient's abilities, degree of independence, and special needs so they can determine the type of assistance he requires
- Plans of care—usually evolve from an interdisciplinary approach to care and should always be based on the patient's health problems, nursing diagnoses, and expected outcomes
- Discharge and transfer forms—must include the reason for discharge as well as the patient's destination and mode of transportation

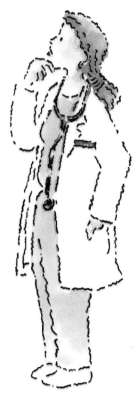

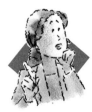

Quick quiz

1. The two levels of care in long-term care settings are:
   A.   skilled and intermediate.
   B.   acute and critical.
   C.   geriatric and special need.

Answer: A. Skilled and intermediate care, the two levels of care in long-term care settings, differ in the amount and type of nursing skills provided.

2. The MDS is required by:
   A.   Medicare.
   B.   Medicaid.
   C.   OBRA.

Answer: C. Under the federal law known as OBRA, an initial assessment must be documented on an MDS form.

3. In a long-term care facility, you must write an interdisciplinary plan of care within:
   A.   14 days of the completion of the MDS.
   B.   7 hours of the completion of the MDS.
   C.   7 days of the completion of the MDS.

Answer: C. You must complete the plan of care within 7 days of the completion of the MDS and update and review it every 3 months.

4. A tool for assessing the patient's mental status is:
   A.   Katz index.
   B.   Lawton scale.
   C.   PASARR form.

Answer: C. A PASARR, or Preadmission Screening Annual Resident Review, form is required by Medicare and Medicaid for reimbursement.

5. Medicare and Medicaid require nursing assessment summaries to be completed:
   A.   weekly.
   B.   monthly.
   C.   daily.

Answer: B. In addition, nursing care summaries must be completed at least once a week for patients receiving skilled care and every 2 weeks for those receiving intermediate care.

6.   Patients in long-term care facilities must be seen by the doctor at least once:

    A.   every 60 days.

    B.   a month.

    C.   every 6 months.

Answer: A. Patients are seen by doctors on an as-needed basis; however, they must be seen at least every 60 days.

Scoring

⭐⭐⭐   If you answered all six items correctly, outasight! You're PASARR (Perfectly Amazing, Stupendous, and Artful at Records and Reports)!

⭐⭐   If you answered four or five correctly, unreal! No doubt about it, you're the RAP (Really Awesome Paperwork) expert!

⭐   If you answered fewer than four correctly, keep plugging! You're an ADL (Admirably Dedicated Learner).

Part III

Special topics

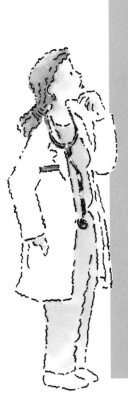

Enhancing your charting

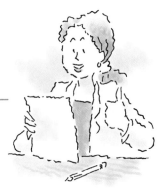

Just the facts

In this chapter, you'll learn:

♦ seven rules of clear charting and how to follow them

♦ different types of doctor's orders and how to clarify them

♦ the nurse's role in documenting doctor's orders.

A look at expert charting

Charting like a pro can be simple, but it requires adherence to seven fundamental rules:

    Document care completely, concisely, and accurately.

    Record observations objectively.

    Document information promptly.

    Write legibly.

    Use approved abbreviations.

    Use the proper technique to correct written errors.

    Sign all documents as required.

Following these rules enhances communication between all members of the health care team and ensures reimbursement for your facility.

Charting completely, concisely, and accurately

Here are a few quick tips for expressing yourself as well as you possibly can:

• Write clear sentences that get right to the point.
• Use simple, precise language.

- Clearly identify the subject of each sentence.
- Don't be afraid to use the word *I*.

Don't be shy, say "I."

Say what?

Without these tips, a rambling, vague, and ultimately meaningless note might be written such as *Communication with patient's home initiated today to delineate progression of disease process and describe course of action.* That's mind-boggling.

Instead, put the four tips to work for you, and your charting savvy will show. Here's how this note should be written: *I contacted Andrea Sovak's daughter by phone at 1300 hours; I explained that Mrs. Sovak's respiratory status had worsened and that she would be moved to the ICU for monitoring.* This clearly differentiates your actions from those of the patient, doctor, or other staff member. (See *Tell it like it is.*)

Don't be wishy-washy

Because we are taught that nurses don't make diagnoses, many of us qualify our observations with words like *appears* or *apparently*. However, using vague language in a patient's chart tells the

> **Art of the chart**
>
> ## Tell it like it is
>
> In the examples below, the first is incomplete, leaving the reader wondering what really happened. The second is both complete and precise.

The wrong way

Not clear who this is

Date	Time	Sign entries	
1/20/02	0200	Patient deceased at 0150. Next of kin notified.	Ann Pine, RN

Vague wording

The right way

This concisely states what occurred.

Date	Time	Sign entries	
1/20/02	0150	Patient pronounced dead by Dr. Ted Burns.	Ann Pine, RN
1/20/02	0155	Dr. Ted Burns notified Mary Ritt, sister of patient, via telephone of patient's death.	Ann Pine, RN

This clearly states who was notified and by whom.

reader that you aren't sure what you're describing or doing. The right approach is to clearly and succinctly describe what occurred without sounding tentative.

Maintaining objectivity

Knowing what to chart is important, too. Record just the facts—exactly what you see, hear, and do—not your opinions or assumptions. Chart only relevant information relating to patient care and reflecting the nursing process.

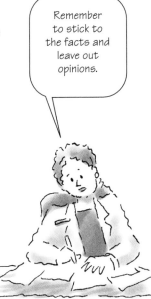

Remember to stick to the facts and leave out opinions.

Don't put words in other people's mouths

Avoid subjective statements such as *Patient's level of cooperation has deteriorated since yesterday.* Instead, use the patient's exact words to describe the facts that led you to this conclusion. You might write: *The patient stated, "I don't want to learn how to inject insulin. I tried yesterday, but I'm not going to do it today."* (See *Quotations are key,* page 206.)

You may also want to chart your subjective conclusion about the patient's condition. This is okay, as long as you also record the objective assessment data that supports it. For example, *Pt sad and tearful with flat affect; states "I miss my family."*

Secondhand data

Document only data that you collect or observe yourself or data from a reliable source, such as the patient or another nurse. When you include data reported by someone else, always cite your source. For example, you may write, *Nurse Ray found pt attempting to climb OOB. Pt was assisted to the bathroom, then back to bedside chair.*

Ensuring timeliness

Timely charting includes these essentials:
- charting as soon as possible
- noting exact times
- charting chronologically
- handling late entries correctly.

Chart ASAP

Record information on the patient's chart as soon as possible after you make an observation or provide care. Information charted immediately is more likely to be accurate and complete. If you leave your charting until the end of the shift, you might forget important details.

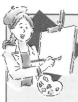

► *Art of the chart*

Quotations are key

Using the patient's exact words makes your charting accurate and objective. The notes below show how.

> Use the patient's own words as much as possible.

> Special instructions are documented precisely.

> Here's proof of patient teaching.

Date	Time	Sign entries
12/10/02	1300	Pt states she has been voiding drops of bloody urine every 5 to 10 minutes for the last hour. She states she feels "pressure" and a "burning pain" with voiding. Pt states pain is a 7 on a scale of 1 to 10, in which 10 is the most severe. Dr. Jones was called. Dr. Jones's answering service responded. Dr. Jones will call back. —————— Tina Clark, RN
	1310	Dr. Jones returned call; was informed of pt's symptoms. Order given for Bactrim DS, one, P.O.
12/10/02	1320	now and Pyridium 200 mg P.O. now. Dr. Jones will see pt this afternoon. —— Tina Clark, RN
12/10/02	1320	Bactrim DS, one P.O. and Pyridium 200 mg P.O. given. —————— Tina Clark, RN
	1420	I gave pt instructions regarding medication uses and adverse effects; encouraged her to drink plenty of fluids. I explained that Pyridium may stain clothing, and turn urine orange-red. Pt stated "I understand" and had no further questions. —————— Tina Clark, RN
		Pt states she has no pain with voiding and that "pressure is also gone." ——— Tina Clark, RN

One way to chart on time is by keeping charting materials at the patient's bedside. However, this system can threaten confidentiality. (See *Keeping it confidential.*)

If your facility uses computerized charting, remember that most computerized programs record the date and time that entries are made. Therefore, it's important to specifically state in the body of your note the time that events occurred and the action taken.

Give them the time of day

Be specific about times in your charting, especially the exact time of sudden changes in the patient's condition, significant events, and nursing actions. Don't chart in blocks of time such as 0700 to 1500. This looks vague, implies inattention to the patient, and makes it hard to determine when specific events occurred. (See *Marking time.*)

Most facilities require nurses to chart in military time, which expresses time as 24 one-hour-long periods per day, rather than 2 sets of 12 one-hour periods. (See *Time marches on,* page 208.)

Put your chart in order

Most assessments and observations are useful only as parts of a whole picture. Isolated assessments reveal very little but, in chronological order, they tell the patient's story over time and reveal a pattern of improvement or deterioration.

Charting in chronological order is easy if you jot down your observations and assessments when they occur. Too often, however, nurses chart at the end of a shift, and then record groups of assessments that fail to accurately reflect variations in the patient's condition over time. (See *Correct and chronological.*)

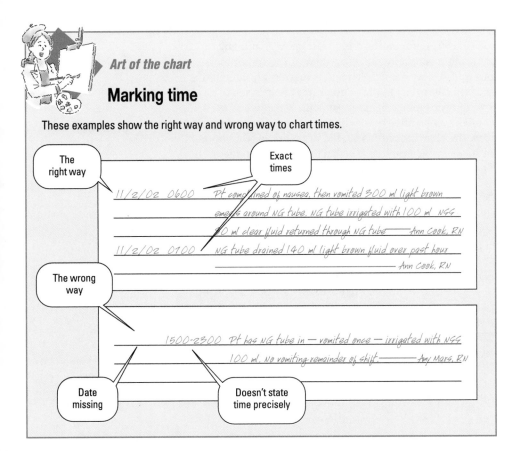

Art of the chart

Marking time

These examples show the right way and wrong way to chart times.

The right way / **Exact times**

11/2/02 0600   Pt complained of nausea, then vomited 300 ml light brown
                 emesis around NG tube. NG tube irrigated with 100 ml NSS
                 0 ml clear fluid returned through NG tube———Ann Cook, RN
11/2/02 0100   NG tube drained 140 ml light brown fluid over past hour
                                                    ——— Ann Cook, RN

The wrong way

1500-2300   Pt has NG tube in — vomited once — irrigated with NSS
             100 ml. No vomiting remainder of shift.———Amy Mars, RN

Date missing / **Doesn't state time precisely**

Advice from the experts

Keeping it confidential

Bedside computers are the ultimate in easy charting, and bedside flow sheets or progress notes run a close second. However, facility policy must be followed to ensure compliance with confidentiality protocols and regulations.

One solution is to keep confidential records in a locked, fold-down desk outside the patient's room. Having a handy writing surface also makes it easier to chart promptly. If your facility doesn't use bedside forms or computers, keep a worksheet or pad in your pocket for note keeping. Jot down key phrases and times, and then transcribe the information onto the chart later.

Time marches on

Many facilities use military time because it alleviates confusion over a.m. and p.m. entries. Here's how it works.

0100 hours = 1 a.m.	1300 hours = 1 p.m.
0200 hours = 2 a.m.	1400 hours = 2 p.m.
0300 hours = 3 a.m.	1500 hours = 3 p.m.
0400 hours = 4 a.m.	1600 hours = 4 p.m.
0500 hours = 5 a.m.	1700 hours = 5 p.m.
0600 hours = 6 a.m.	1800 hours = 6 p.m.
0700 hours = 7 a.m.	1900 hours = 7 p.m.
0800 hours = 8 a.m.	2000 hours = 8 p.m.
0900 hours = 9 a.m.	2100 hours = 9 p.m.
1000 hours = 10 a.m.	2200 hours = 10 p.m.
1100 hours = 11 a.m.	2300 hours = 11 p.m.
1200 hours = 12 noon	2400 hours = 12 midnight

If you're using computerized records, know that many software programs require nurses to answer predetermined questions or fields with multiple choice answers. Although this approach will capture core data and prompt responses to key issues, it will never replace a patient-specific narrative note. If possible, combine a narrative note with the prompted charting.

Review the charting entries for the previous 24 to 48 hours. If the charting is so generic that you can't identify the patient, then you'll need to incorporate narrative notes in your charting.

Better late than never

You may occasionally need to add a late entry in certain situations, such as:
• when the chart is unavailable at the time of the event
• if you forgot to document something
• if you need to add important information.

Bear in mind, however, that late entries can look suspicious during a malpractice trial. Find out if your facility has a protocol for late entries. If not, add the entry on the first available line and label it *late entry* to indicate that it's out of sequence. Then record the date and time of the entry as well as the date and time when the entry should have been made.

► *Art of the chart*

Correct and chronological

Here's an example of charting that's done correctly in chronological order

> Events are documented in correct time sequence.

11/14/02	0800	Neuro: Pt AAO x 3, follows commands, moves all extremities, speech clear and appropriate. Jane Klass, RN	
		CV: Afebrile; skin warm, dry and intact; palpable pulses; no edema. ———— Jane Klass, RN	
		Resp: Bilateral breath sounds, no SOB lungs clear, on room air. ———— Jane Klass, RN	
11/14/02	0915	Pt complaining of sudden shortness of breath, O_2 2 L/minute applied. Stat chest X-ray obtained, MD notified. ———— Jane Klass, RN	
11/14/02	0920	Lasix 40 mg I.V. provided to pt per Dr. Jones's order. ———— Jane Klass, RN	
11/14/02	0930	Shortness of breath continues, pulse oximetry 81%, O_2 increased to 50% face mask. ———— Jane Klass, RN	
11/14/02	0935	Pt transferred to ICU, report provided to Sally Brown, RN. Pt's family notified by MD. — Jane Klass, RN	

Ensuring legibility

One of the main reasons to document your nursing care is to communicate with other members of the health care team. Trying to decipher sloppy handwriting wastes people's time and puts the patient in jeopardy if critical information is misinterpreted. (See *Neatness counts!* page 210.)

Use printing instead of cursive writing because it's usually easier to understand. If you don't have room to chart something legibly, leave that section blank, put a bracket around it, and write *See progress notes*. Then record the information fully and legibly in the notes.

No pencils, please

Because it's a permanent document, the clinical record should be completed in ink or by computer. Use only black or blue ink. Red and green ink — which are traditionally used on evening and night shifts — don't photocopy clearly. Also, don't use felt-tipped pens on forms with carbon copies because these pens usually don't hold up under the pressure needed to produce copies, and the ink

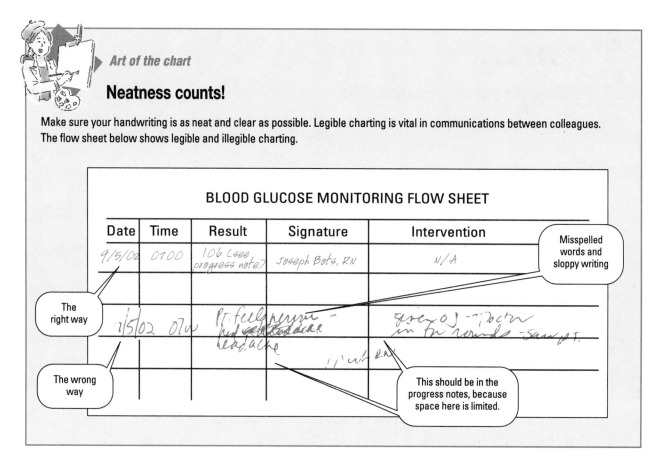

Art of the chart

Neatness counts!

Make sure your handwriting is as neat and clear as possible. Legible charting is vital in communications between colleagues. The flow sheet below shows legible and illegible charting.

BLOOD GLUCOSE MONITORING FLOW SHEET

Date	Time	Result	Signature	Intervention
9/5/02	0100	106 (see progress note)	Joseph Bots, RN	N/A
9/5/02				

The right way

The wrong way

Misspelled words and sloppy writing

This should be in the progress notes, because space here is limited.

is more likely to bleed through to another page or smear if the paper gets wet.

Spelling counts

Notes filled with misspelled words and incorrect grammar create the same negative impression as illegible handwriting. Try hard to avoid these errors; information can be misrepresented or misconstrued if an error-filled medical record ends up in court. (See *Tips for improving spelling and grammar.*)

Using abbreviations appropriately

Standards set by the Joint Commission on Accreditation of Healthcare Organizations (JCAHO) and many state regulations stipulate that health care facilities develop a list of approved abbreviations to use during charting. (See *Avoid these abbreviations!*) Make sure you know and use your facility's approved abbreviations. When you have doubts about an abbreviation's meaning, spell it out.

Avoid these abbreviations!

The Joint Commission on Accreditation of Healthcare Organizations requires every health care facility to develop a list of approved abbreviations for staff use. Certain abbreviations should be avoided because they're easily misunderstood, especially when handwritten. Here's a list of those to avoid.

Abbreviation	Intended meaning	Correction
Apothecaries' symbols		
℥	fluid ounce	Use the metric equivalents.
ʒ	fluid dram	Use the metric equivalents.
♏	minim	Use the metric equivalents.
℈	scruple	Use the metric equivalents.
Drug names		
MTX	methotrexate	Use the complete spelling for drug names.
CPZ	Compazine (prochlorperazine)	Use the complete spelling for drug names.
HCl	hydrochloric acid	Use the complete spelling for drug names.
DIG	digoxin	Use the complete spelling for drug names.
MVI	multivitamins *without* fat-soluble vitamins	Use the complete spelling for drug names.
HCTZ	hydrochlorothiazide	Use the complete spelling for drug names.
ara-a	vidarabine	Use the complete spelling for drug names.

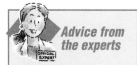

Advice from the experts

Tips for improving spelling and grammar

Want to look smart when you chart? Here are a few pointers:
• Keep both standard and medical dictionaries in charting areas and refer to them as needed.
• Post a list of commonly misspelled or confusing words, especially terms and medications regularly used on the unit. Many medications have very similar names but extremely different actions.
• If your computer system includes a spelling or grammar check, use it. Understand, however, these are far from foolproof and don't replace careful proofreading.

(continued)

Avoid these abbreviations! *(continued)*

Abbreviation	Intended meaning	Correction
Dosage directions		
a U	each ear	Write it out.
Mg	microgram	Use "mcg."
OD	once daily	Write it out. Don't abbreviate "daily."
OJ	orange juice	Write it out.
Per os	orally	Use "P.O.," "by mouth," or "orally."
qn	nightly or at bedtime	Use "h.s." or "nightly."
subq	subcutaneous	Use "S.C." or write it out
U or *U*	unit	Write it out.

Using unapproved or ambiguous abbreviations can endanger a patient. For example, if you use *o.d.* for "once a day," another nurse might think you mean "oculus dexter" (right eye) and instill medication into the patient's eye instead of giving it orally. (See *Acceptable vs. unacceptable abbreviations.*)

Correcting errors properly

When you make a mistake on a chart, correct it immediately by drawing a single line through the entry and writing *mistaken entry* above or beside it, along with the date and time. Then sign your name. Never erase a mistake, cover it with correction fluid, or completely cross it out because this looks as if you're trying to hide something. Also, writing *oops* or *sorry* or drawing a happy or sad face anywhere on a document is unprofessional and inappropriate. (See *Correct correctly!* page 214.)

Art of the chart

Acceptable vs. unacceptable abbreviations

These examples show approved and unapproved abbreviations.

This is an example of the proper use of approved abbreviations.

Date	Time	
11/9/02	1620	The pt's medical history includes IDDM, CVA, and COPD.————————Susan Rig, RN
11/2/02	0200	The pt's medical history includes cataracts ou, Cereb. Vas. Acc., and Chr. Obs. Pul. Dis.————————Linda May, RN

These aren't accepted abbreviations.

Changing a record in any way is illegal and constitutes tampering. If the chart ends up in court, the plaintiff's lawyer will be looking for red flags that cast doubt on the chart's accuracy. So heed the following list of five don'ts:

Don't add information at a later date without indicating that you did so.

Don't date the entry so that it appears to have been written at an earlier time.

Don't add inaccurate information.

Don't omit information.

Don't destroy records.

If your facility uses computerized records, follow the protocols for the correction of entries made in the chart. Once notes are entered into the computer, they become the permanent record and shouldn't be deleted or edited at a later time without an explanation that's documented, signed, and dated.

An important charting rule: Never erase a mistake.

Signing documents

Sign each entry you make in your progress notes with your first name or initial, last name, and professional licensure, such as RN or LPN. Your employer may also re-

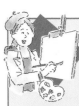

Art of the chart

Correct correctly!

When you make a mistake on the clinical record, correct it by drawing a single line through the entry and writing the words *mistaken entry* above or beside it (don't use an abbreviation like *m.e.*, which could be someone's initials). Follow this with your initials and the date. If appropriate, briefly explain why the correction was necessary.

   Make sure that the mistaken entry is still readable. This indicates that you're only trying to correct a mistake, not cover something up.

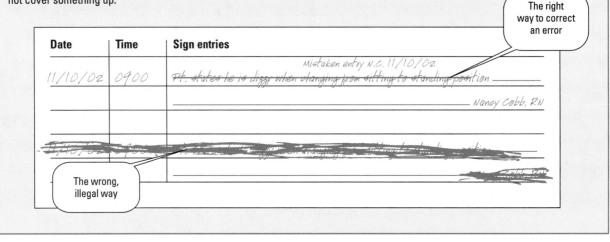

quire that you include your job title. If you find the last entry unsigned, immediately contact the nurse who made the entry and have her sign her name. If you can't locate her, simply write and sign your progress notes. The difference in charting times and handwriting should make it clear who the author was. (See *Charting do's and don'ts.*)

To be continued...

When charting continues from one page to the next, sign the bottom of the first page. At the top of the next page, write the date, time, and *continued from previous page.* Make sure that each page is stamped or labeled with the patient's identifying information.

   Never leave blank spaces on forms. This could imply that you failed to give complete care or to assess the patient completely. If information listed on a form doesn't apply to your patient, write *N/A* (not applicable) in the space. If your charting doesn't fill the designated space, draw a line through the empty space until you reach your signature.

Art of the chart

Charting do's and don'ts

The samples below illustrate some important rules about charting care.

> Do draw a line through the blank space to your signature. This discourages anyone from adding a note to yours.

> Don't skip lines or leave blank spaces.

> Don't forget to provide the caregiver's name.

> Do make clear the identity of key caregivers.

Date	Time	Sign entries
11/5/02	1200	I.V. of NSS absorbing at 125 ml/hr Site of insertion observed — no adverse effects noted. ——————————— Tim Smith, RN
11/14/02	0600	Pt assisted to bathroom by nurse's aide. ———— Mary Rob, RN
12/10/02	0810	Loud noise heard in pt's room. Pt found lying on floor by Brian Sim, nurse technician. Pt awake, confused; one inch laceration noted above right eyebrow. ——————————— James Born, RN

What you didn't see can hurt you

If you need to chart the actions of nursing assistants or technicians, write the caregiver's full name — not just his initials. Many nurses worry about countersigning care that they didn't actually see performed. If this is the case, you may refer to your facility's policy, contact your state board of nursing, or discuss the issue with your nurse-manager. Remember, your signature makes you responsible for everything in the notes.

If your facility uses computerized records, know that most software programs establish an electronic signature based on your personal user password. It's extremely important to guard your password and not share it with others. This is your legal signature! Always be sure to log off when leaving the computer station. Don't allow anyone else to use the computer with your password logged in. Any entries they make will be stamped with your electronic signature.

Doctors' orders

Almost every treatment you give a patient requires a doctor's order, so accurate documentation of these orders is critical. Doctors' orders fall into four categories:

- written orders
- preprinted orders
- verbal orders
- telephone orders.

Written orders

No matter who transcribes a doctor's order—an RN, LPN, or unit secretary—a second person must double-check the transcription for accuracy. An effective method used by many facilities is the "chart check"—rechecking orders from the previous shift once per shift.

Checking for transcription errors at least once every 24 hours is also a good idea. These checks are usually done on the night shift. A line is placed across the order sheet to indicate that all orders above the line have been checked. Then the sheet is signed and dated to verify that the check was done.

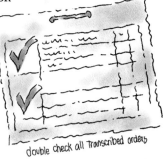

double check all transcribed orders

Heading off mistakes

When checking a patient's order sheet, make sure that the orders were written for the right patient. An order sheet might be stamped with one patient's identification plate and then inadvertently placed in another patient's chart. Double-checking averts potential mistakes.

If an order is unclear, call the doctor who wrote the order for clarification. Don't ask other people for their interpretation; they'll only be guessing, too. If a doctor is notorious for his poor handwriting, ask him to read his orders to you before he leaves the unit.

If you use computerized charting, be aware that some programs allow you to select more than one patient at a time. Be sure to double-check the patient's name on the computer screen before charting.

Some facilities that use a computerized system require the doctors to enter all of their orders into the computer system. This greatly reduces errors because it eliminates transcription.

Preprinted orders

Many health care facilities use preprinted order forms for specific procedures, such as cardiac catheterization, or admission to certain units such as the coronary care unit. As with other standardized documents, blank spaces are used for information that must be individualized according to the patient's needs.

If your facility uses these forms, don't assume that they're flawless just because they're preprinted. You may still need to clarify an order by discussing it with the doctor who gave it. (See *Preprinted orders*.)

> *Art of the chart*

Preprinted orders

The following is an example of a preprinted form for charting doctors' orders. This form specifies the treatment for a patient who is about to undergo cardiac catheterization.

DOCTOR'S ORDERS

Allergies: *None known*

> Blanks are left for information that should be individualized according to the patient's needs.

Date/Time	PRECARDIAC CATHETERIZATION ORDERS:
12/1/02 0130	1. NPO after _midnight_ except for medications.
	2. Shave and prep right and left groin areas.
	3. Premedications:
	Benadryl _25_ mg ⎫
	Xanax _0.5_ mg ⎬ P.O. on call to Cath lab
	4. Have ECG, PT, PTT, creatinine, Hgb, Hct, and platelet count
	on chart prior to sending the patient to the Cath lab.
	5. Have patient void before leaving for the Cath lab.
12/1/02 0200	*John Smith, MD*
12/1/02 0200	*Mona Jones, RN*

Verbal orders

Verbal orders are easy to misinterpret. Errors in understanding or documenting such orders can cause mistakes in patient care and liability problems for you and your facility. Try to take verbal orders only in an emergency when the doctor can't immediately attend to the patient. As a rule, do-not-resuscitate and no-code orders should *not* be taken verbally.

From words to paper

Carefully follow your facility's policy for documenting verbal orders, using a special form if one exists. Here's the usual procedure:

• Record the order on the doctor's order sheet as soon as possible. Note the date and time.

• On the first line, write *V.O.* for verbal order. Then write the doctor's name and your name as the nurse who received and read the order back to the doctor.

• Record the order verbatim.

• Sign your name.

• Draw lines through any space between the order and your verification of the order.

• Write in ink the type of drug, the dosage, the time you administered it, and any other information. (See *Charting verbal orders.*)

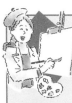

Art of the chart

Charting verbal orders

This form shows the correct way to chart verbal orders. Make sure that the doctor countersigns the order.

Date/time	Sign entries
11/16/02 1500	V.O. Dr. Marks to Mary Jones, RN
	Lasix 40 mg I.V. now and daily starting in a.m. ————
	———————————————————— Mary Jones, RN

Make sure the doctor countersigns the order within the time limits set by your facility. Without his countersignature, you may be held liable for practicing medicine without a license.

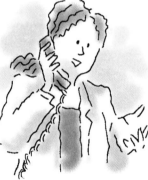

When charting verbal or telephone orders, make sure that the doctor later reads and countersigns the forms.

Telephone orders

Ideally, you should accept only written orders from a doctor. However, telephone orders are permissible when:
• the patient needs immediate treatment and the doctor isn't available to write an order
• you're providing care to the patient at home (If so, the orders must be signed by the doctor according to state nursing practice regulations. Under Medicare guidelines, verbal orders must be signed within 30 days. Other agencies impose their own, stricter rules. Failure to obtain a signed order could jeopardize reimbursement.)
• new information (laboratory data, for example) has become available and the telephone order will enable you to expedite care. (See *Taking telephone orders*.)

From phone to paper

Telephone orders should be given directly to you; they should never go through a third party. Carefully follow your facility's policy for documenting these orders. Usually, you'll follow this procedure:

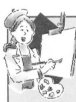

Art of the chart

Taking telephone orders

This form shows the correct way to chart telephone orders. Make sure that the doctor countersigns the order.

Date/Time	Sign entries
12/4/02 0900	T.O. Dr. Bartholomew White to Cathy Phillips, RN
	Demerol 75 mg and vistaril 50 mg I.M. now for pain.
	———————————————— Cathy Phillips, RN

• Record the order on the doctor's order sheet as soon as possible. First, note the date and time. On the next line, write *T.O.* for telephone order. (Don't use *P.O.* for phone order — it could be mistaken for "by mouth.") Then write the doctor's name and sign your name.

• Write the order verbatim.

• If you're having trouble understanding the doctor, ask another nurse to listen in as the doctor gives you the order. Then have her sign the order, too.

• Draw lines through any blank spaces in the order.

• Make sure that the doctor countersigns the order within the time limits set by your facility. Without his signature, you may be held liable for practicing medicine without a license.

• To save time and avoid errors (and if permitted by your facility's confidentiality policy), ask the doctor to fax you a copy of the order. Make sure that you wait at the fax machine for the transmission to protect the patient's right to confidentiality.

Questioning doctors' orders

Although the unit secretary may transcribe orders, you're ultimately responsible for the transcription's accuracy. Only you have the authority and the knowledge to question the validity of orders and to spot errors. This is why a chart check is so important.

Stop, question, and chart

What if an order seems vague or even wrong? Refuse to carry it out until you talk to the doctor. (See *When in doubt, check it out.*) Your facility should have a written procedure for clarifying orders. If it doesn't, take these steps:

• Contact the prescribing doctor for clarification.

• Document that you did this.

• Document whether you carried out the order.

• If you refuse to carry out an order, document your refusal, including the reasons why you refused and your communications with the doctor. Inform your immediate supervisor.

• Ask your nursing administrator for a step-by-step policy to follow so you'll know what to do if the situation recurs.

Sometimes an order is correct when it's given, and it later becomes incorrect because the patient's status changes. When this occurs, delay the treatment until you have contacted the doctor for clarification.

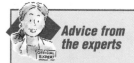

Advice from the experts

When in doubt, check it out

An order may be correct when issued but incorrect later because of changes in the patient's status. When this occurs, delay the treatment until you have contacted the doctor and clarified the situation.

Failure to question

In *Poor Sisters of Saint Francis Seraph of the Perpetual Adoration, et al. v. Catron (1982)*, a hospital was sued for negligence because a nurse failed to question a doctor's order regarding an endotracheal tube.

The doctor ordered that the tube be left in place for 5 days instead of the standard 2 to 3 days. The nurse knew that 5 days was exceptionally long but, instead of clarifying the doctor's order and documenting her actions, she followed the order. As a result, the patient's larynx was irreparably damaged, and the court ruled the hospital negligent.

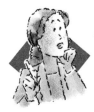

Cheat sheet

Review of charting tips

Seven fundamental rules
• Chart completely, concisely, and accurately.
• Avoid using opinions; stick to the facts.
• Chart as soon as possible, making sure the information is in chronological order and noting exact times.
• Make sure your charting is legible (use printing instead of cursive and use black or blue ink).
• Use only accepted abbreviations.
• Follow protocols for correcting written errors and adding late entries.
• Sign your notes with your first name or initial, last name, and licensure.

Doctor's orders
• Written—double-check all orders and clarify them, if necessary
• Preprinted—must be individualized according to the patient's needs; don't assume they're flawless; you may still need to clarify an order
• Verbal—take only in an emergency and make sure the doctor countersigns in time
• Telephone—take only under certain circumstances and make sure to take the order yourself

Quick quiz

1. When documenting objectively, you should chart:
   A. what you see, hear, and do.
   B. the opinions of the health care team.
   C. what you think the patient's response will be.

Answer: A. Objective statements include facts, not opinions or assumptions.

2. When documenting events in a patient's chart, you should chart:
   A. the period of time the shift covers such as 0700 to 1500 hours.
   B. the specific time of each event.
   C. every hour on the hour.

Answer: B. Chart the exact time of all sudden changes in a patient's condition, significant events, and nursing actions.

3. Assessments and observations should be charted in chronological order because:
- A. they'll reveal a pattern of improvement or deterioration.
- B. it's more convenient to chart this way.
- C. JCAHO requires it.

Answer: A. Usually, an isolated assessment tells us very little about a patient.

4. If you make a mistake on a chart, correct it by immediately:
- A. covering it with correction fluid.
- B. crossing it out completely so it can't be read and adding the date, time, and your signature.
- C. drawing a single line through the entry, writing "mistaken entry," and adding the date, the time, and your signature.

Answer: C. Incorrect entries shouldn't look as if you're trying to hide something. A single line through an incorrect entry is sufficient, along with a note stating "mistaken entry" and the date, the time, and your signature.

Scoring

☆☆☆ If you answered all four items correctly, wow! Your charting is complete, concise, accurate, and all that good stuff. Turn to the next chapter and keep mastering the art of the chart.

☆☆ If you answered three items correctly, that's great! Your charting skills are definitely in order.

☆ If you answered fewer than three items correctly, don't worry! In keeping with the tenets of good charting, we'll keep it confidential.

Avoiding legal pitfalls

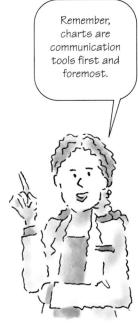

Just the facts

In this chapter, you'll learn:

♦ the legal significance of the medical record

♦ how to chart defensively

♦ the relationship between charting and risk management

♦ how to handle eight charting pitfalls.

A look at legal pitfalls in charting

As your professional responsibility grows, so does your legal accountability. Complete, accurate documentation proves that you're giving quality care and meeting the standards set by the nursing profession, your health care facility, and the law. It's your best protection if you're named in a malpractice lawsuit. (See *What sways the jury?* page 224.)

The aim is communication

Faulty charting is a pivotal issue in many malpractice cases. Medical records are reviewed by health care experts and can be presented in court case trials. Think of the medical record as a communication tool and document accordingly. Focus on the facts, be objective, and document chronologically.

Legal standards

What and how you chart on the medical record is controlled by:
• nurse practice acts
• American Nurses Association (ANA) credentialing committee certification requirements
• malpractice litigation
• your facility's policies and procedures.

Remember, charts are communication tools first and foremost.

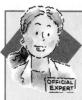

Advice from the experts

What sways the jury?

The outcome of every malpractice trial boils down to one question: Whom will the jury believe? The answer depends on the credibility of the evidence. Jurors usually view the medical record as the best evidence of what really happened. It's often the hinge on which the verdict swings.

A general overview
In a nutshell, here's what happens in court: The plaintiff's (patient's) lawyer presents evidence showing that the patient was harmed because care provided by the defendant (in this case, the nurse) failed to meet accepted standards. The defendant's (nurse's) lawyer presents evidence showing that his client provided a standard of care that would be used by other nurses given the same circumstances.

   If the nurse wasn't negligent, the medical record will provide evidence of quality care. However, if she *was* negligent and didn't document her care, the medical record is the plaintiff's best evidence. The jury will almost certainly rule in favor of the patient. Don't believe the myth that all cases settle out of court. Some do, but you don't want to be the exception.

Nurse practice acts

Nurse practice acts are state laws that designate what a nurse can do in that state. Today, nurses are considered managers of care as well as practitioners; states revise their laws and documentation requirements to keep up with changes like this in the nursing profession.

In a confused state? Read on...

The range of a nurse's legal responsibilities may vary from state to state—perhaps only to a small degree in certain cases. However, if licensed in more than one state, you must take care to follow precisely the specific guidelines of the state you're practicing in at the time. Always be familiar with your scope of practice. You'll be held liable if you're found practicing outside of your designated scope of practice.

ANA credentialing

What you write in a medical record shouldn't be dictated by the courts; it should be guided by the nursing profession's own standards. Charting that meets these standards describes the patient's status, medical treatment, and nursing care. The ANA sets standards for most nursing specialties. It says that documentation must be:

- systematic
- continuous
- accessible
- communicated
- recorded
- readily available to all members of the health care team.

Going with the flow sheet

Although documentation goals haven't changed much over the years, documentation methods have. Nurses now use flow sheets, graphic records, and checklists in place of long narrative notes. In malpractice cases, the charting method used isn't important, as long as it's used consistently and provides comprehensive, factual information that's relevant to the patient's care.

Malpractice litigation

When charting, your main goal is to convey information. However, keep the legal implications in the back of your mind. If the care you provide and your charting are both top-notch, the records may be used to refute a plaintiff's accusation of nursing malpractice.

A malpractice verdict depends on three factors:

- breach of duty

- damage

- causation.

Every relationship brings with it responsibility

The courts have ruled that it's your duty to provide an appropriate standard of care once a nurse-patient relationship is established — even if the relationship takes place over the phone. Breach of duty means that your care didn't meet that standard.

Proving that a nurse was guilty of breach of duty is difficult because her duties overlap with those of other health care providers. The court will ask, "How would a reasonable, prudent nurse with comparable training and experience have acted in the same or a similar circumstance?"

Once the plaintiff establishes a breach of duty, he must then prove that the breach caused the patient's injury (damage and causation).

Facility policies and procedures

How you chart is also controlled by the policies and procedures in your facility's employee and nursing manuals. Straying

> When you establish a relationship with a patient, you take on a legal responsibility.

from these rules suggests that you failed to meet the facility's standards of care.

Although the courts have yet to decide whether these policies actually establish a legal standard of care, there are legal standards in place. In each nursing malpractice case, the courts compare a nurse's actions with regularly updated, national minimum standards established by professional organizations and accrediting bodies such as the Joint Commission on Accreditation of Healthcare Organizations (JCAHO).

> Establishing a strong nurse-patient relationship may help reduce legal risks.

The ties that bind

According to insurance company data, lawsuits naming nurses as defendants are increasing. Why? Two reasons are a nurse's expanding role and the breakdown of the nurse-patient relationship due to shorter hospital stays.

Developing a rapport with your patients, even on a short-term basis, can help decrease errors and foster a nurse-patient relationship — both of which help prevent lawsuits. Patients who feel their nurse attempted to do all in her power to provide care — often despite short staffing — typically don't sue the nurse. However, they may sue the facility as the responsible party.

Charting defensively

In the world of nursing and malpractice, a defensive attitude has become necessary — that is, chart factually but defensively as well. This involves knowing:

- how to chart
- what to chart
- when to chart
- who should chart.

How to chart

A skilled nurse charts with possible litigation in mind and knows that how she charts is just as important as what she charts.

Rule #1: Stick to the facts

Record only what you see, hear, smell, feel, measure, and count — not what you suppose, infer, conclude, or assume. For example, if a patient pulled out his I.V. line, but you didn't witness it, write *Found pt, arm board, and bed linens covered with blood. I.V. line and venipuncture device were untaped and hanging free.* If the patient says he pulled out his I.V. line, record that.

Don't chart your opinions. If the chart is used as evidence in court, the plaintiff's lawyer might attack your credibility and the medical record's reliability.

Rule #2: Avoid labeling

Objectively describe the patient's behavior instead of subjectively labeling it. For example, *Pt found pacing back and forth in his room, muttering phrases such as, "I'll take care of him my way" while punching one hand into the other.* Avoid using expressions such as *appears spaced out, flying high, exhibiting bizarre behavior,* or *using obscenities,* which can mean different things to different people. Ask yourself, could you define these terms in court? Objectivity in charting will increase your credibility with the jury.

Rule #3: Be specific

Your charting goal is to present the facts clearly and concisely. To do so, use only approved abbreviations and express your observations in quantifiable terms. (See *Specifics are terrific!* page 228.)

For example, writing *output adequate* isn't as helpful as writing *output 1,200 ml.* And *Pt appears to be in pain* is vague compared with *Pt requested pain medication after complaining of lower back pain radiating to his Ⓡ leg, which he rated 7 out of 10 on the visual analogue scale.* Also, avoid catch-all phrases such as *Pt comfortable.* Instead, describe how you know this. For instance, is the patient resting, reading, or sleeping?

Rule #4: Use neutral language

Don't use inappropriate comments or language in your notes. This is unprofessional and can cause legal problems.

In one case, an elderly patient developed pressure ulcers and his family complained that he wasn't receiving adequate care. The patient later died, probably of natural causes. Because family members were dissatisfied with the patient's care, they sued. The insurance company questioned the abbreviation *PBBB* in the chart, which the doctor had written under prognosis. After learning that this stood for "pine box by bedside," the family was awarded a significant sum.

Rule #5: Eliminate bias

Don't use language that suggests a negative attitude toward the patient. Examples include *obstinate, drunk, obnoxious, bizarre,* or *abusive.* The same goes for what you say out loud and then

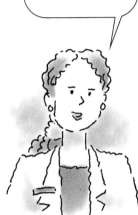

Remember, facts speak for themselves. Never chart subjective information.

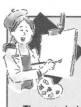

Art of the chart

Specifics are terrific!

The note below is clear and concise because it uses approved abbreviations and specific measurements.

5/16/02	1100	Complaining of pain at ⓛ antecubital I.V. site at 1000. Pain rated on VAS
		3/10. Dressing removed. Redness 2 cm wide around I.V. insertion site. No
		drainage. Quarter-sized area of edema above insertion site. I.V. removed; site
		cleaned with povidone-iodine and sterile dressing applied. Warm compress ap-
		plied to site X 20 min. Dr. Smith notified. Acetaminophen 650 mg given P.O.
		at 1015. Pt reports relief. ———————— Margaret Doherty, RN

document. Disparaging remarks, accusations, arguments, or name calling could lead to a defamation of character or libel suit. In court, the plaintiff's lawyer might say, "This nurse called my client 'rude, difficult, and uncooperative.' It's right here in her own handwriting! No wonder she didn't take good care of him—she didn't like him." *Remember:* The patient has a legal right to see his chart. If he spots a derogatory reference, he'll be hurt, angry, and more likely to sue.

If a patient is difficult or uncooperative, document the behavior objectively and let the jurors draw their own conclusions. (See *Polite and to the point.*)

Rule #6: Keep the record intact

Be sure to keep the patient's chart complete. Discarding pages, even for innocent reasons, raises doubt in a lawyer's mind.

Let's say that you spill coffee on a page and blur several entries. Don't discard the original! Copy it and put the copy and the original in the chart. Then cross-reference the pages by writing *Recopied from page___* on the copy and *Recopied on page___* on the original.

What to chart

Caring for patients seems more important than documenting every detail, doesn't it? However, legally speaking, an incomplete chart reflects incomplete nursing care. Neglecting to record every detail is such a serious and common charting error that malpractice lawyers have coined the expression "Not charted, not done."

This doesn't mean that you have to document everything. Some information, like staffing shortages and staff conflicts, is definitely off limits. (See *Charting don'ts*, page 230.)

Rule #1: Chart significant situations

Learn to recognize legally dangerous situations as you give patient care. Assess each critical or out-of-the-ordinary situation, and decide whether your actions might be significant in court. If they could be, chart them as well as every other detail of the situation in the progress notes. (See *A case of negligence*, page 231, and *Out of the ordinary*, page 232.)

Art of the chart

Polite and to the point

The note below describes a difficult situation dispassionately, while still getting the point across.

6/11/02	1300	I attempted to perform the daily abdominal dressing change, but pt stated,
		"This doesn't need to be done every day. It doesn't hurt and I don't want you
		to touch it. Leave me alone." I explained the importance of monitoring and
		cleaning the incision and offered an analgesic to be given 20 min before
		dressing would be changed. Pt became agitated and still refused. Dr. Humbert
		notified that incisional site was not assessed nor was dressing changed and
		that pt is agitated. ————————————————— Mary Marley, RN

Advice from the experts

Charting don'ts

Negative language and inappropriate information don't belong in a medical record and can return to haunt you in a lawsuit. The charting mistakes below are legal land mines. Avoid them.

1. Don't record staffing problems

True, staff shortages may affect patient care or contribute to an incident. But don't mention this in a patient's chart; it can be used as legal ammunition against you if the chart lands in court. Instead, write a confidential memo to your nurse-manager, and review your facility's policy and procedure manuals to see how you're expected to handle this situation.

2. Don't record staff conflicts

Don't chart:
- disputes with other nurses (including criticisms of their care)
- questions about a doctor's treatment
- a colleague's rude or abusive behavior.

   Personality clashes aren't legitimate patient care concerns. In the event of a lawsuit, the plaintiff's lawyer will exploit conflicts among codefendants.

   Instead of charting these problems, talk with your nurse-manager, or consult with the doctor directly if an order puzzles you. If another nurse writes personal accusations or charges of incompetence in a chart, talk to her about the implications of doing this. Remember, you're responsible for your actions.

3. Don't mention incident reports

Incident reports are confidential and filed separately from the patient's chart. Document only the facts of an incident in the chart, and never write "incident report" or indicate that you filed one.

   For example, write: *Found pt lying on the floor at 1250 hours. Vital signs BP 110/70, P 82, R 20, T 98.6° F. No visible bleeding or*

trauma. *AA Ox3, PERLA, + ROM to all extremities. Pt returned to bed with all side rails up and bed in low position. Pt stated, "I must have been sleepwalking." Notified Dr. Gary Dietrich at 1253 hours, and he saw pt at 1300 hours.*

4. Don't use words associated with errors

Terms like "by mistake," "accidentally," "somehow," "unintentionally," "miscalculated," and "confusing" are bonus words to the plaintiff's attorney. Steer clear of words that suggest an error was made or a patient's safety was jeopardized. Let the facts speak for themselves.

   For example, suppose you gave a patient 100 mg of Demerol instead of 50 mg. Here's how to chart this without calling undue attention to it: *Pt was given Demerol 100 mg I.M. at 1300 hours for abdominal pain VAS 7/10. Dr. Smith was notified but gave no orders. Pt's vital signs remained stable.*

5. Don't name a second patient

Naming a second patient in a patient's chart violates confidentiality. Instead, write *roommate*, the patient's initials, or his room and bed number.

6. Don't chart casual conversations with colleagues

Telling your nurse-manager in the elevator or restroom about a patient's deteriorating condition doesn't qualify as informing her. She's likely to forget the details, or may not even realize you expect her to intervene. Before notifying someone, clearly state why you're notifying the person so she can focus on the facts and take appropriate action. Otherwise, you can't chart that you informed her.

Rule #2: Chart complete assessment data

Failing to perform and document a complete physical assessment is a key factor in many malpractice suits. During your initial assessment, focus on the patient's reason for seeking care, and then follow up on all other problems he mentions. Be sure to chart everything you do as well as why.

A case of negligence

Here's a fictional case that exemplifies how negligence may be interpreted in court.

Seventeen-year old Tommy York was partially paralyzed and severely brain damaged after an accident. He was admitted to the hospital for an intensive rehabilitation program.

Soon afterward, his parents told the nurse that a support from the right side of his wheelchair was missing and that they saw scratches on his right arm. Although the nurse also noticed this, she didn't record it.

Failure to document

Later, the patient's hip became red, swollen, and increasingly painful. His mother also reported these symptoms to the nurse, who again failed to record them in the medical record.

When the patient was finally diagnosed with a broken hip, his parents sued. The court ruled the hospital negligent and awarded the plaintiff $250,000.

A matter of duty

Inadequate observation of patients that leads to misdiagnosis or injury is a common cause of lawsuits involving nurses. Most of these lawsuits involve issues of negligence—the failure to exercise the degree of care that a person of ordinary prudence would exercise under the same circumstances. A claim of negligence requires that there be a duty owed by one person to another, that the duty be breached, and that injury resulted.

Malpractice is a more restricted, specialized type of negligence, defined as a violation of professional duty to act with reasonable care and in good faith. Several states have begun to recognize nursing negligence as a form of malpractice.

Avoid negligence cases by documenting any and all unusual patient events.

After completing the initial assessment, write a well-constructed plan of care. This gives you a clear approach to the patient's problems and helps defend your care if you're sued.

Phrase each problem statement clearly, and modify them as you gather new assessment data. State the plan of care for solving each problem; then identify the actions you intend to take.

Rule #3: Document discharge instructions

Because of insurance constraints, facilities are now discharging patients earlier than they once did. This means that patients and family members are changing dressings, assessing wounds, and tackling other tasks that nurses traditionally performed.

Patient and family teaching is your responsibility. If a patient receives inadequate or incorrect instructions and an injury results, you could be held liable.

Many facilities give patients printed instruction sheets that describe treatments and home care procedures. In court, these materials may be used as evidence that instruction took place. To

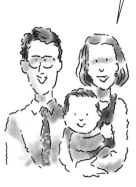

Family teaching is part of your professional responsibility.

Art of the chart

Out of the ordinary

This note shows the right way to chart atypical information.

1/18/02	1900	Furosemide 40 mg P.O. not given because of
		impending upper GI series. Dr. Wenger notified
		that Furosemide was not given. Dr. Wenger
		gave order for Furosemide 20 mg I.V. Adminis-
		tered at 0915. ——— Charles Cashman, RN

support testimony, they should be tailored to each patient's specific needs and contain any verbal or written instructions you provided. Documentation of referrals to home health care agencies or other community providers is another essential component of discharge planning.

When to chart

Finding time to chart can be hard during a busy shift. However, the timeliness of entries is a major issue in malpractice suits.

Don't get ahead of yourself

Document nursing care when you perform it or shortly afterward. Never document ahead of time—your notes will be inaccurate and you'll leave out information about the patient's response to treatment. Even if you did what you charted, a lawyer might ask, "Do you occasionally chart something before doing it?" If you answer "yes," the jury won't see the chart as a reliable indicator of what you actually did, which wrecks your credibility.

Who should chart

State nurse practice acts have strict rules about who can chart. Breaking these rules can cause you to have your nursing license suspended.

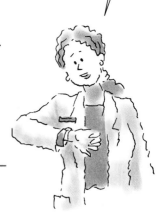

Document ahead of time? Never! My credibility is at stake.

Finish what you started

No matter how busy you are, never ask another nurse to complete your charting (and never complete another nurse's charting). Doing so is a dangerous practice that may be specifically prohibited by your state's nurse practice act. If the other nurse makes an error or misinterprets information, the patient can be harmed. Then, if he sues you for negligence, both you and your facility will be held accountable because delegated documentation doesn't meet nursing standards.

Delegating charting has another consequence: It destroys the credibility and value of the medical record both in the facility and in court. Judges give little, if any, weight to medical records containing secondhand observations or hearsay evidence.

Risk management and documentation

A health care facility's reputation for safe, reliable, and effective service is its main defense against liability claims. Well-coordinated risk management and performance improvement programs show the public that the facility is being managed in a legally responsible manner. If complaints arise, a good program ensures that they're handled promptly to contain the damage and minimize liability claims. (See *Understanding risk management and performance improvement.*)

Mining the records for potential risk

Sometimes documentation reveals potential problems within a health care facility. For example, a certain procedure may repeatedly lead to patient injury or another type of accident. Risk management programs help reduce injuries and accidents and thereby minimize financial loss.

In the past, the focus of risk management and performance improvement programs was to maintain and improve facilities and equipment and ensure employee, visitor, and patient safety. Today, the focus is on identifying, evaluating, and reducing patient injury in specialty units that have the greatest malpractice risks.

Preventing adverse events

Risk management has three main goals:

☝ decreasing the number of claims by promptly identifying and following up on adverse events (early warning systems)

Understanding risk management and performance improvement

Do the terms *risk management* and *performance improvement* confuse you? Here's how to tell them apart: Risk management focuses on the patient's and family members' perceptions of the care provided; performance improvement focuses on the role of the health care provider.

Two for one

Many facilities combine these two programs in their educational efforts. They place a high priority on teaching new medical residents and nurses about malpractice claims, staff members' reporting obligations, proper informational and reporting channels, and principles of risk management and performance improvement.

✌️ reducing the frequency of preventable injuries and accidents leading to lawsuits by maintaining or improving the quality of care

✌️ controlling costs related to claims by pinpointing trouble spots early and working with the patient and his family.

Early warning systems

Early warning systems can pinpoint much useful information. However, to be effective they need:
• a strong organizational structure
• cooperation between risk management and performance improvement departments
• the commitment of all staff members to report adverse events to the appropriate clinical chairperson, so he can study the medical records more closely or talk to the staff member involved and recommend remedial education, monitoring, or restricted privileges
• the commitment of key staff members—such as nurses, doctors, administrators, and chiefs of high-risk services—to analyze the information
• the commitment of all staff members to be compliant with policies and procedures in order to maintain and maximize quality patient care.

The most commonly used early warning systems are occurrence reporting and occurrence screening.

Reporting the out of the ordinary

An occurrence or incident report refers to the documentation of events that are inconsistent with a health care facility's ordinary routine, regardless of whether injury occurs. Doctors, nurses, or other staff are responsible for reporting such events when they're observed or shortly afterward. Examples include the unplanned return of a patient to the operating room or a medication error.

Let's review

Occurrence screening involves reviewing medical records to find adverse events. Both general indicators of adverse events (such as a nosocomial infection or medication error) and more specific indicators (such as an incorrect sponge count during surgery) are considered.

Reducing injuries and accidents

Many health care facilities coordinate educational efforts to help prevent injuries and accidents that may lead to lawsuits.

> Occurrence screening requires careful review of medical records.

Making sure everyone is on the same page

The facility may reach out to a specific employee, such as a nurse or doctor, who has been identified as having a particular problem, or to a larger population, such as new nurses or residents, that may face the same types of problems. Required teaching topics for new employees include malpractice claims, reporting obligations, proper informational and reporting channels, and principles of risk management and performance improvement.

Cost control

Systematic, well-coordinated risk management and performance improvement programs demonstrate to the public that the facility is managed in a legally responsible way. When complaints do arise, risk managers handle them promptly to contain the damage and minimize liability claims.

Managing incidents

Despite risk management programs, adverse events still occur. Health care facilities rely on the following sources to identify dangerous situations or trends:

• *Incident reports*, also called occurrence reports, are a primary source of information for lawyers. They use the reports when researching potential lawsuits and in court as evidence.

• *Nurses* are usually the first ones to recognize potential problems because they spend so much time with patients and families. They know which patients are dissatisfied with their care and which ones have complications that may lead to injuries.

• *Patient-representatives* keep files of patient complaints, identify litigious patients, and maintain contact with the patient and his family after an incident has occurred.

• *The business office and medical records department* may be alerted to potential lawsuits when a patient threatens to sue after he receives his bill or when a patient or a lawyer requests a copy of the medical record.

• *Other sources* can also help. For example, the engineering department has information on the safety of the hospital environment; purchasing, biomedical engineering, and the pharmacy can report on the safety and adequacy of products and equipment; and social workers, hospital clergy, volunteers, and patient escorts often know about highly dissatisfied patients. *Remember:* Whenever you get a report from one of these sources, document it thoroughly on the patient's medical record and fill out an incident report.

The claim chain reaction

Once the risk manager learns of a potential or actual lawsuit, he notifies the medical records department and the facility's insurance company. The medical records department makes copies of the patient's chart and files the original in a safe place to prevent tampering.

A claim notice should also trigger a performance improvement peer review of the medical record. This review measures the health care provider's conduct against the professional standards of conduct for the particular situation. This information is used by the risk manager to investigate the claim's merit and the facility's responsibility. The standard required for a successful defense isn't always as high as the facility's optimal standard.

Eight legal hazards

Every day, you face patient care situations that could land you in court. Your challenge is to watch out for potential pitfalls and know how to chart them defensively when they arise. The section that follows describes eight volatile legal situations.

Hazard #1: Incident reports

Whenever you witness an adverse event, file an incident report. Some things to report are injuries from restraints, burns, or other causes; falls (even if the patient wasn't injured); and a patient's insistence on being discharged against medical advice. If an incident report form doesn't leave enough space to fully describe an incident, attach an additional page of comments. (See *Completing an incident report.*)

The form's function

An incident report isn't part of the patient's chart, but it may be used later in litigation. A report has two functions:

It informs the administration of the incident so the risk management staff can work on preventing similar incidents.

It alerts the administration and the facility's insurance company to a potential claim and the need for further investigation.

> Following the guidelines here will reduce your legal risks.

Art of the chart

Completing an incident report

When you witness a reportable event, you must fill out an incident report. Forms vary, but most include the following information.

INCIDENT REPORT

Name _Greta Manning_
Address _1 Worth Way, Boston, MA_
Phone _(617) 555-1122_

| 9. DATE OF INCIDENT | 10. TIME OF INCIDENT |
| _11-14-02_ | _1442_ |

11. EXACT LOCATION OF INCIDENT (Bldg., Floor, Room No., Area)
4-Main, Rm. 441

Addressograph if patient

12. TYPE OF INCIDENT (CHECK ONE ONLY) ☐ PATIENT ☐ EMPLOYEE ☑ VISITOR ☐ VOLUNTEER ☐ OTHER (Specify)

13. DESCRIPTION OF THE INCIDENT (WHO, WHAT, WHEN, WHERE, HOW, WHY) (Use Back of Form if Necessary)

Wife of pt found on floor next to bed. States "I was trying to put siderail of bed down to sit on pt's bed and I fell do...

> **Describe relevant conditions.**

> **State only what you saw or heard.**

14. ☑ CLEAN & SMOOTH ☐ OTHER _____ ☐ SLIPPERY (WET)   FRAME OF BED ☑ LOW ☐ HIGH   NIGHT LIGHT ☑ NO

PATIENT FALL INCIDENTS

15. WERE BED RAILS PRESENT? ☐ NO ☐ 1 UP ☐ 2 UP ☐ 3 UP ☑ 4 UP   **17. OTHER RESTRAINTS** (TYPE & EXTENT) _N/A_

18. AMBULATION PRIVILEGE ☐ UNLIMITED ☐ LIMITED WITH ASSISTANCE ☐ COMPLETE BEDREST ☐ OTHER _____

19. WAS NARCOTICS, ANALGESICS, HYPNOTICS, SEDATIVES, DIURETICS, ANTIHYPERTENSIVES OR ANTICONVULSANTS GIVEN DURING LAST 4 HOURS? ☐ YES ☑ NO

DRUG _____ AMOUNT _____ TIME _____

PATIENT INCIDENTS

20. PHYSICIAN NOTIFIED NAME OF PHYSICIAN _J. Reynolds, MD_   DATE _11-14-02_   TIME _1445_   COMPLETE IF APPLICABLE

21. DEPARTMENT _____ **22. JOB TITLE** _____ **23. SOCIAL SECURITY #** _____

EMPLOYEE INCIDENTS

24. MARITAL STATUS _____

27. SUPERVISOR NOTIFIED NAME OF SUPERVISOR _C. Jones, RN_   DATE _11-14-02_   TIME _1500_   **28. LOCATION** (WHERE TREATMENT WAS RENDERED) _____

29. NAME, ADDRESS AND TELEPHONE NUMBER OF WITNESS(ES) OR PERSONS FAMILIAR WITH INCIDENT - WITNESS OR NOT
Connie Smith, RN (617)555-0912 1 Main St., Boston, MA

ALL INCIDENTS

> **List the name, telephone number, and address of anyone involved.**

SIGNATURE OF PERSON PREPARING REPORT _Connie Smith_   TITLE _RN_   **31. DATE OF REPORT** _11-14-02_

- To be completed for all cases involving injury or illness (DO NOT USE ABBREVIATIONS) (Use back of Form if necessary)

...ent in Emergency Department after reported fall in husband's room. 12 cm x 12 cm ecchymotic area noted on right hip. X-rays negative for fracture. Good range of motion, no c/o pain. VAS 0/10. Ice pack applied. — J. Reynolds, MD

33. DISPOSITION _sent home, written instructions provided_

34. PERSON NOTIFIED OTHER THAN HOSPITAL PERSONNEL NAME AND ADDRESS _R. Manning (daughter) address same as pt_   **35. DATE** _11-14-02_   **36. TIME** _1500_

37. PHYSICIAN'S SIGNATURE _J. Reynolds, MD_   **38. DATE** _11-14-02_

It's an eyewitness report

Only people who witnessed an incident should fill out and sign an incident report, and each witness should file a separate report. Once the report is filed, it may be reviewed by the nursing supervisor, the doctor who examined the patient after the incident, various department heads and administrators, the facility's attorney, and the insurance company.

Because incident reports will be read by many people and may even turn up in court, you must follow strict guidelines when completing them. (See *Tips for reporting incidents.*)

Facilities are continually revising their incident report forms; some have begun to use computerized forms. Incident reports are also processed by computer, which permits classifying and counting of incidents to indicate trends.

Charting incidents in progress notes

When documenting an incident in the medical record, follow these guidelines:

• Write a factual account of the incident, including treatment and follow-up care as well as the patient's response. This shows that the patient was closely monitored after the incident. Make sure the descriptions in the chart match those in the incident report.

• Don't write *incident report completed* after charting the event. This destroys the confidential nature of the report and may result in a lawsuit. For the same reason, the doctor shouldn't write an order for an incident report in the chart.

• In charting the incident, include everything the patient or family member says about his role in the incident. For example, you might write *Pt stated, "The nurse told me to ask for help before I went to the bathroom, but I decided to go on my own."* In a negligence lawsuit, this information may help the defense lawyer show that the incident was entirely or partially the patient's fault. If the jury finds that the patient was partially at fault, the concept of

The information I document in the incident report...

...has to match the information in the medical record.

Advice from the experts

Tips for reporting incidents

In the past, a plaintiff's lawyer wasn't allowed to see incident reports. Today, however, many states allow lawyers access to incident reports if they make their requests through proper channels. So, when writing an incident report, keep in mind who may read it and follow these guidelines:
• Include essential information, such as the identity of the person involved in the incident, the exact time and place of the incident, and the name of the doctor you notified.
• Document any unusual occurrences that you witnessed.
• Record the events and the consequences for the patient in enough detail that administrators can decide whether or not to investigate further.
• Write objectively, avoiding opinions, judgments, conclusions, or assumptions about who or what caused the incident. Tell your opinions to your supervisor or the risk manager later.
• Describe only what you saw and heard and the actions you took to provide care at the scene. Unless you saw a patient fall, write *Found pt lying on the floor.*
• Don't admit that you're at fault or blame someone else. Steer clear of statements such as *Better staffing would have prevented this incident.*
• Don't offer suggestions about how to prevent the incident from happening again.
• Don't include detailed statements from witnesses and descriptions of remedial action; these are normally part of an investigative follow-up.
• Don't put the report in the medical record. Send it to the person designated to review it according to your facility's policy.

contributory negligence may be used to reduce or even eliminate the patient's recovery of damages.

Hazard #2: Informed consent

A patient must sign a consent form before most treatments and procedures. Informed consent means that he understands the proposed therapy and its risks and agrees to undergo it. The doctor performing the procedure is legally responsible for explaining the procedure and its risks and obtaining consent. However, he may ask you to witness the patient's signature. Some facilities may specifically require the person who informs the patient of the treatment or procedure to be the one to obtain the consent. Check with your facility's legal counsel if you have any questions. (See *Sign here: Witnessing a consent form*, page 240.)

Advice from the experts

Sign here: Witnessing a consent form

After the doctor informs the patient about a medical procedure, he may ask you to obtain the patient's signature on the consent form and then sign as a witness. Before doing this, review the checklist below.

• Make sure that the patient is competent, awake, alert, and aware of what he's doing. He should not be under the influence of alcohol, illicit drugs, or prescribed medications that impair his understanding or judgment.

• Ask the patient if the doctor explained the diagnosis, proposed treatment, and expected outcome to his satisfaction. Also ask if he understands all that was said.

• Ask the patient if he has been told about the risks of the treatment or procedure, the possible consequences of refusing it, and alternative treatments or procedures.

• Ask the patient if he has any concerns or questions about his condition or the treatment. If he does, help him get answers from the doctor or other appropriate sources.

• Tell the patient that he can refuse the treatment without having other care or support withdrawn, and that he can withdraw his consent after giving it.

• Notify your nurse-manager and the doctor immediately if you suspect that the patient has doubts about his condition or the procedure, hasn't been properly informed, or has been coerced into giving consent. Performing a procedure without voluntary consent may be considered battery.

• Objectively document your assessment of the patient's understanding in the chart, noting the situation, his responses, and actions you took.

• When you're satisfied that the patient is well informed, have him sign the consent form including the date and time, and then sign your name as a witness.

• Remember that you're responsible for obtaining oral informed consent for any procedures that you'll be performing, such as inserting an I.V. line or a urinary catheter, even though a general treatment consent was signed upon admission.

Waive it good-bye

The legal requirement for obtaining informed consent can be waived only if:

• a mentally competent patient says that he doesn't want to know the details of a treatment or procedure.

• an urgent medical or surgical situation occurs (many facilities specify how you should document such an emergency).

Most facilities use a standard consent form that lists the legal requirements for consent. If the patient doesn't understand the doctor's explanation or asks for more information, answer all questions that fall within the scope of your practice. Be sure to document your interaction with the patient. (See *Informed consent*.)

Art of the chart

Informed consent

If the patient signs a consent form, this implies that he understands the risks of a procedure and agrees to undergo it. Here's a typical form.

CONSENT FOR OPERATION AND RENDERING OF OTHER MEDICAL SERVICES

1. I hereby authorize Dr. _____Wesley_____ to perform upon _____Joseph Smith_____ (Patient name), the following surgical and/or medical procedures: (State specific nature of the procedures to be performed) _____Exploratory laparotomy_____

2. I understand that the procedure(s) will be performed at Valley Medical Center by or under the supervision of Dr. _____Wesley_____, who is authorized to utilize the services of other doctors, or members of the house staff as he or she deems necessary or advisable.

> **The form should state the specific procedure under consideration.**

3. ~~explained~~ to me that during the course of the operation, unforeseen conditions may be revealed that necessitate an ex-~~tra~~nal procedure(s) or different procedure(s) than those set forth in Paragraph 1, I therefore authorize and request ~~said~~ doctor, and his or her associates or assistants, perform such medical surgical procedures as are necessary ~~in the~~ exercise of professional judgment.

4. ~~I understand the~~ nature and purpose of the procedure(s), possible alternative methods of diagnosis or treatment, the possibility of complications, and the consequences of the procedure(s). I acknowledge that no guarantee made as to the results that may be obtained.

> **The patient acknowledges that he understands therapy and its risks and agrees to undergo it.**

5. I authorize the above named doctor to administer local or regional anesthesia (for all other anesthesia mana~~gement~~ sent must be signed by the patient or patient's authorized representative).

6. I understand that if it is necessary for me to receive a blood transfusion during this procedure or this hospital~~...~~ supplied by sources available to the hospital and tested in accordance with national and regional regulations. I understand that there are risks in transfusion, including but not limited to allergic, febrile, and hemolytic transfusion reactions, and the transmission of infectious diseases, such as hepatitis and AIDS (Acquired Immune Deficiency Syndrome). I hereby consent to blood transfusion(s) and blood derivative(s).

7. I hereby authorize representatives from Valley to photograph or videotape me for the purpose of research or medical education. It is understood and agreed that patient confidentiality shall be preserved.

8. I authorize the doctor named above and his or her associates and assistants and Valley Medical Center to preserve for scientific purposes or to dispose of any tissue, organs, or other body parts removed during surgery or other diagnostic procedures in accordance with customary medical practice.

9. I certify that I have read and fully understand the above consent statement. In addition, I have been afforded an opportunity to ask whatever questions I might have regarding the procedure(s) to be performed and they have been answered to my satisfaction.

_____Joseph Smith_____   _____11/15/02_____   _____C. Gurney, RN_____
Legal Patient or Authorized Representative   Date   Witness
(State Relationship to Patient)

> **Signing indicates only that you're witnessing the patient's signature.**

If the patient is unable to consent on his or her own behalf, complete the following:

Patient _____ is unable to consent because _____

_____

Legally Responsible Person _____ Doctor Obtaining Consent _____M. Wesley, MD_____

Hazard #3: Advance directives

The Patient Self-Determination Act requires health care facilities to provide information about the patient's right to choose and refuse treatment. Facilities must also ask patients if they have advance directives, which are documents that state a patient's wishes regarding life-sustaining medical care in case the patient is no longer able to indicate his own wishes. Your job is to document that the patient received the required information and whether he brought an advance directive with him. (See *Tips for dealing with advance directives.*)

A change may be in order

When a patient's advance directive is given to the doctor, the nurse's orders may change, depending on the patient's wishes. For example, if the patient's family submits an advance directive that includes the information that the patient doesn't want to be resuscitated, a do-not-resuscitate (DNR) order may be written.

Don't forget this

DNR orders are instructions not to attempt to resuscitate a patient who has suffered cardiac or respiratory failure. A DNR order may be appropriate if the patient has a terminal illness, is permanently unconscious, or won't respond to cardiopulmonary resuscitation (CPR). A terminally ill patient may ask not to be resuscitated if he experiences sudden cardiac arrest, or he may write this request into his advance directive.

A DNR order should be reviewed periodically or whenever a significant change occurs in the patient's clinical status. (See *Charting last wishes*, page 244.)

Who else can give a DNR order?

If the patient doesn't ask for a DNR order, or if no policies exist, the doctor may write the order if it's medically appropriate and the patient understands the impact of the DNR order. If the patient is incompetent, an appropriate surrogate must give consent for the doctor to write the DNR order.

A patient's right

The patient has the right to change advance directives at any time. Because the patient's requests may differ from what the family or doctor wants, document discrepancies carefully. Use social services or the legal department for advice on how to proceed. (See *Check this out: Advance directive checklist*, page 245.)

Two common types of advance directives are:
• living will
• durable power of attorney for health care.

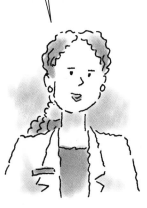

When the patient's wishes with regard to life-sustaining care clash with the doctor's or family members', document the discrepancy.

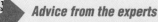

Advice from the experts

Tips for dealing with advance directives

Many patients wait until they're hospitalized to consider an advance directive or to make significant legal decisions. So, be prepared to offer information and advice and to record the patient's wishes in a legally appropriate manner. Here are some important points to remember.

Legal competence

Only a competent adult can execute a legally binding document. To prevent a patient's relatives from raising questions about his competence later, discuss his mental status with the doctor and, possibly, a psychiatrist. Be sure to document his mental status assessment in the chart before he signs any legal document.

Living will and durable power of attorney

If a patient has a living will or durable power of attorney for health care, a copy should be in his chart. Also, you should know how to contact the person with decision-making power. If the patient doesn't have the document with him, ask a family member to bring it to the health care facility. As your patient's advocate, you must ensure that his wishes are properly executed. If conflicts arise, discuss them with your nurse-manager as well as with a risk manager.

If a patient wants to execute a living will during his hospital stay, you aren't required, or even allowed in some states, to sign as a witness. Many facilities have the social service or

risk management department oversee this process. Find out who is responsible in your facility. The person who acts as witness can be held accountable for the patient's competence. Place the signed and witnessed document in the chart.

Last will and testament

In some facilities, dictating a patient's last will and testament is so commonplace that special forms have been designed for it. If this situation occurs often in your facility, discuss creating a form with your manager.

If no form exists in your facility, and a patient wants to dictate his last will and testament to you, document his request and what has been done to facilitate it; for example, who has been contacted and when.

If an administrator isn't available, two nurses should be present during dictation of the will. One should record the information in the chart, and both should sign it. In most instances, the patient's family will obtain their own legal representatives to process the recording of the will.

Living will

In making a living will, a legally competent person declares what medical care he wants or doesn't want if he develops a terminal illness. Living wills may apply only to treatment decisions made after a terminally ill patient becomes comatose and has no reasonable chance of recovery. They usually authorize the doctor to withhold or discontinue lifesaving measures.

State-ments

Most states recognize living wills as valid legal documents. Although the legal requirements vary from state to state, most states specify:
- circumstances under which a living will applies
- who is authorized to make a living will (usually only competent adults)

Advice from the experts

Charting last wishes

Do-not-resuscitate (DNR) orders are extremely tricky. On the one hand, if a terminally ill patient asks not to be resuscitated, you must abide by his wishes if he goes into cardiac or respiratory arrest. Calling a code (initiation of emergency treatment by doctors and nurses to resuscitate a patient after cardiac or respiratory arrest) violates his right to refuse treatment. On the other hand, if you don't call a code, you could be accused of negligence and be found liable for his death. Without a DNR order, you're obligated to call a code if warranted.

Now what?

So how should you proceed? First, document the patient's wishes and chart his degree of awareness and orientation. Then contact your nurse-manager and request help from administration, legal services, or social services. Don't place yourself in the middle. Let the doctor, the patient, and the patient's family make the decisions.

If the doctor knows about the patient's wish but still refuses to write a DNR order, document this in your notes. Like you, the doctor must abide by the patient's wishes and may be found liable if he doesn't. If the patient has prepared an advance directive, make sure that the doctor has seen it.

- limitations or restrictions on care that can be refused (for example, some states don't allow refusal of food and water)
- elements the will must contain to be considered a legal document, including witnessing requirements
- who is immune from liability for following a living will's directions
- procedure for rescinding a living will.

Durable power of attorney

A durable power of attorney for health care enables a person to state what type of care he does or doesn't want. However, it also names another person to make health care choices if the patient becomes legally incompetent. This person is usually a family member or friend or, in rare instances, the doctor.

Hazard #4: Patients who refuse treatment

You're also responsible for helping patients make informed decisions about continuing treatment. When treatment is refused, important patient care, safety, and documentation issues come into play.

Art of the chart

Check this out: Advance directive checklist

The Joint Commission on Accreditation of Healthcare Organizations requires that information on advance directives be charted on the admission assessment form. However, many facilities also use a checklist like the one below.

ADVANCE DIRECTIVE CHECKLIST

Check appropriate boxes.

I. DISTRIBUTION OF ADVANCE DIRECTIVE INFORMATION

  A. Advance directive information was presented to the patient: .... ☑

    1. At the time of preadmission testing .... ☑

    2. Upon inpatient admission .... ☐

    3. Interpretive services contacted .... ☐

    4. Information was read to the patient .... ☐

  B. Advance directive information was presented to the next of kin as the patient is incapacitated .... ☐

  C. Advance directive information was not distributed as the patient is incapacitated and no relative or next of kin was available .... ☐

        <u>Mary Barren, RN</u>   <u>11/15/02</u>

        RN   **DATE**

	Upon admission		Upon transfer to Critical Care Unit	
II. ASSESSMENT OF ADVANCE DIRECTIVE UPON ADMISSION	YES	NO	YES	NO
A. Does the patient have an advance directive?	☐	☑	☐	☐
If yes, was the attending physician notified?	☐		☐	
B. If no advance directive, does the patient want to execute an advance directive?	☑	☐	☐	☐
If yes, was the attending physician notified?	☑		☐	
Was the patient referred to resources?	☑		☐	

Sign and date.

    <u>Mary Barren, RN</u>   **RN**

    RN   **RN**

    <u>11/15/02</u>

    DATE   **DATE**

III. RECEIPT OF AN ADVANCE DIRECTIVE AFTER ADMISSION

  A. The patient has presented an advance directive after admission and the attending physician has been notified.

Sign here if the patient brought an advance directive and presented it after admission.

    RN   **DATE**

Refusing treatment

Any mentally competent adult can legally refuse treatment if he has been fully informed about his medical condition and the likely consequences of his refusal. This means he can refuse mechanical ventilation, tube feedings, antibiotics, fluids, and other treatments that are needed to keep him alive.

When a patient refuses treatment, chart his exact words.

The patient who says "no"

When your patient refuses treatment, chart his exact words. Inform him of the risks involved in refusing treatment, preferably in writing. If he still refuses treatment, chart that you didn't provide the prescribed treatment, and then notify the doctor. The doctor will explain the risks to the patient again. If he continues to refuse treatment, the doctor will ask him to sign a refusal-of-treatment release form, which you may need to sign as a witness. (See *Witnessing refusal of treatment.*)

If the patient won't sign this form, document this, too. For extra protection, your facility may require you to have the patient's spouse or closest relative sign another refusal-of-treatment release form.

Get to them early

More and more facilities are informing patients soon after admission about their future treatment options. Discuss the patient's wishes at your first opportunity, and document the discussion in case he becomes incompetent later. It may be helpful to use a chaplain or someone from social services to speak with the patient to verify his wishes.

Legal guidelines

Failure to respond appropriately to a patient's refusal to accept treatment may have serious legal consequences. To prevent problems, take these steps:

• Confirm the patient's condition and prognosis with the doctor and record them in the medical record.
• Make sure that the doctor documented the patient's understanding of the consequences of his refusal, such as pain or decreased life expectancy or quality of life.
• Search the medical record for a living will, a durable power of attorney for health care, or letters from people who heard the patient express his wishes.
• Search the medical record for documentation of conversations between the patient and health care providers, including the conversation about the patient's final decision to withhold treatment.

> **Art of the chart**

Witnessing refusal of treatment

To prevent misunderstandings and lawsuits if a patient refuses treatment, the doctor must explain the risks involved in making this choice. If the patient still refuses treatment, the doctor will ask him to sign a refusal-of-treatment release form, such as the one below, which you may need to witness.

REFUSAL-OF-TREATMENT RELEASE FORM

I, _Joseph Arden_ , refuse to allow anyone to _administer parenteral nutrition_
    (patient's name)   (insert treatment)

The risks attendant to my refusal have been fully explained to me, and I fully understand the benefits of this treatment. I also understand that my refusal of treatment seriously reduces my chances for regaining normal health and may endanger my life.

I hereby release ___Memorial General___ , its nurses and employees, together with all doctors in any way
                    (name of facility)
connected with me as a patient, from liability for respecting and following my express wishes and direction.

___Donna Burns___   ___Joseph Arden___
(Witness's signature)   (Patient's or legal guardian's signature)

___12/11/02___   ___76___
(Date)   (Patient's age)

> The patient acknowledges that he understands the risks of refusing treatment.

Documentation should include the dates of conversations, the full names of people involved, the circumstances, and what treatments and medical conditions were discussed.

• DNR orders should be reviewed every 48 to 72 hours, or according to your facility's policy.

• DNR orders must be written; they can't be provided as verbal orders or telephone orders.

• Refuse written or spoken orders for "slow codes," such as calling the doctor before resuscitating a patient, doing CPR but withholding drugs, giving oxygen but withholding CPR, or not putting a patient on a ventilator. These orders are unethical and illegal.

• Suggest that your facility set up an ethics committee to resolve problems about withholding treatment.

Hazard #5: Documenting for unlicensed personnel

Anyone reading your notes assumes these notes are a firsthand account of care provided—unless you chart otherwise. In some settings, nursing assistants and technicians aren't allowed to make formal chart entries. In such cases, determine what care was provided, assess the patients and the tasks performed (for example, a dressing change), and document your findings. Be sure to record the full names and titles of unlicensed personnel who provided care. Don't just record their initials.

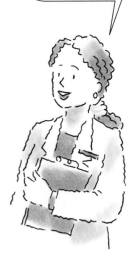

If you're charting care provided by unlicensed personnel, assess the patient and the task performed and document your findings.

Countersign-language

If your facility allows unlicensed personnel to chart, you may have to countersign their notes. If your facility's policy states that the unlicensed person must provide care in your presence, don't countersign unless you actually witness her actions. If the policy says that you don't have to be there, your countersigning indicates that the notes describe care that other people had the authority and competence to perform and that you verified that the procedures were performed. You can specifically document that you reviewed the notes and consulted with the technician on certain aspects of care. Of course, you must document any follow-up care you provide.

Hazard #6: Using restraints

When physical restraints are ordered for a patient, your job is to check the patient frequently for problems associated with the restraints, perform comfort measures, perform range-of-motion exercises on all extremities, and then document your care. Most facilities have a policy outlining the proper procedure for using restraints. You may also recommend to the doctor that he order physical restraints for a patient and chart your observations in the progress notes. The doctor must reevaluate the need for physical restraints and rewrite orders for them every 24 hours. (See *Physical restraint order.*)

Unrestrained? Get a release

If a competent patient refuses physical restraints, a facility may require him to sign a release absolving everyone involved of liability if he's injured as a result. (See *Charting the need for restraints,* page 250.)

Hazard #7: Patients who request to see their charts

A patient has a legal right to read his medical record. He may ask to see it because he's confused about the care he's receiving. First,

Art of the chart

Physical restraint order

A form such as the one below must be in the patient's chart before physical restraints are applied.

Date: _____3/5/02_____   Time: ____0315____

Reason for restraint use (circle all that apply):
To prevent:
1. High risk for self-harm
2. High risk for harm to others _____® subclavian CV line_____
3. High potential for removing tubes, equipment, or invasive lines
4. High risk for causing significant disruption of the treatment environment
5. Other _____

Duration of restraint (Not to exceed 24 hr): _____24_____

Type of restraint (circle all that apply):
   Vest
   Left mitt   Right mitt
   Left wrist   Right wrist
   Left ankle   Right ankle
   Other _____

Doctor's signature _____J. Donnelly, MD_____

---

ask him if he has questions about his treatment and try to clear up any confusion.

If he still wants to see the record, check your facility's policy to see whether he has to read it in your presence. Document questions the patient asks about the record or statements he makes about it as well as what you say to him.

Don't just hand it over

Never release medical records to unauthorized people, including family members and police officers. Refer all requests from insurance companies to the appropriate administrator, and refer other requests to your nurse-manager. Be sure to notify your nurse-manager if you have any doubts about the validity of a request — she may want to notify the facility's administrator.

Art of the chart

Charting the need for restraints

The following progress note entry documents the need for restraints to ensure patient safety.

12/2/02	0100	Pt found at 2345 holding onto ET tube and subclavian line and pulling at
		them. I explained the necessity of the ET tube and the subclavian line and not
		to pull on them. At 0045 pt sleeping; ET tube and lines intact.
		———————————————————————————— Barbara Brogan, RN
		Pt again found pulling at ET tube. Dr. Smith notified. (L)and (R)mitt restraints
12/2/02	0200	ordered and applied. ————————————————— Barbara Brogan, RN

Hazard #8: Patients who leave against medical advice

The law says that a mentally competent patient can leave a facility at any time. Having the patient sign an against medical advice (AMA) form protects you, the doctors, and the facility if problems arise from his unapproved discharge.

Taking aim at the AMA form

The AMA form should clearly document that the patient knows he's leaving against medical advice, that he has been advised of and understands the risks of leaving, and that he knows he can come back. Use his own words to describe his refusal.

Here's what to include on the AMA form:
• names of relatives or friends notified of the patient's decision and the dates and times of the notifications
• explanation of the risks and consequences of the AMA discharge, as told to the patient, and the name of the person who provided the explanation
• other places the patient can go for follow-up care
• names of people accompanying the patient at discharge and the instructions given to them
• patient's destination after discharge.

If the patient leaves without anyone's knowledge or if he refuses to sign the AMA form, check your facility's policy; you most likely have to fill out an incident report in either situation.

Relate the patient's state

In the progress notes, document statements and actions that reflect the patient's mental state at the time he left your facility. This helps protect you, the doctor, and security; and the facility against a charge of negligence if the patient later claims that he was mentally incompetent at the time of discharge and was improperly supervised while in that state. (See *The patient's progress.*)

The case of the missing patient

Suppose a patient never says anything about leaving but, on rounds, you discover he's missing? If you can't find him in the facility, notify your nurse-manager, hospital security, and the doctor; then try to contact the patient's home. If he isn't there, call the police if you think the patient might hurt himself or others, especially if he left the hospital with any medical devices.

Chart the time you discovered the patient missing, your attempts to find him, the people you notified, and other pertinent information.

Art of the chart

The patient's progress

When a patient leaves against medical advice, document it in the progress notes as shown below.

11/5/02	1300	Pt found in room dressed in own clothes with coat on. When asked why he was
		dressed, he stated, "They still don't know why I keep getting dizzy, and nothing
		is turning up in any of the tests. I don't want any more tests and I'm going
		home." Dr. McCarthy notified and came to speak with pt and his son. Pt willing
		to sign AMA form. AMA form signed. Pt told of the possible risks of his leaving
		the hospital with dizziness and hypertension. Pt agrees to see Dr. McCarthy
		in office tomorrow. Discussed appointment with pt and son. Pt going to son's
		home after discharge. Accompanied pt in wheelchair to main lobby with son. Pt
		left at 1245. ———————————————— Lola Caudullo, RN

Cheat sheet

Avoiding legal pitfalls review

Basics
- Complete, accurate documentation proves that you're providing quality care and meeting standards.
- Faulty charting is a pivotal issue in many malpractice cases.

Legal standards
- Nurse practice acts—state laws that designate nursing scope of practice
- ANA requirements—standards set by the nursing profession
- Malpractice litigation—previous rulings, which are influenced by breach of duty, damage, and causation
- Facility policies and procedures—rules that are developed by each facility to identify standards of care

Defensive charting
How to chart
- Stick to facts.
- Avoid labeling.
- Be specific.
- Use neutral language.
- Eliminate bias.
- Keep the chart intact.

What to chart
- Significant situations
- Complete assessment data and plan of care
- Discharge instructions

Other charting tips
- Always document care when it's performed or shortly after.
- Never delegate your charting.

Risk management goals
- Decreasing claims
- Reducing preventable accidents
- Controlling costs related to claims

Eight legal hazards
- Incident reports
- Informed consent
- Advance directives
- Patients who refuse treatment
- Documentation for unlicensed personnel
- Restraints
- Patients who request to see their charts
- Patients who leave AMA

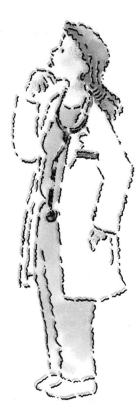

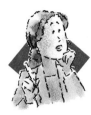

Quick quiz

1. Failure to provide patient care and to follow appropriate standards is called:
    A.   breach of duty.
    B.   breach of promise.
    C.   negligent duty.

Answer: A. When investigating breach of duty, the courts ask, How would a reasonable, prudent nurse with comparable training and experience have acted in the same or similar circumstances?

2. Professional standards for most nursing specialties are set by which of the following bodies?
    A.   The court system
    B.   ANA
    C.   JCAHO

Answer: B. ANA sets standards for most nursing specialties.

3. If you spill something on a page of the medical record, you should:
    A.   throw the old page away after copying it.
    B.   copy it and leave both pages in the chart.
    C.   leave the stained page in the chart and write a note explaining what happened.

Answer: B. Discarding pages from the medical record, even for innocent reasons, will raise doubt in the jury's mind if the chart ends up in court.

4. If your facility uses flow sheets, checklists, and graphic forms, you still need to chart in the progress notes if:
    A.   you filled out an incident report.
    B.   there's any out-of-the-ordinary information.
    C.   there are staff conflicts.

Answer: B. Anticipate litigation, and include in the progress notes anything that needs further explanation or clarification.

5. One way to expedite the charting process is to:
    A.   ask another nurse to help with some of your charting.
    B.   chart before you perform care, if you have more time then.
    C.   chart your care as close to the time of the event as possible.

Answer: C. If you chart care right away, you'll be able to record it faster because events will be fresh in your mind.

Scoring

☆☆☆ If you answered all five items correctly, way to go! Document your achievement on an AMA—amazingly meticulous attitude—form.

☆☆ If you answered three or four items correctly, terrific! Document your score on a DNR—definitely nice results—form.

☆ If you answered fewer than three items correctly, don't worry. Draw a line through your test score, initial it, and try again.

Documenting procedures

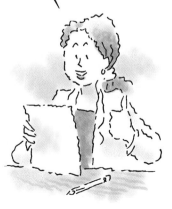

Just the facts

In this chapter, you'll learn:

♦ how to chart routine nursing procedures

♦ how to chart on a medication administration record

♦ extra steps to take when charting drug administration and I.V. therapy

♦ what to chart when you're assisting a doctor with a procedure.

Guidelines for charting nursing procedures

Your notes about routine nursing procedures usually appear in the patient's chart, on flow sheets, or graphic forms. Whatever your health care facility's requirements are, you need to include this information in your documentation:

• what procedure was performed
• when it was performed
• who performed it
• how it was performed
• how well the patient tolerated it
• adverse reactions to the procedure, if any.

The section that follows outlines information that must be documented for several nursing procedures.

> Take the time to document accurately, objectively, thoroughly, consistently, and legibly — both in routine and exceptional situations.

Drug administration

A medication administration record (MAR) is part of most documentation systems. It may be included in the medication Kardex, or it may be on a separate sheet. In either case, it's the central record of medication orders and their execution and is part of the patient's permanent record.

You chart MARvelously

When charting on the MAR, follow these guidelines:
• Follow your facility's policies and procedures for recording drug orders and administration.
• Record the patient's full name, medical record number, and allergy information on each MAR.
• Immediately document the drug's name, dose, route of administration, frequency, the number of doses ordered or the stop date (if applicable), and the administration time for doses given.
• Write legibly.
• Use only standard abbreviations. When in doubt, write out the word or phrase.
• After administering the first dose, sign your full name, licensure status, and initials in the appropriate space.
• Record drug administration immediately so that another nurse doesn't inadvertently repeat the dose.
• If you chart by computer, do so right after giving each drug—especially if you don't use printouts as a backup. This gives all team members access to the latest drug administration data.
• If a specific assessment parameter must be monitored during administration of a drug, document this requirement on the MAR. For example, when digoxin is administered, the patient's pulse rate needs to be monitored and charted on the MAR.
• If you didn't give a drug, circle the time and document the reason for the omission.
• If you suspect that a patient's illness, injury, or death was drug-related, report this to the pharmacy department, who will relay the information to the Food and Drug Administration.

> Can't remember the standard abbreviation? When in doubt, write it out.

P.r.n. medications

Chart all p.r.n. (as needed) drugs when administered, including reason for giving and the patient's response. For specific drugs given p.r.n., follow these guidelines:
• For eye, ear, or nose drops, chart the number used as well as the administration route.
• For suppositories, chart the type (rectal, vaginal, or urethral) and how the patient tolerated it.
• For dermal drugs, chart the size and location of the area where you applied the drug and the condition of the skin or wound.
• For dermal patches, chart the location of the patch.

- For I.V., I.M., or subcutaneous medications, chart the dose given and the location of administration.

No room for exceptions

If you administer p.r.n. drugs according to accepted standards, you don't need to chart more specific information. However, if your MAR doesn't have space to document, for example, a patient's response to a drug or refusal to take a drug, document that information in the progress notes.

Drug abuse or refusal

If the patient refuses or abuses medications, describe the event in his chart. Here are some situations needing careful documentation:

- You discover nonprescribed drugs at the patient's bedside. Document the type of medication (pill or powder), the amount of medication, and its color and shape. (You may wish to send the drug to the pharmacy for identification.) Follow your facility's policy regarding the completion of the appropriate report.
- You find a supply of prescribed drugs in the patient's bedside table, indicating that he isn't taking each dose. Record the type and amount of medication.
- You notice a sudden change in the patient's behavior after he has visitors, and you suspect them of giving him narcotics or other drugs. Document how the patient appeared before the visitors came and afterward. Notify the doctor immediately and follow your facility's policy.
- You offer prescribed medications and the patient refuses to take them. Document the refusal, the reason for it (if he tells you), and the medication. This prevents the refusal from being misinterpreted as an omission or a medication error on your part. Note the example below.

12/15/02	1100	Pt refused K-Dur tabs, stating that they were too big and made her feel like she was choking when she tried to swallow one. Dr. Boyle notified. K-Dur tabs D/C. KCl elixir ordered and given. ——— Kathy Collins, RN

Paging the doctor...

Report any medication abuse or refusal to the doctor. When you do so, document the name of the doctor and the date and time of notification.

Narcotic administration

Whenever you give a narcotic, you must document it according to federal, state, and facility regulations. These regulations require you to:
- sign out the drug on the appropriate form
- verify the amount of drug in the container before giving it
- have another nurse document your activity and observe you if you must waste or discard part of a narcotic dose
- count narcotics after each shift.

Double team

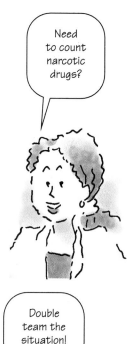

Two nurses should be present to count narcotic drugs — preferably the oncoming and off-going nurse. If you discover a discrepancy in the narcotic count, report it, following your facility's policy. Also, file an incident report. An investigation will follow.

I.V. therapy

More than 80% of hospitalized patients receive some form of I.V. therapy, such as fluid or electrolyte replacement, total parenteral nutrition (TPN), drugs, or blood products. Document all facets of I.V. therapy carefully, including subsequent complications. Your facility may have you document in the progress notes, on a special I.V. therapy sheet, in a flowchart, or in another format.

Basic charting

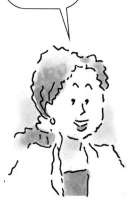

After establishing an I.V. route, document:
- date, time, and venipuncture site
- equipment used, such as the type and gauge of the catheter or needle
- number of venipuncture attempts made and the type of assistance required (if applicable).
    Once per shift, document:
- type, amount, and flow rate of I.V. fluid
- condition of the I.V. site
- fact that you flushed the I.V. line as well as what medication you used.
    Update your records each time you change the insertion site, venipuncture device, or I.V. tubing. Also, document the reason you

changed the I.V. site, such as extravasation, phlebitis, occlusion, patient removal, or a routine change.

Getting complicated

Document complications precisely. For example, record if extravasation occurs and what interventions you took, such as stopping the I.V., assessing the amount of fluid infiltrated, and notifying the doctor.

If a chemotherapeutic drug extravasates, stop the I.V. immediately and follow the procedure specified by your health care facility. Document the appearance of the I.V. site, the treatment you gave (especially antidotes), and the kind of dressing you applied. Document the amount of any discarded medication.

If the patient has an allergic reaction during I.V. therapy, stop the infusion and notify the doctor immediately. Then document all pertinent information about the reaction as well as your interventions and the patient's response.

Don't forget the family

Last, record patient and family teaching, such as explaining the purpose of I.V. therapy, describing the procedure itself, and discussing possible complications.

Total parenteral nutrition

If a patient is receiving TPN, document:
- type and location of the central line
- condition of the insertion site
- volume and rate of the solution infused.

We interrupt this service...

When you discontinue a central or peripheral I.V. line for TPN, record:
- date and time
- type of dressing applied
- appearance of the administration site.

Blood transfusions

Whenever you administer blood or blood components—such as packed cells, plasma, platelets, or cryoprecipitates—use proper identification and crossmatching procedures. Also, check the expiration date of the product and clearly document that you matched the label on the blood bag to:
- patient's name
- patient's medical record number
- patient's blood group or type

- patient's and donor's Rh factor
- crossmatch data
- blood bank identification number.

  In addition, the blood or blood component must be identified by two health care professionals, both of whom sign the slip that comes with the blood and verify that the information is correct.

For the (transfusion) record

Once you determine that the information on the blood bag label is correct, you may administer the transfusion. On the transfusion record, document:
- dates and times the transfusion was started and completed
- name of the health care professional who verified the information
- type and gauge of the catheter used
- total amount of the transfusion
- patient's vital signs before, during, and after the transfusion
- infusion device used, if any, and its flow rate
- blood warming unit used, if any.

Accounting for autotransfusions

If the patient receives his own blood, document the amount retrieved and reinfused in the intake and output records. Document the results of laboratory tests performed during and after the autotransfusion, paying special attention to the coagulation profile, hematocrit, and arterial blood gas, hemoglobin, and calcium levels. Also chart the patient's pretransfusion and posttransfusion vital signs.

Reacting to a transfusion reaction

If the patient develops a transfusion reaction, stop the transfusion immediately and notify the doctor. On a transfusion reaction form or in the progress notes, document:
- time and date of the reaction
- type and amount of infused blood or blood products
- times you started and stopped the transfusion
- clinical signs in order of occurrence
- patient's vital signs per facility protocol
- whether urine specimens and blood samples were sent to the laboratory for analysis
- treatment you gave and the patient's response to it.

  You may need to send the noninfused blood and tubing back to the blood bank. Follow your facility policy. An example of a note documenting a reaction is shown on the next page.

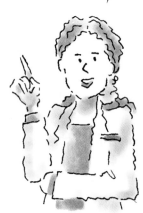

Proper identification procedures are key to charting blood transfusions.

11/16/02	1130	Pt reports nausea and chills. Transfusion started at 1030 hr. Cyanosis of the lips noted at 1100 hr with first unit of PRBCs transfusing. Stopped infusion. Approximately 100 ml infused. Tubing changed. I.V. of 1,000 ml NSS infusing at 40 ml/hr in left hand. Dr. Dunn notified. BP 170/90; P 110; R 28; T 99.4° F. Blood sample taken from PRBCs. Remaining blood discarded. Two red-top tubes of blood drawn from pt and sent to lab. Urine specimen obtained and sent to lab for UA. Pt given diphenhydramine 50 mg I.M. Two blankets placed on pt —— Anne Grasso, RN
	1145	Pt reports he's getting warmer and less nauseated. BP 164/86; P 100; R 24; T 99.2° F. ——————Anne Grasso, RN
	1200	Pt without chills or nausea. I.V. 1,000 ml NSS infusing at 80 ml/hr in left hand. BP 156/82; P 92; R 22; T 98.9° F.——————— Anne Grasso, RN

Surgical incision care

When a patient returns from surgery, document his vital signs and level of consciousness (LOC) and carefully record information about his surgical incision, drains, and the care you provide. An example of a progress note documenting surgical incision care is shown below.

11/11/02	1030	Dressing removed from right mastectomy incision; dime-sized area of serous sanguineous drainage on dressing. Incision well-approximated with staples intact. Site cleaned with sterile NSS. 4" x 4" sterile dressing applied. Teaching given to pt regarding dressing change and signs and symptoms of infection. Verbalized understanding. ——————— Deborah Liu, RN

Records that get around

Study the records that travel with the patient from the postanesthesia care unit. (See *Roaming records*, page 262.)

Who is up first?

Look for a doctor's order stating whether you or he will perform the first dressing change. If you'll be performing it, document:
• type of wound care performed

Advice from the experts

Roaming records

When your patient recovers from anesthesia, he'll be transferred from the postanesthesia care unit (PACU) to his assigned unit for ongoing recovery and care. As his nurse, you're responsible for the four-part document that travels with the patient. Make sure the PACU report is complete by checking for the following information.

Part 1: History
This section of the report should describe the patient's pertinent medical and surgical history, including drug allergies, medication history, chronic illnesses, significant surgical history, hospitalizations, and smoking history.

Part 2: Operation
This section describes the surgery itself and should include:
- the procedure performed
- the type and dosage of anesthetics
- how long the patient was anesthetized
- the patient's vital signs throughout surgery
- the volume of fluid lost and replaced
- drugs administered
- surgical complications
- tourniquet time
- drains, tubes, implants, or dressings used during surgery and removed or still in place.

Part 3: Postanesthesia period
This part of the record includes information about:
- pain medications and pain control devices that the patient received and how he responded to them
- interventions that should continue on the unit, such as frequent circulatory, motor, and neurologic checks if the patient underwent leg surgery and had a tourniquet on for a long time
- a flow sheet showing the patient's postanesthesia recovery scores on arrival and discharge in the areas of activity level, respiration, circulation, and level of consciousness (LOC).
- unusual events or complications that occurred in the PACU; for example, nausea or vomiting, shivering, hypothermia, arrhythmias, central anticholinergic syndrome, sore throat, back or neck pain, corneal abrasion, tooth loss during intubation, swollen lips or tongue, pharyngeal or laryngeal abrasion, and postspinal headache.

Part 4: Current status
This section should describe the patient's status at the time of transfer back to the unit. Information should include his vital signs, LOC, sensorium, and the condition of the surgical site.

- wound's appearance (size, color, condition of margins, presence of wound closure devices, and necrotic tissue); odor, if any; location of drains; and drainage characteristics (type, color, consistency, and amount)
- type and amount of dressing and whether a pouch was applied
- additional wound care procedures, such as drain management, irrigation, and packing, or application of a topical medication
- how the patient tolerated the dressing change
- any teaching provided to the patient (or family, if applicable).

Detailed care and discharge data

Document special or detailed wound care instructions and pain management measures on the nursing plan of care. Also, chart the color and amount of measurable drainage on the intake and output form.

If the patient needs wound care after discharge, provide patient teaching and document it. Chart that you explained aseptic technique, described how to examine the wound for infection or other complications, demonstrated how to change the dressing, and gave written instructions for home care. Also, document whether the patient demonstrates an understanding of the instructions and is able to perform wound care measures.

Pacemaker care

If the patient has a temporary pacemaker inserted, record:
- date and time of placement
- reason for placement
- pacemaker settings
- patient's response
- patient's LOC and vital signs, including which arm you used to obtain the blood pressure reading
- complications, such as chest pain or signs of infection
- interventions such as X-ray studies to verify correct electrode placement
- medications that may have been given before or during the procedure.

Make sure the rhythm strip includes the patient's name and the date and time of placement. An example of a progress note documenting pacemaker care is shown on the next page.

If the patient has a transcutaneous pacemaker, document the reason for this kind of pacing, the time pacing started, and the locations of the electrodes.

12/1/02	1315	Pt with temporary transvenous pacemaker in right sub-
		clavian vein. Heart rate 60. Monitor showing 100%
		ventricular paced rhythm. ECG obtained. Pacemaker
		sensing and capturing correctly. Site without redness
		or swelling. Dressing dry and intact. Anne Galata, RN

Get a rhythm going

Document the information obtained from a 12-lead electrocardiogram (ECG). Put rhythm strips in the medical record before, during, and after pacemaker placement; any time pacemaker settings change; and any time the patient receives treatment for a pacemaker complication.

As ECG monitoring continues, record capture, sensing rate, intrinsic beats, and competition of paced and intrinsic rhythms.

Peritoneal dialysis

If your patient is receiving peritoneal dialysis, monitor and document his response to treatment during and after the procedure. Be sure to chart:
- vital signs per facility protocol
- abrupt changes in the patient's condition and your notification of the doctor
- amount of dialysate infused and drained and medications added (Complete a dialysis flowchart every 24 hours.)
- effluent's characteristics (color and clarity) and the assessed negative or positive fluid balance at the end of each infusion-dwell-drain cycle
- patient's daily weight (immediately after the drain phase) and abdominal girth, noting the time of day and variations in the weighing and measuring technique
- physical assessment findings
- fluid status
- equipment problems, such as kinked tubing or mechanical malfunction, and your interventions
- condition of the patient's skin at the catheter site
- patient's reports of unusual discomfort or pain and your interventions
- any break in aseptic technique and notification of the doctor

• whether the patient or family member performs the peritoneal dialysis procedure.

An example of a progress note documenting peritoneal dialysis is shown below.

12/20/02	0300	Pt receiving exchanges q2h of 1,500 ml 4.25 dialysate with 500 units
		heparin and 2 mEq. KCl; infused over 15 min. Dwell time 15 min. Drain
		time 30 min. Drainage clear, pale yellow fluid. Pt tolerating procedures
		without complications or discomfort. LLQ catheter site nonreddened.
		Site cleaned and dressed per protocol. Pt weight after dialysis 205 lb.
		Abdominal girth 45 1/2". ———————————— Amanda Taylor, RN

Peritoneal lavage

For the patient recovering from peritoneal lavage, document:
• vital signs and symptoms of shock, such as tachycardia, decreased blood pressure, diaphoresis, dyspnea, or vertigo
• condition of the incision site
• type and size of the peritoneal dialysis catheter used
• type and amount of solution instilled into the peritoneal cavity
• amount and color of the fluid withdrawn from the peritoneal cavity and whether it flowed freely in and out
• what specimens were obtained and sent to the laboratory for analysis
• complications that occurred and your interventions.

An example of a progress note documenting peritoneal lavage is shown below.

12/21/02	0400	#16 Fr. Foley catheter inserted without incident. NG tube inserted via right
		nostril to low intermittent suction. Dr. Byrne inserted # 15 Fr. peritoneal
		catheter below umbilicus via trocar; 20 ml clear fluid withdrawn. 150 ml warm
		NSS instilled as ordered and clamped. Pt turned from side to side. NSS dwell
		time 10 min, then drained freely from abdomen. Fluid samples sent to lab as
		ordered. Peritoneal catheter removed and incision closed by Dr. Byrne. 4" x 4"
		gauze pad with povidone-iodine ointment applied to site. Pt tolerated
		procedure well and is in no distress. ———————— Lois Testa, RN

Thoracic drainage

If your patient has thoracic drainage, initially record:
- date and time the drainage began
- type of system used
- amount of suction applied to the pleural cavity
- presence or absence of bubbling or fluctuation in the water-seal chamber
- amount and type of drainage
- patient's respiratory status.
  At the end of each shift, record this information:
- how frequently you inspected the drainage system
- presence or absence of bubbling or fluctuation in the water-seal chamber
- patient's respiratory status
- condition of the chest dressings
- type, amount, and route of pain medication you gave
- complications and subsequent interventions.

The charting goes on and on

Ongoing documentation should include:
- color, consistency, and amount of thoracic drainage in the collection chamber as well as the time and date of each observation
- patient-teaching sessions and activities you taught the patient to perform, such as coughing and deep breathing exercises, sitting upright, and splinting the insertion site to minimize pain
- rate and quality of the patient's respirations and your auscultation findings
- complications, such as cyanosis, rapid or shallow breathing, subcutaneous emphysema, chest pain, or excessive bleeding, and the time and date you notified the doctor
- dressing changes and the patient's skin condition at the chest tube site.

An example of a progress note documenting thoracic drainage is shown below.

12/22/02	0100	Right anterior chest tube intact to 20 cm H₂0
		suction. 100 ml bright red bloody drainage noted
		since 0300. No air leak noted. + water chamber
		fluctuation. Chest tube site dressing dry and in-
		tact; no crepitus palpated. Resp. assessment
		unchanged as per flow sheet.
		———————— Nancy Siegfried, RN

Cardiac monitoring

For the patient receiving cardiac monitoring, include in your notes:
• date and time the monitoring began
• monitoring leads used
• rhythm strip readings labeled with the patient's name and room number and the date and time
• changes in the patient's condition.

An example of a progress note documenting cardiac monitoring is shown below.

12/24/02	1315	At 1245 monitor showing ST (HR 150s)
		with multifocal PVCs. Pt complaining of
		SOB and palpitations. O₂ 2 L via nasal
		cannula placed. BP 178/96. ECG done.
		Dr. Corcoran notified and he administered
		Lopressor 5 mg I.V. at 1250. Blood drawn
		for serum electrolytes and sent to lab.
		Monitor presently showing NSR with
		occasional multifocal PVCs. Pt without
		SOB, chest pain, or palpitations at present.
		—————————————— Nancy Shwan, RN

Keep on chartin'

If the patient is to continue cardiac monitoring after discharge, document:
• which caregivers can interpret dangerous rhythms and perform cardiopulmonary resuscitation
• patient and family teaching, including troubleshooting techniques to use if the monitor malfunctions
• referrals to equipment suppliers, home health agencies, and other community resources.

Chest physiotherapy

Whenever you perform chest physiotherapy, document:
• date and time of your interventions

- patient's positions for secretion drainage and how long he remains in each
- chest segments you percussed or vibrated
- characteristics of the secretion expelled, including color, amount, odor, viscosity, and the presence of blood
- patient's tolerance of the chest physiotherapy
- complications and your interventions.

    An example of a progress note documenting chest physiotherapy is shown below.

12/28/02	1130	Pt placed on right side of bed in
		Trendelenburg position. Chest physiotherapy and
		postural drainage performed for 10 min from lower
		to middle then upper lobes as ordered. Produc-
		tive cough produced large amount yellow tenacious
		sputum Pt tolerated procedure without difficulty;
		lungs clear to auscultation. —— Harry Moppert, RN

Mechanical ventilation

For patients receiving mechanical ventilation, initially chart:
- date and time the mechanical ventilation began
- type of ventilator used and its settings
- patient's responses to mechanical ventilation, including vital signs, breath sounds, use of accessory muscles, secretions, intake and output, and weight.

Take a deep breath — then chart!

Throughout mechanical ventilation, chart:
- complications and subsequent interventions
- pertinent laboratory data, including results of arterial blood gas (ABG) analyses and oxygen saturation findings
- duration of spontaneous breathing and the ability to maintain the weaning schedule for patients receiving pressure support ventilation or those using a T-piece or tracheostomy collar
- rate of controlled breaths, the time of each breath rate reduction, and the rate of spontaneous respirations for patients receiving intermittent mandatory ventilation, with or without pressure support ventilation
- adjustments made in ventilator settings as a result of ABG levels

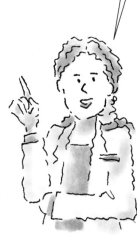

Don't forget to document the patient's responses to mechanical ventilation.

- adjustments of ventilator components, such as draining condensate into a collection trap and changing, cleaning, or discarding the tubing
- interventions to increase mobility, protect skin integrity, or enhance ventilation; for example, active or passive range-of-motion exercises, turning, or positioning the patient upright for lung expansion
- presence and characteristics of secretions
- type and frequency of oral care provided
- assessment findings related to LOC, peripheral circulation, urine output, decreased cardiac output, fluid volume excess, or dehydration
- patient's sleep and wake periods, noting significant trends
- patient and family teaching in preparation for the patient's discharge, especially that associated with ventilator care and settings, artificial airway care, communication, nutrition, and therapeutic exercise
- teaching discussions and demonstrations related to signs and symptoms of infection and equipment functioning
- referrals to equipment vendors, home health agencies, and other community resources.

An example of a progress note documenting mechanical ventilation is shown below.

12/29/02	1100	ventilator wean started, placed 40%
		T-piece from 0930 to 1030. O₂ sat. remained
		above 90% during the entire weaning period.
		Resp. assessment unchanged from flow sheet; pt in
		no distress at present. ———— John Devine, RN

Nasogastric tube insertion and removal

After you insert a nasogastric (NG) tube, record:
- type and size of the NG tube
- date, time, and insertion route (left naris, right naris, oral)
- type and amount of suction
- amount, color, consistency, and odor of the drainage
- how the patient tolerated the insertion procedure
- signs and symptoms of complications, such as nausea, vomiting, and abdominal distention

• method of placement verification (for example, auscultation of air in gastric cavity or X-ray)
• subsequent irrigation procedures and problems occurring afterward, if any.

Record information about irrigations on an input and output sheet. An example of a progress note documenting NG tube replacement is shown below.

| 12/30/02 | 2100 | #12 Fr. NG tube placed in right naris. Placement verified and tube attached to low intermittent suction, as ordered. Drainage dark brown; heme +. Dr. Cohen notified. Hypoactive bowel sounds in all 4 quadrants. Pt tolerated procedure well. ————————————————— Diane Harris, RN |
| | | |

The tube is removed — so chart some more!

After you remove an NG tube, record:
• date and time of removal
• how the patient tolerated the procedure
• unusual events accompanying tube removal, such as nausea, vomiting, abdominal distention, and food intolerance.

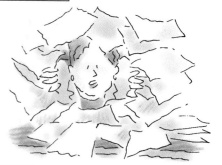

Seizure management

If your patient had a seizure while hospitalized, document:
• what seizure precautions you took
• date and time the seizure began and its duration
• precipitating factors, including auralike sensations reported by the patient
• involuntary behavior occurring before the seizure, such as lip smacking, chewing movements, or hand and eye movements
• incontinence during the seizure
• patient's vital signs (response to the seizure)
• what medications you gave
• complications resulting from the medications or the seizure and your interventions
• your assessment of the patient's postseizure mental status
• what and when you reported to the doctor.

An example of a progress note documenting seizure management is shown below.

| 12/30/02 | 1615 | At 1500 pt observed with generalized tonic-clonic seizure activity lasting 3 min. Awake at time of onset and stated, "Here it comes!" + urinary incontinence during seizure. Siderail pads in place prior to seizure. Placed on left side, airway patent. Dr. DeFabio notified of seizure. Diazepam 10 mg given I.V. as ordered. Pt sleeping at present. Vital signs stable (see graphic form). No further seizure activity noted. |
| | | ———————————————— Barbara Chao, RN |

Suture and staple removal

If the doctor writes an order for you to remove sutures or staples, document:
• date and time the sutures were removed
• appearance of the suture line
• appearance of the wound site, including the presence of purulent drainage
• if and when you notified the doctor
• if and when you collected a specimen and sent it to the laboratory for analysis.

Tube feedings

When documenting your care of a patient receiving tube feedings, write down:
• patient's tolerance of the procedure and the feeding formula
• kind of tube feeding the patient is receiving (such as duodenal or jejunal feedings or a continuous drip or bolus)
• amount, rate, route, and method of feeding (with continuous feedings, document the rate hourly)
• dilution strength if you need to dilute the formula (for example, half-strength or three-quarters strength)
• time you flushed the tube and the type and amount of solution used, if applicable

When giving tube feedings, be sure to document the patient's tolerance of the feeding formula.

• time you replaced the tube and how the patient tolerated the procedure, if applicable
• amount of gastric residual, if applicable
• description of the patient's gastric function, including prescribed medications or treatments to relieve constipation or diarrhea
• urine and serum glucose, serum electrolyte, and blood urea nitrogen levels as well as serum osmolality values
• feeding complications, such as hyperglycemia, glycosuria, and diarrhea
• patient and family teaching if the patient will continue receiving tube feedings after discharge
• referrals to suppliers or support agencies.

Obtaining an arterial blood sample

When you obtain blood for ABG analysis, record:
• patient's vital signs and temperature
• arterial puncture site
• results of Allen's test
• indications of circulatory impairment, such as swelling, discoloration, pain, numbness, or tingling in the bandaged arm or leg, and bleeding at the puncture site
• time you drew the blood sample
• how long you applied pressure to the site to control bleeding
• type and amount of oxygen therapy that the patient was receiving (if applicable).

An example of a progress note documenting obtainment of an arterial blood sample is shown below.

12/31/02	0930	Blood drawn from left radial artery after + Allen's test,
		brisk capillary refill. Pressure applied to site for
		5 min and pressure dressing applied. No swelling,
		bleeding, or hematoma noted. Hand pink and warm,
		with brisk capillary refill. Dr. Smith notified of
		ABG results; O_2 increased to 40% nonrebreather
		mask at 0845. Pt in no resp. distress. ————
		———————— Karen Andrews, RN

Need an ABG analysis? That's another form!

When filling out a laboratory request form for ABG analysis, include:
- patient's current temperature and respiratory rate
- his most recent hemoglobin level
- fraction of inspired oxygen and tidal volume if he's receiving mechanical ventilation.

Charting assisted procedures

When you assist a doctor during a procedure, you have the added responsibilities of providing patient support and teaching, evaluating the patient's response, and carefully documenting the procedure.

Procedures may change, but the charting remains the same

Regardless of the procedure, you must always document:
- date, time, and name of the procedure
- doctor who performed it
- how it was performed
- how the patient tolerated it
- adverse reactions to the procedure, if any
- any teaching provided to the patient.

The section that follows describes documentation for several procedures during which you may assist the doctor.

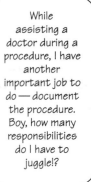

While assisting a doctor during a procedure, I have another important job to do — document the procedure. Boy, how many responsibilities do I have to juggle!?

Bone marrow aspiration

After assisting the doctor with bone marrow aspiration, document:
- date and time of the procedure
- name of the doctor performing the procedure
- appearance of the specimen aspirated
- how the patient responded to the procedure
- location and appearance of the aspiration site, including bleeding and drainage
- patient's vital signs after the procedure
- teaching provided to the patient.

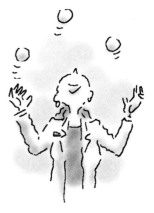

An example of a progress note documenting assistance during bone marrow aspiration is shown below.

| 12/3/02 | 1015 | Bone marrow aspiration explained to pt with questions answered. Bone marrow aspiration on left iliac crest performed by Dr. Wallace at 0945. No bleeding at site. Specimens sent to lab as ordered. Maintaining bed rest. Vital signs stable. Pt tolerated procedure well. ———— |
| | | ————————————— Pamela Clark, RN |

Esophageal tube insertion and removal

After assisting with esophageal tube insertion or removal, document:
- date and time that you assisted in the insertion or removal
- name of the doctor who performed the procedure
- intragastric balloon pressure, amount of air injected into the gastric balloon port, amount of fluid used for gastric irrigation, and color, consistency, and amount of gastric return before and after lavage (if applicable)
- baseline intraesophageal balloon pressure, which varies with respirations and esophageal contractions
- patient's tolerance of the insertion and removal procedures
- vital signs before, during, and after the procedure.

An example of a progress note documenting esophageal tube insertion is shown below.

| 11/4/02 | 1320 | Sengstaken-Blakemore tube placed without difficulty by Dr. Weathers via left naris. 50 cc air injected into gastric balloon, then 500 cc air injected into gastric balloon after abdominal X-ray confirmed placement. Tube secured to football helmet traction. Large amount of bright red blood drainage noted. Tube irrigated with 1,800 ml of iced NSS until clear. Esophageal balloon inflated to 30 mm Hg and clamped. Vital signs stable. Equal breath sounds bilat. Pt tolerated procedure well. Emotional support given.——— |
| | | ————————— James Carr, RN |

Arterial line insertion and removal

When assisting the doctor who is inserting an arterial line, record:
• date and time
• doctor's name
• insertion site
• type, gauge, and length of the catheter
• patient's response to the procedure, including circulation to the involved extremity.

An example of a progress note documenting insertion of an arterial line is shown below.

11/5/02	0820	20G arterial catheter placed in left radial artery
		by Dr. Watson after + Allen's test. Transducer
		leveled and zeroed. Readings accurate to cuff
		pressures. Site without redness, swelling, or
		ecchymosis. Dressed as per protocol. Left hand and
		wrist taped and secured to armboard. Line flushes
		easily. Arterial waveform visible on monitor. Hand
		warm and pink with brisk capillary refill. ————
		———————————— Harry Nguen, RN

The arterial line's work may be done, but not yours...

After removing the arterial line, record:
• date and time
• doctor's name
• length of the catheter
• condition of the insertion site
• specimens that were obtained from the catheter for culture
• patient's response to the procedure
• amount of time pressure was held at site.

Central venous line insertion and removal

When you help the doctor insert a central venous (CV) line, you need to document:
• time and date of insertion
• doctor's name
• length and location of the catheter

- solution infused
- patient's response to the procedure
- time that X-rays were done to confirm correct placement, the results, and when you notified the doctor of them. Also document if more than one attempt was made to insert the catheter.

An example of a progress note documenting insertion of a CV line is shown below.

11/6/02	1030	Procedure explained to pt and consent obtained by Dr. Rafferty.
		Triple-lumen catheter placed by Dr. Rafferty on 2nd attempt in left subclavian.
		Catheter sutured in place and dressing applied as per protocol. All lines
		flushed with 5 ml NSS. Portable chest X-ray obtained to confirm placement. Pt.
		tolerated procedure well. Vital signs stable. ————————— Eva Ryan, RN

See ya CV line, it's time to document...

After assisting with removal of a CV line, record:
- time and date of removal
- type of dressing applied
- condition of the insertion site
- catheter specimens you collected for culture or other analysis.

Lumbar puncture

During a lumbar puncture, observe the patient closely for signs of complications, such as a change in LOC, dizziness, or changes in vital signs. Report these to the doctor immediately and document them carefully.

Also document:
- color and clarity of the fluid obtained
- number of test tubes sent to the lab for analysis
- how the patient tolerated the procedure
- observations about the patient's condition and your interventions, including keeping him in a supine position for 6 to 12 hours, encouraging fluid intake, and assessing for headache and leaking cerebrospinal fluid around the puncture site.

Paracentesis

When caring for a patient during and after paracentesis, document:
- date and time of the procedure

- puncture site
- whether the site was sutured
- amount, color, viscosity, and odor of the initially aspirated fluid (also, record this in the intake and output record).

With responsibility comes more charting

If you're responsible for ongoing patient care, document:
- running record of the patient's vital signs
- frequency of drainage checks per facility protocol
- patient's response to the paracentesis
- characteristics of the drainage, including color, amount, odor, and viscosity
- patient's daily weight and abdominal girth measurements (taken at about the same time every day)
- what fluid specimens were sent to the laboratory for analysis
- peritoneal fluid leakage, if any. (Be sure to notify the doctor and chart the time and date.)

An example of a progress note documenting paracentesis is shown below.

3/15/02	1300	Procedure explained to pt and consent
		obtained. Dr. Wolf performed paracentesis
		in LLQ as per protocol. 1,800 ml of straw-
		colored fluid drained and sent to lab as
		ordered. Site sutured with two 3-0 silk
		sutures. Sterile 4" x 4" gauze pad
		applied. No leakage noted at site. Abdominal
		girth 48" preprocedure and 45 1/4" post-
		procedure. Weight 210 lb preprocedure
		and 205 lb postprocedure. Pt tolerated
		procedure. ——————— Owen Starr, RN

Thoracentesis

When assisting with thoracentesis, you need to chart:
- date and time of the procedure
- name of the doctor who performed it
- amount and characteristics of fluid aspirated
- patient's response to the procedure

• if the patient had sudden or unusual pain, faintness, dizziness, or changes in vital signs and when you reported these problems to the doctor

• symptoms of pneumothorax, hemothorax, subcutaneous emphysema, or infection as well as when you reported them to the doctor along with your interventions

• when you sent a fluid specimen to the laboratory for analysis.

An example of a progress note documenting thoracentesis is shown below.

9/2/02	1100	Procedure explained to pt and consent obtained by Dr. McCall. Pt positioned over secured bedside table. RLL thoracentesis performed by Dr. McCall without incident. Sterile 4" x 4" gauze dressing applied to site; site without redness, edema, or drainage. 900 ml straw-colored fluid aspirated and specimens sent to lab as ordered. Vital signs stable. Lungs clear to auscultation. ———————————— Donna Taylor, RN

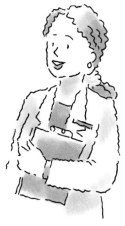

When charting a diagnostic test, begin by recording your preliminary assessment findings.

Charting miscellaneous procedures

Documentation isn't limited to procedures you perform or help the doctor perform. You'll also chart in other situations, including the ones described here.

Diagnostic tests

Before receiving a diagnosis, most patients undergo testing, which can be as simple as a blood test or as complicated as magnetic resonance imaging. Record in the medical record all tests and how the patient tolerated them.

Chart your first impressions

Start your documentation by recording preliminary assessments you made of the patient's condition. For example, chart if she's pregnant or has allergies because these conditions might affect the way a test is performed or the test's result. If the patient's age, illness, or disability requires special preparation for a test, record this information as well.

Also chart what you taught the patient about the test and follow-up care, the administration or withholding of drugs and preparations, special diets, food or fluid restrictions, enemas, and specimen collection.

An example of a progress note documenting a diagnostic test is shown below.

5/14/02	0600	24-hr test for urine protein started. Pt
		instructed on purpose of test and how to collect
		urine. Demonstrated correct technique. Sign placed
		on pt's door and in bathroom. Specimen container
		placed on ice in bathroom. ———— Mary Brady, RN

Pain control

In your quest to eliminate or minimize your patient's pain, you may use a number of assessment tools to determine the degree of pain. When you use these tools, always document the results. (See *Chart pain three ways,* page 280.)

When charting pain levels and characteristics, determine whether the pain is internal, external, localized, or diffuse, and whether it interferes with the patient's sleep or other activities of daily living. Describe the pain in the patient's own words and enter them in the chart.

Translating body language

Be aware of the patient's body language and behaviors associated with pain. Does he wince or grimace? Does he move or squirm in bed? What positions seem to relieve or worsen the pain? What other measures—such as heat, cold, massage, or drugs—relieve or heighten the pain? Also, note if the pain appears to worsen or improve when visitors are present. Document all of this information as well as your interventions and how the patient responded.

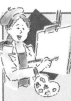

Art of the chart

Chart pain three ways

Some facilities use standardized questionnaires, such as the McGill-Melzack Pain Questionnaire or the Initial Pain Assessment Tool. Other facilities have devised their own pain measurement tools, such as the flow sheet and rating scales shown below. Whichever pain assessment tool you choose, remember to document its use and put the graphic form in your patient's chart.

Pain flow sheet

Flow sheets are convenient tools for pain assessment because they allow you to reevaluate the patient's pain at regular intervals. They're also useful when patients and families feel too overwhelmed to answer a long, detailed questionnaire.

    Try to incorporate pain assessment into the flow sheet you're already using. The easier it is to use the flow sheet, the more likely you and your patient will be to use it.

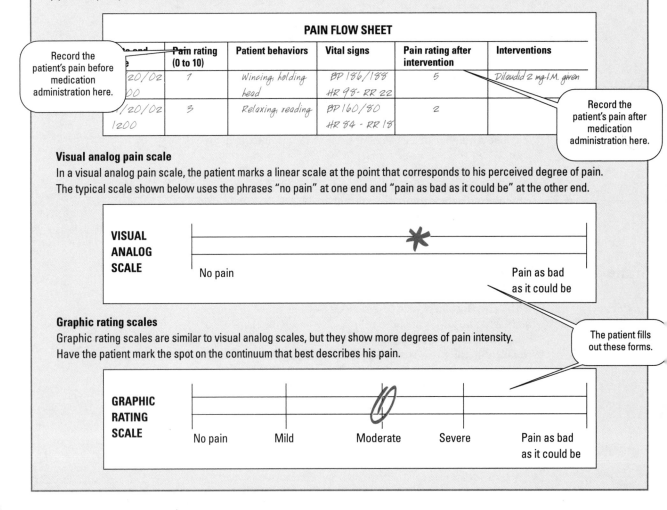

PAIN FLOW SHEET

Date and time	Pain rating (0 to 10)	Patient behaviors	Vital signs	Pain rating after intervention	Interventions
1/20/02 00	7	Wincing, holding head	BP 186/188 HR 98- RR 22	5	Dilaudid 2 mg I.M. given
1/20/02 1200	3	Relaxing, reading	BP 160/80 HR 84 - RR 18	2	

> Record the patient's pain before medication administration here.

> Record the patient's pain after medication administration here.

Visual analog pain scale

In a visual analog pain scale, the patient marks a linear scale at the point that corresponds to his perceived degree of pain. The typical scale shown below uses the phrases "no pain" at one end and "pain as bad as it could be" at the other end.

VISUAL ANALOG SCALE

No pain   Pain as bad as it could be

Graphic rating scales

Graphic rating scales are similar to visual analog scales, but they show more degrees of pain intensity. Have the patient mark the spot on the continuum that best describes his pain.

GRAPHIC RATING SCALE

No pain   Mild   Moderate   Severe   Pain as bad as it could be

> The patient fills out these forms.

An example of a progress note documenting care for a patient with pain is shown below.

| 3/2/02 | 0800 | Pt admitted with osteosarcoma and severe lower back pain. Took ibuprofen 800 mg q6h at home without relief last night or this morning. Dr. Kobb notified. Morphine 2 mg ordered and given I.V. at 0715. Vital signs stable. Pt states relief given.———————— |
| | | ———————— Sarah Bane, RN |

Intake and output

Many patients, including surgical and burn patients, those receiving I.V. therapy, and those with fluid and electrolyte imbalances, hemorrhage, or edema need 24-hour intake and output monitoring. To expedite documentation, you'll probably keep intake and output sheets at the bedside or by the bathroom door. If the patient is incontinent, document this as well as tube drainage and irrigation volumes.

Taking the intake charting challenge

Keeping track of foods and fluids that are premeasured is easy. You can list the volumes of specific containers for quick reference and use infusion devices to more accurately record enteral and I.V. intake.

Keeping track of intake that isn't premeasured is harder. For example, measuring and recording a food like gelatin that's fluid at room temperature requires the cooperation of the patient and other caregivers. You'll also need to teach family members and friends to record or report to you all snacks and soft drinks they bring the patient and all meals they help him eat.

Don't forget these types of intake

Don't forget to document as intake I.V. piggyback infusions, drugs given by I.V. push, patient-controlled analgesics, and irrigation solutions that aren't withdrawn. Also, chart oral or I.V. fluids that the patient receives when he's not on your unit. This requires the cooperation of the patient and staff members in other departments. In addition, remind ambulatory patients to use a urinal or a commode.

Fluid loss through the GI tract is normally 100 ml or less daily. However, if the patient's stools become excessive or watery, you

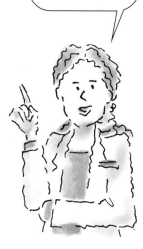

Keeping track of intake is a group effort! It requires the cooperation of the patient, his family and friends, and your colleagues.

must document them as output. Vomiting, drainage from suction devices and wound drains, and bleeding are other measurable sources of fluid loss that require documentation.

Transferring a patient to a specialty unit

If your patient's condition deteriorates and he requires transfer to a specialty unit, make sure to record:

• date and time of the transfer as well as the name of the unit receiving the patient
• that you received transfer orders
• patient's condition at the time of transfer, including vital signs, descriptions of incisions and wounds, and locations of any tubes or medical devices still in place as well as any significant events during the hospital stay, noting whether the patient has advanced directives and any special factors such as allergies, special diet, sensory deficits, and language or cultural issues
• medications, treatments, and teaching needs, noting which goals were and weren't met
• time that you gave a report to the receiving unit, including the name of the nurse who received the report
• how the patient was transported to the specialty unit along with who accompanied him
• any patient teaching related to the transfer such as the reason for transfer. (Some facilities use a transfer form to record this information.)

An example of a progress note documenting a patient transfer is shown below.

5/24/02	1430	Pt is a 63 y.o. white English-speaking female, with early Alzheimer's disease, being transferred from medical unit to
		MICU, by stretcher, accompanied by daughter and medical resident. Report given to Sue Riff, RN. Advance directives
		in chart. Pt unresponsive to verbal stimuli, opens eyes to painful stimuli. Prior to this episode, daughter reports
		pt. was alert and oriented to name but not always to place and time. Daughter states that pt's forgetfulness and
		confusion has recently gotten worse. Found alone in her apartment 2 days ago, unresponsive, no food eaten or dishes
		used since last groceries purchased for pt 5 days ago. Pt is severely dehydrated despite 2,000 ml over last 24
		hrs. Currently NPO. I.V. with #18 catheter in ®antecubital with 0.45% NSS at 75 ml/hr. HR 124 irregular, BP
		84/palp, R 28, rectal T 100 F, weight 78 lb, height 64". Allergies to molds, pollen, and mildew. Lungs clear,
		normal heart sounds. Skin intact, pale, cool, poor skin turgor. Radial pulses weak, pedal pulses not palpable. Foley
		catheter in place draining approximately 30 ml/hr. Dr's orders written. Medical record, MAR, and nursing Kardex
		transferred with pt. ———————————————————————— Diana Starr, RN

Termination of life support

According to the right-to-die laws of most states, a patient has the right to refuse extraordinary life-supporting measures if he has no hope of recovery. If the patient can't make the decision, the patient's next of kin is usually permitted to decide if life support should continue. A written statement of the patient's wishes is always preferable.

Advanced warning

Because of the Patient Self-Determination Act, each health care facility is required to ask the patient upon admission if he has an advance directive. An advance directive is a statement of the patient's wishes if he's unable to make decisions for himself. An advance directive may include a living will, which goes into effect when the patient is unable to make decisions for himself, as well as a durable power of attorney, which names a designated person to make these decisions when the patient can't. The act also states that the patient must receive written information concerning his right to make decisions about his medical care.

Match the patient's wishes to the situation

If life support is to be terminated, read the patient's advance directive to ensure that the present situation matches the patient's wishes and verify that the risk manager has reviewed the document. Check that the appropriate consent forms have been signed. Ask the family whether they would like to see the chaplain and if they would like to be with the patient before, during, and after life-support termination.

Charting directions for directives

If your patient has an advance directive, you need to record:
• if the patient's advance directive matches his present situation and life support wishes
• that your facility's risk manager has reviewed the advance directive
• that a consent form has been signed to terminate life support, according to facility policy
• the names of persons who were notified of the decision to terminate life support and their responses
• types of physical care for the patient before and after life-support termination
• whether the family was with the patient prior to, during, and after termination of life support as well as whether a chaplain was present

> The Patient Self-Determination Act requires that the patient be asked upon admission if he has an advance directive.

- time of termination, name of the doctor who turned off equipment, and names of people present
- vital signs after extubation, the time the patient stopped breathing, the time he was pronounced dead, and who made the pronouncement
- family's response, your interventions for them, and after-care for the patient.

An example of a progress note documenting the terminating of life support is shown below.

6/02/02	1800	Advance directive provided by pt's wife. Document reviewed by risk manager who
		verified that it matched the pt's present situation. Wife signed consent form to
		terminate life support. Wife spent approximately 10 min alone with pt before ter-
		mination of life support. Declined to have anyone with her during this time. Life
		support terminated at 1730 by Dr. Brown, with myself, Chaplain Greene, and pt's
		wife present. VS after extubation: P 50, BP 50/20, no respiratory effort not-
		ed. Pronounced dead at 1731. Pt's wife tearful. Chaplain Greene and myself
		stayed with her, listening to her talk about her 35 years with her husband. Pt
		bathed and dressed in pajamas for family visitation. ————Lucy Danios, RN

Codes

Guidelines established by the American Heart Association direct you to keep a written, chronological account of a patient's condition throughout CPR. If you're the designated recorder, document therapeutic interventions and the patient's responses *as* they occur. Don't rely on your memory later.

Getting up to code

The form used to chart a code is the *code record*. It incorporates detailed information about your observations and interventions as well as drugs given to the patient. (See *Charting CPR*.)

A helpful critique

Some facilities use a *resuscitation critique* form to identify actual or potential problems with the resuscitation process. This form tracks personnel responses and response times as well as the availability of appropriate drugs and functioning equipment. Make sure a copy of the completed critique form is submitted to the performance improvement department for analysis.

During CPR, the designated recorder should document events as they occur.

Art of the chart

Charting CPR

A completed code record like the one below should be included in your patient's chart.

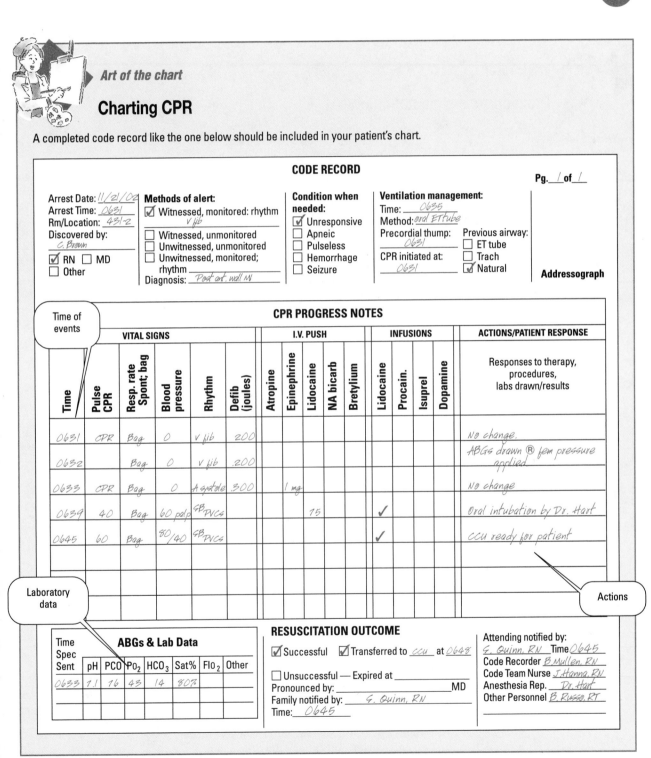

CODE RECORD

Pg. _/_ of _/_

Arrest Date: 11/21/02
Arrest Time: 0631
Rm/Location: 431-2
Discovered by: C. Brown
☑ RN ☐ MD
☐ Other

Methods of alert:
☑ Witnessed, monitored: rhythm _V fib_
☐ Witnessed, unmonitored
☐ Unwitnessed, unmonitored
☐ Unwitnessed, monitored; rhythm _Post ant. wall MI_
Diagnosis: _Post ant. wall MI_

Condition when needed:
☑ Unresponsive
☐ Apneic
☐ Pulseless
☐ Hemorrhage
☐ Seizure

Ventilation management:
Time: _0635_
Method: _oral ET tube_
Precordial thump: _0631_
CPR initiated at: _0631_

Previous airway:
☐ ET tube
☐ Trach
☑ Natural

Addressograph

CPR PROGRESS NOTES

Time of events

Laboratory data

Actions

Time	VITAL SIGNS						I.V. PUSH					INFUSIONS				ACTIONS/PATIENT RESPONSE
	Pulse CPR	Resp. rate Spont; bag	Blood pressure	Rhythm	Defib (joules)	Atropine	Epinephrine	Lidocaine	NA bicarb	Bretylium	Lidocaine	Procain.	Isuprel	Dopamine	Responses to therapy, procedures, labs drawn/results
0631	CPR	Bag	0	V fib	200										No change.
0632		Bag	0	V fib	.200										ABGs drawn ® fem pressure applied.
0633	CPR	Bag	0	Asystole	300		1 mg								No change
0639	40	Bag	60 palp	GB PVCs				15			✓				Oral intubation by Dr. Hart
0645	60	Bag	80/40	GB PVCs							✓				CCU ready for patient

Time Spec Sent	ABGs & Lab Data						
	pH	PCO	PO₂	HCO₃	Sat%	FIO₂	Other
0633	7.1	16	43	14	80%		

RESUSCITATION OUTCOME

☑ Successful ☑ Transferred to _CCU_ at _0648_

☐ Unsuccessful — Expired at _____
Pronounced by: _____ MD
Family notified by: _G. Quinn, RN_
Time: _0645_

Attending notified by:
G. Quinn, RN Time _0645_
Code Recorder _B. Mullen, RN_
Code Team Nurse _J. Hanna, RN_
Anesthesia Rep. _Dr. Hart_
Other Personnel _B. Russo, RT_

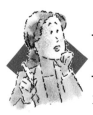

Cheat sheet

Procedure documentation review

What to include
- What procedure was performed
- When it was performed
- Who performed it
- How it was performed
- How well the patient tolerated it
- Adverse reactions to the procedure, if any

Drug administration charting guidelines
Basics
- Follow facility policy.
- Record the patient's full name, medical record number, and allergy information on each MAR.
- Immediately document the drug's name, dose, route of administration, frequency, the number of doses ordered or the stop date (if applicable), and the administration time for doses given.
- Write legibly.
- Use only standard abbreviations.
- Record drug administration immediately so that another nurse doesn't inadvertently repeat the dose.

- If you didn't give a drug, circle the time and document the reason for the omission.

P.r.n. medications
- Chart all p.r.n. drugs when administered, including reason for giving and the patient's response.
- If your MAR doesn't have space to document a patient's response to a drug or refusal to take a drug, document that information in the progress notes.

Drug abuse or refusal
- If the patient refuses or abuses medication, describe the event in his chart.

I.V. therapy
- Document all facets of I.V. therapy carefully, including subsequent complications.
- Also document in the progress notes, on a special I.V. therapy sheet or in a flowchart, or in another format (as required by your facility).

Quick quiz

1. When using an MAR, you need to:
   A. use abbreviations that only people on your unit understand.
   B. squeeze in as much information as possible.
   C. record drugs immediately after you give them.

Answer: C. Recording a drug immediately after you give it prevents other nurses from inadvertently giving the drug again.

2. After you establish an I.V. route, document:

    A.   each time you check the I.V. setup.

    B.   the condition of the patient's veins.

    C.   the number of venipuncture attempts if more than one is made.

Answer: C. Chart the number of attempts you made and the type of assistance required.

3. In charting about mechanical ventilation, include:

    A.   only the ventilator adjustments you make.

    B.   your assessment findings.

    C.   only the patient's objective responses.

Answer: B. Document assessment findings related to peripheral circulation, urine output, decreased cardiac output, fluid volume excess, or dehydration.

4. When assisting a doctor with procedures, document:

    A.   only what you did.

    B.   why you think the patient is having the procedure done.

    C.   the doctor's name and the patient's response.

Answer: C. Also, record the date and time, pertinent information about the procedure, the patient's response, and your patient teaching.

5. Before giving a blood transfusion:

    A.   ask another health professional to identify and document the blood or blood component.

    B.   ask the patient if he'd rather receive his own blood.

    C.   try to figure out if he'll develop a reaction.

Answer: A. You also need to match the patient's name, medical record number, blood group or type, Rh factor (patient's and donor's), crossmatch data, and blood bank identification number with the label on the blood bag—and then document that you did so.

6. Which of the following tools is used for documenting pain?

    A.   French scale

    B.   Graphic rating scale

    C.   Analogous graphic sheet

Answer: B. The graphic rating scale allows the patient to chart his degree of pain on a linear scale.

Scoring

☆☆☆ If you answered all six items correctly, gadzooks! You're able to complete tall stacks of medical records in a single round!

☆☆ If you answered four or five correctly, leaping lizards! You've performed your purpose: polishing off a plethora of paperwork!

☆ If you answered fewer than four correctly, don't worry! You can go back and review this chapter, take this book to work, and feel confident knowing you have a reference that makes charting incredibly easy.

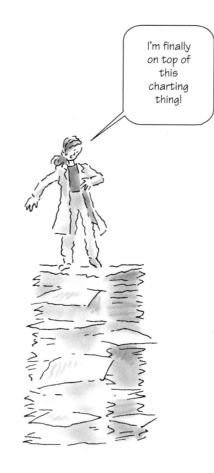

Appendices and index

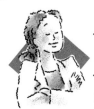

Practice makes perfect

1.   A 68-year-old patient was just admitted to your unit. She's tired and wants to know why she has to answer so many questions. You explain to her that nursing documentation is necessary because:
> A.   it's a state-mandated requirement.
> B.   it's a mode of communication.
> C.   the nurse-manager told you to do it.

2.   A 67-year-old patient on your unit recently had abdominal surgery and requires several dressing changes per day. He expresses concern about whether Medicare will pay for all the supplies being used. You explain to him that:
> A.   nurses accurately document the number of supplies used, which aids reimbursement.
> B.   the government has plenty of money to pay for supplies.
> C.   you'll try and cut back on the number of dressing changes.

3.   One of your patients overheard hospital personnel discussing the hospital's recent accreditation. He wants to know how a hospital becomes accredited. You explain that to receive accreditation the hospital must do all of the following except:
> A.   maintain accurate records that reflect standards of care.
> B.   provide quality of care in all areas of the hospital.
> C.   maintain accurate doctor documentation only.

4.   You tell your patent that you must attend your hospital's performance improvement committee meeting and that another nurse will be caring for her while you're gone. The patient wants to know what performance improvement is. Which description is most appropriate?
> A.   A committee in which the members are chosen based on the quality of care they deliver
> B.   A method used to develop, implement, and evaluate quality measures in your hospital
> C.   A method used to identify problems that occur within the hospital

5.   A 65-year-old patient is admitted to your unit with an exacerbation of chronic obstructive pulmonary disease. After the patient is settled into bed, you begin asking about his health history. A health history should include all the following information except:
> A.   discharge planning.
> B.   cultural information.
> C.   your best advice on the patient's illness.

6.   A 72-year-old patient is admitted to your unit with a fever of unknown origin. You complete the health history and the admission assessment. From this data, you begin making your nursing diagnosis. Which components should be included in the nursing diagnosis?

A. Human response or problem

B. Medical diagnosis

C. Expected outcome

7. The nurse caring for your patient on the previous shift identified *Impaired physical mobility* as a nursing diagnosis for the patient. One of the expected outcomes states, "The patient will ambulate unassisted by 11/12/02." Which element of the outcome hasn't been included?

A. Behavior

B. Measure

C. Condition

8. A 68-year-old patient with type 2 diabetes mellitus is admitted to your unit with a diagnosis of unstable angina. Which type of plan of care would best meet this patient's needs?

A. Standardized

B. Traditional

C. Both standardized and traditional

9. You need to develop a medication teaching plan for a patient with angina and type 2 diabetes mellitus. You must include instructions about when to take each medication. Which type of learning outcome is required for this patient?

A. Cognitive domain

B. Affective domain

C. Psychomotor domain

10. During an admission assessment, the patient states that she enjoys reading. You observe numerous books and magazines at her bedside. Based on this information, which type of learning materials are most appropriate for this patient?

A. Videotapes

B. Brochures and pamphlets

C. Computers

11. You're developing a teaching plan for a patient with coronary artery disease. Which of the following learning outcomes is in the psychomotor domain?

A. The patient will state when to take each prescribed medication.

B. The patient will demonstrate willingness to comply with lifestyle changes.

C. The patient will demonstrate how to measure his heart rate.

12. A 45-year-old patient comes to the short procedure unit for a hernia repair; his stay is uneventful. Which charting method is best for this patient?

A. Narrative

B. Problem-oriented medical record

C. FOCUS charting

13. When using narrative charting, you document the following statements for a patient who recently underwent exploratory abdominal surgery: *Pt states that incisional pain is unrelieved 30 min. after administration of analgesic. He's grimacing and holding incision site.* This documented observation is an example of:

    A.   change in the patient's condition.
    B.   patient's response to a treatment or medication.
    C.   lack of improvement in the patient's condition.

14. A 52-year-old patient was admitted 3 days ago with acute myocardial infarction. One of the problems on her problem-oriented medical record (POMR) problem list has been resolved. This should be indicated by:

    A.   assigning a different number to the problem.
    B.   placing the problem at the bottom of the list.
    C.   retiring the problem number.

15. A patient underwent colon resection 2 days ago. During his dressing change, you notice an increase in serosanguineous drainage from his incision. Because this is a deviation from written guidelines, you document this observation on the nursing and medical order flow sheet. This type of charting system is called:

    A.   charting by exception.
    B.   problem-intervention-evaluation.
    C.   narrative.

16. You've been teaching a patient with recently diagnosed diabetes about monitoring his blood glucose. To document this in the progress notes, you record the data, action, and evaluation of his response to the teaching. This type of charting format is called:

    A.   POMR.
    B.   Core.
    C.   FACT.

17. A 29-year-old patient is admitted to your unit after sustaining a femur fracture in a motor vehicle accident. You're performing your admission assessment and compiling the data on a form that contains a checklist. Which type of form are you using?

    A.   Open-ended
    B.   Closed-ended
    C.   Integrated

18. Because of your patient's deteriorating condition, you were unable to complete the admission database form. You report this information at change of shift. An initial admission assessment must be completed within how many hours after admission?

    A.   8 hours
    B.   12 hours
    C.   24 hours

19. You withhold your patient's blood pressure medication because his blood pressure is below the specified parameters needed to administer the medication. You circle the omitted dose on the medication Kardex; however, there's no space on the medication Kardex to document why the dose was withheld, so you must also document this information in:

    A.   progress notes.

    B.   patient care Kardex.

    C.   plan of care.

20. Your patient has an oral temperature of 103.2° F (39.6° C). You document this finding on the graphic flow sheet. In addition, you should do which of the following?

    A.   Document this finding on the patient care Kardex.

    B.   Document this finding and your interventions in narrative form in the progress notes.

    C.   Nothing. You only need to document on the graphic flow sheet.

21. An 82-year-old patient admitted with heart failure is scheduled for discharge. Your facility combines discharge summaries and patient instructions in one form. The patient receives one copy and the other remains with the medical record. Which of the following traits isn't an advantage of this form?

    A.   It provides useful data and additional teaching needs.

    B.   It establishes compliance with JCAHO requirements.

    C.   It's a narrative discharge summary.

22. A 73-year-old patient is referred to your home health agency. As you assess his condition, using OASIS, he states, "Why do you have to ask so many questions?" Which of the following is an appropriate response?

    A.   "The government requires this paperwork."

    B.   "My agency is required by the Health Care Financing Administration (HCFA) to complete this form for reimbursement purposes."

    C.   "My agency has always required this paperwork."

23. A patient is admitted to your long-term care facility. Her son, who is with her, asks you what the difference is between a skilled care unit and an intermediate care unit. Which is your best response?

    A.   "It depends on what part of the country you live in."

    B.   "A skilled facility provides specialized nursing skills and an intermediate facility provides less complex care."

    C.   "A skilled facility provides less complex care and an intermediate facility provides specialized nursing skills."

24. An 86-year-old patient is being admitted to your skilled care facility. Her son asks, "How does Medicare know how to reimburse for my mother's care?" You reply that Medicare requires:

    A.   daily documentation.

    B.   weekly documentation.

    C.   monthly documentation.

25. You're completing a nursing summary for a patient who is receiving skilled nursing care. How often must you complete this summary?

    A.   Every 3 months

    B.   Every 2 to 4 weeks

    C.   Once, on admission only

26. A patient who suffered a closed head injury in a motor vehicle accident is admitted to your skilled care facility. You're now working on this patient's interim plan of care. This plan of care should be completed:

    A.   within 7 days of admission.

    B.   within 48 hours of admission.

    C.   within 24 hours of admission.

27. A patient needs to be assessed for his ability to perform activities of daily living (ADLs). Which assessment tool helps evaluate six basic ADLs?

    A.   Katz index

    B.   Lawton scale

    C.   Barthel index and scale

28. While documenting in your patient's progress notes, you notice that you've made a mistake. How should you proceed?

    A.   Cross out the error completely.

    B.   Use white-out and continue to document.

    C.   Draw a single line through the entry.

29. You're concerned about your patient's sleeping patterns. How should you document your findings?

    A.   *Pt sleeps a lot.*

    B.   *Pt appears to sleep a lot.*

    C.   *Pt appears to have slept from 10 p.m. to 6 a.m.*

30. Your facility has started to use military time. Your patient received a one-time dose of furosemide 40 mg I.V. at 3 p.m. How should you document the administration time?

    A.   *Pt received furosemide 40 mg I.V. at 1500 hours.*

    B.   *Pt received furosemide 40 mg I.V. at 0300 hours.*

    C.   *Pt received furosemide 40 mg I.V. at 2300 hours.*

31. A nursing assistant was assigned to give morning care to your patient. How should you document the care he received from the assistant?

    A.   *Morning care given by Nancy Jones, NA.*
    B.   *Morning care given.*
    C.   *Morning care given by nurse's aide.*

32. A doctor gives you a verbal order for digoxin 0.25 mg P.O. stat for your patient with heart failure. When documenting the verbal order you should:
    A.   record the order on the doctor's order sheet.
    B.   include the doctor's prescriber number in the order.
    C.   sign the doctor's name.

33. Your patient told you that he isn't happy with the care he has been receiving at your facility and that he's thinking of suing. How should you proceed?
    A.   Notify the patient's family members and discuss the problem.
    B.   Fill out an incident report.
    C.   Chart factually and defensively.

34. An 83-year-old patient got out of bed by himself and fell. Which information should you include in your documentation?
    A.   Mention that an incident report was completed.
    B.   Describe what you saw and heard and the actions you took when you arrived at the patient's bedside.
    C.   Describe what you think occurred.

35. A patient is to undergo surgery in the morning and the doctor asks you to witness the patient's signing of the consent form. What should you do?
    A.   Make sure the patient is competent, awake, and alert before he signs the consent form.
    B.   Make sure that the doctor explained the procedure.
    C.   Console the patient because patients are typically anxious before surgery.

36. A 19-year-old patient who was recently diagnosed with diabetes mellitus asks to see his chart. What should you do first?
    A.   Immediately allow the patient to view his chart.
    B.   Ask the patient if he has questions about his treatment.
    C.   Check with your nurse-manager and the doctor first.

37. Your patient refuses to take his 10 a.m. medication. How should you document this on his medication administration record?
    A.   Cross out the time the drug was to be administered.
    B.   Circle the time the drug was to be administered.
    C.   Leave the space blank where you would typically sign your initials.

38. An 81-year-old patient admitted with dehydration requires I.V. therapy. After establishing I.V. access, you should document:
    A.   the number of venipuncture attempts made.
    B.   the date, time, and venipuncture site as well as the type and gauge of the catheter and the number of venipuncture attempts made.
    C.   the name of the catheter used.

39. A patient diagnosed with lower GI bleeding is ordered a transfusion of 1 U of packed red blood cells. What information should you document about this procedure?
    A   Confirmation that you alone verified the blood label information
    B.   Patient's vital signs before the transfusion
    C.   Patient's vital signs before, during, and after the transfusion as well as the total volume of blood transfused

40. While assisting the doctor with chest tube insertion, which of the following actions should you perform?
    A.   Provide support to the patient.
    B.   Tell the patient that he's going to be fine.
    C.   Update the doctor on your other patients' conditions.

Answers

1. B. The medical record is the main source of information and communication among nurses, doctors, physical therapists, social workers, and other caregivers. It helps provide the patient with better care.

2. A. Reimbursement from Medicare depends heavily on accurate nursing documentation.

3. C. Patient's medical records are evaluated by accrediting organizations for medical orders and progress notes by doctors as well as for assessment and plans of care completed by nursing personnel.

4. B. Individual states and the Joint Commission on Accreditation of Healthcare Organizations (JCAHO) require all health care facilities to regularly monitor, evaluate, and seek ways to improve the quality of care for their patients.

5. C. Giving advice implies that you know what's best for the patient. Instead, encourage him to participate in health care decisions.

6. A. A nursing diagnosis usually has three components—the human response or problem, related factors, and signs and symptoms.

7. B. The four elements of an outcome statement are behavior, measure, condition, and time. Measure should include criteria for measuring the behavior and should specify how much, how long, or how far.

8. C. The standardized plan (especially those classified by medical diagnosis or diagnosis-related groups [DRGs]), which takes into account the patient's multiple diagnoses, and the traditional plan, which allows for a more individualized plan of care for a patient with multiple diagnoses, would both meet this patient's needs.

9. A. Cognitive learning outcomes are related to understanding.

10. B. When choosing learning materials, you should focus on which material is best for the individual patient. Be sure to keep the patient's abilities and limitations in mind as you chose learning materials.

11. C. The psychomotor domain involves manual skills; therefore, demonstrating heart rate measurement is within the psychomotor domain.

12. C. FOCUS charting works best in acute care settings and on units where the same care and procedures are frequently repeated; this is the case in a short procedure unit.

13. B. When documenting a patient's response to a treatment or medication in a narrative note, be sure to include the patient's stated response and your observations.

14. C. Once you've resolved a problem, draw a line through it or show that it's inactive by retiring the problem number and highlighting the problem with a colored felt-tip pen. Don't use that number again for the same patient.

15. A. The charting by exception (CBE) format requires documentation of abnormal findings only. Guidelines for each body system are printed on CBE forms.

16. B. In the Core system, which focuses on the nursing process, the progress notes are recorded using DAE: data (D), action (A), and evaluation (E).

17. B. A closed-ended admission database form comes with preprinted headings, checklists, and questions with specific responses that you simply check off for the appropriate response.

18. C. JCAHO requires an initial nursing assessment to be completed within 24 hours of admission. Check your facility's policy, however, because your facility may require the form to be completed in a shorter time frame.

19. A. If your medication administration record or medication Kardex doesn't have space to explain why a dose was omitted, you need to document the reason in the progress notes.

20. B. Using flow sheets doesn't exempt you from narrative charting, in which you should describe your observations, patient teaching performed, patient responses, detailed interventions, and any unusual circumstances.

21. C. A narrative-style discharge summary is similar to a progress note; it contains the patient's status at admission and discharge, significant information about the patient's stay, and instructions given to the patient and his family members.

22. B. Explaining government regulations and reimbursement to the patient will increase his knowledge and cooperation.

23. B. Skilled patient care includes I.V. therapy, parenteral nutrition, respiratory care, and mechanical ventilation. Intermediate care includes care of patients who have chronic illnesses and those who need less complex care such as assistance with activities of daily living.

24. A. Medicare provides reimbursement for patients who require skilled care, such as chemotherapy and tube feedings. They require daily documentation to justify that the service is needed.

25. B. Usually, you must complete a standard nursing summary at least once every 2 to 4 weeks for patients with specific problems who are receiving skilled nursing care.

26. C. The interim plan of care must be in place within 24 hours of admission.

27. A. The Katz index ranks the patient's ability in six basic ADLs — bathing, dressing, toileting, moving from wheelchair to bed and returning, continence, and feeding.

28. C. When you make a mistake in charting, correct it immediately by drawing a single line through the entry and writing "error" above or beside it, along with your initials, the date, and the time.

29. C. Record just the facts, exactly what you see, hear, and do — not your opinions or assumptions.

30. A. Most facilities require the nurse to chart in military time, which expresses time as a continuous 24-hour period.

31. A. If you need to chart the actions of nursing assistants or technicians, write the caregiver's full name, not just her initials.

32. A. When documenting a verbal order, first write V.O. on the first line (indicating that it's a verbal order), then write the doctor's name and your name as the nurse who received the order, and then write the order. It's the doctor's responsibility to countersign this order within your facility's time limit.

33. C. Document the patient's complaints using his own words, and record the specific care given to the patient in direct response to his complaints. When a patient threatens to sue, notify your nurse-manager or nursing supervisor immediately. She'll contact the risk management department, which may be able to offer advice about how to handle this difficult situation.

34. B. When a patient falls, document what you saw and heard. Also document the accounts given by witnesses. Avoid documenting what you think may have occurred. Documenting that an incident report was completed may open up you and the hospital to a lawsuit.

35. A. Before witnessing a patient's consent, make sure that the patient is competent, awake, and alert and is aware of what he's doing. Also make sure that the patient understands the procedure and the associated risks. Simply giving the patient an explanation doesn't ensure that he understands. Notify your nurse-manager and the doctor immediately if you suspect that that patient has doubts about the procedure or his condition. Performing a procedure without voluntary consent may be considered battery.

36. B. Your patient has a legal right to see his chart. However, if he asks to see it, you should first ask him if he has any questions about his treatment and try to clear up any confusion. The patient may just be confused about his care.

37. B. Circle the time and document the reason for omission.

38. B. When documenting I.V. catheter insertion, document the date, time, and venipuncture site. Also document the type and gauge of the catheter and the number of venipuncture attempts made.

39. C. In order to properly document a blood transfusion, include the patient's vital signs before, during, and after the transfusion as well as the total volume of blood transfused. Before administering blood or blood components, the bag must be identified by two health care professionals who verify that the information on the label is correct.

40. A. While assisting the doctor during a procedure, your role is to provide support to the patient, evaluate the patient's response, and document the procedure.

JCAHO nursing care and documentation standards

The 2001 standards for accreditation of hospitals that were developed by the Joint Commission on Accreditation of Healthcare Organizations (JCAHO) include identification of goals, functions, and standards for provision of patient care. The guidelines place emphasis on integration of services from a variety of providers so that goals, functions, and standards reflect the combined responsibilities of those providing patient care. The standards are written to address patient needs rather than identify discrete responsibilities of separate providers.

In addition, the standards stress the value of continuous, rather than episodic, accreditation so that ongoing data collection, assessment, intervention, and evaluation can be performed.

The selected standards presented here address assessment of patients, care of patients, leadership, management of human resources, and nursing.

Assessment of patients

The standards associated with assessment of patients clearly show the focus on performance-improvement processes, while addressing the hospital's responsibility to collect data about each patient's physical and psychosocial status and health history, to analyze that data, and to make patient care decisions based on the following information:

• Each patient's physical, psychological, and social status is assessed.

• Nutritional status is assessed when warranted by the patient's needs or condition.

• Pain is assessed in all patients.

• Functional status is assessed when warranted by the patient's needs or condition.

• Diagnostic testing necessary for determining the patient's health care needs is performed.

• The need for discharge planning assessment is determined.

• Each admitted patient's initial assessment is conducted within a time frame specified by hospital policy.

• Before surgery, the patient's physical examination and medical history, any indicated diagnostic tests, and a preoperative diagnosis are completed and recorded in the patient's medical record.

• Possible victims of abuse are identified using criteria developed by the hospital.

• Pathology and clinical laboratory services and consultation are readily available to meet the patient's needs.

• Each patient is reassessed at points designated in hospital policy.
• Staff members integrate the information from various assessments of the patient to identify and assign priorities to his care needs.
• The hospital has defined patient assessment activities in writing.
• A registered nurse assesses the patient's need for nursing care in all settings where nursing care is provided.
• The assessment process for an infant, a child, or an adolescent patient is individualized.
• The assessment process addresses the special needs of patients who are receiving treatment for emotional or behavioral disorders.
• The assessment process addresses the special needs of patients who are receiving treatment for alcoholism or other drug dependencies.
• The assessment process addresses the special needs of patients who are possible victims of abuse.

Care of patients

The selected standards presented here apply to any organization that provides care to patients, and the standards are to be applied collaboratively to ensure that care is integrated and continuous. The responsibilities of individual providers are determined by their professional credentials, licensure, and scope of practice; the type of care being provided; the experience level of the individual provider; and hospital policies and job descriptions.
• Care, treatment, and rehabilitation are planned to ensure that they're appropriate to the patient's needs and severity of disease, condition, impairment, or disability.
• Care is planned and provided in an interdisciplinary, collaborative manner by qualified individuals.
• Patient care procedures (such as bathing) are performed in a manner that respects privacy.
• The patient's progress is periodically evaluated against care goals and the plan of care and, when indicated, the plan or goals are revised.
• Patients are informed in a timely manner of the need to plan for discharge or transfer to another facility or level of care.
• Continuing care at the time of discharge is based on the patient's assessed needs.
• Medication use processes are organized and systematic throughout the hospital.

- Each patient's nutritional care is planned.
- Functional rehabilitation status is assessed to determine the current level of functioning, self-care, self-responsibility, independence, and quality of life.
- Restraint or seclusion use is limited to situations with adequate, appropriate, clinical justification.
- Patients are educated about pain and pain management.

Leadership

The selected leadership standards presented here clearly show the focus on patient care and the integration of services. JCAHO specifies that leadership should be inclusive, not exclusive; should encourage staff participation in shaping the hospital's vision and values; should develop leaders at every level who help to fulfill the hospital's mission, vision, and values; should accurately assess the needs of patients and other users of the hospital's services; and should develop an organizational culture that focuses on continuously improving performance to meet these needs:

- The leaders provide for hospital planning.
- Each hospital department has effective leadership.
- Patient care services are integrated throughout the hospital.
- The hospital leaders set expectations, develop plans, and manage processes to measure, assess, and improve the quality of the hospital's governance, management, and clinical and support activities.
- All leaders participate in interdisciplinary, interdepartmental performance-improvement activities.
- The leaders allocate adequate resources for measuring, assessing, and improving the hospital's performance.
- The leaders ensure the implementation of an organization-wide patient safety program.

Management of human resources

Efficient management of human resources requires making provisions for the right number of competent staff members to meet the patient needs. Adequate staffing is the responsibility of all hospital leaders, not solely of the human resources department. Hospital leaders are responsible for considering a number of factors when identifying how patient care will be delivered, including: the hospital's mission, the case mix of patients (including degree and complexity of care), the technology used in patient care, and the expectations of the patients:

• The hospital's leaders define the qualifications and performance expectations for all staff positions.

• The hospital provides an adequate number of staff members whose qualifications are consistent with job responsibilities.

• The leaders ensure that the competence of all staff members is assessed, maintained, demonstrated, and improved continually.

• An orientation process provides initial job training and information and assesses the staff's ability to fulfill specified responsibilities.

• Ongoing in-service and other education and training maintain and improve staff competence.

• The hospital assesses each staff member's ability to meet the performance expectations stated in his job description.

• The hospital addresses a staff member's request not to participate in any aspect of patient care.

Nursing

Standards related to the nurse-executive position focus on responsibilities. Qualifications for the position are outlined in the intent statements and include education at the master's level or equivalent. The nurse-executive, registered nurses, and other designated nursing staff members write nursing policies and procedures, nursing standards of patient care, standards of nursing practice, and standards to measure, assess, and improve patient outcomes:

• Nursing services are directed by a nurse-executive who is a registered nurse qualified by advanced education and management experience.

• The nurse-executive has the authority and responsibility for establishing standards of nursing practice.

• Nursing policies and procedures, nursing standards of patient care, and standards of nursing practice are approved by the nurse-executive or a designee.

NANDA taxonomy II codes

The North American Nursing Diagnosis Association (NANDA) endorsed its first nursing diagnosis taxonomic structure, NANDA Taxonomy I, in 1986. This taxonomy has been revised several times, most recently in 2000. The new Taxonomy II has a code structure that is compliant with the recommendations of the National Library of Medicine concerning health care terminology codes. The taxonomy that appears here represents the accepted classification system for nursing diagnosis. The nurse-executive and other nursing leaders participate with leaders from the governing body, management, medical staff, and clinical areas in planning, promoting, and conducting organization-wide performance-improvement activities.

Nursing diagnosis	Taxonomy II codes	Nursing diagnosis	Taxonomy II codes
Imbalanced nutrition: More than body requirements	00001	Risk for imbalanced fluid volume	00025
Imbalanced nutrition: Less than body requirements	00002	Excess fluid volume	00026
		Deficient fluid volume	00027
Risk for imbalanced nutrition: More than body requirements	00003	Risk for deficient fluid volume	00028
Risk for infection	00004	Decreased cardiac output	00029
Risk for imbalanced body temperature	00005	Impaired gas exchange	00030
		Ineffective airway clearance	00031
Hypothermia	00006	Ineffective breathing pattern	00032
Hyperthermia	00007	Impaired spontaneous ventilation	00033
Ineffective thermoregulation	00008	Dysfunctional ventilatory weaning response	00034
Autonomic dysreflexia	00009	Risk for injury	00035
Risk for autonomic dysreflexia	00010	Risk for suffocation	00036
Constipation	00011	Risk for poisoning	00037
Perceived constipation	00012	Risk for trauma	00038
Diarrhea	00013	Risk for aspiration	00039
Bowel incontinence	00014	Risk for disuse syndrome	00040
Risk for constipation	00015	Latex allergy response	00041
Impaired urinary elimination	00016	Risk for latex allergy response	00042
Stress urinary incontinence	00017	Ineffective protection	00043
Reflex urinary incontinence	00018	Impaired tissue integrity	00044
Urge urinary incontinence	00019	Impaired oral mucous membrane	00045
Functional urinary incontinence	00020	Impaired skin integrity	00046
Total urinary incontinence	00021	Risk for impaired skin integrity	00047
Risk for urge urinary incontinence	00022	Impaired dentition	00048
Urinary retention	00023	Decreased intracranial adaptive capacity	00049
Ineffective tissue perfusion (specify type: renal, cerebral, cardiopulmonary, GI, peripheral)	00024	Disturbed energy field	00050
		Impaired verbal communication	00051

Nursing diagnosis	Taxonomy II codes	Nursing diagnosis	Taxonomy II codes
Impaired social interaction	00052	Risk for perioperative-positioning injury	00087
Social isolation	00053	Impaired walking	00088
Risk for loneliness	00054	Impaired wheelchair mobility	00089
Ineffective role performance	00055	Impaired transfer ability	00090
Impaired parenting	00056	Impaired bed mobility	00091
Risk for impaired parenting	00057	Activity intolerance	00092
Risk for impaired parent/infant/child attachment	00058	Fatigue	00093
Sexual dysfunction	00059	Risk for activity intolerance	00094
Interrupted family processes	00060	Disturbed sleep pattern	00095
Caregiver role strain	00061	Sleep deprivation	00096
Risk for caregiver role strain	00062	Deficient diversional activity	00097
Dysfunctional family processes: Alcoholism	00063	Impaired home maintenance	00098
Parental role conflict	00064	Ineffective health maintenance	00099
Ineffective sexuality patterns	00065	Delayed surgical recovery	00100
Spiritual distress	00066	Adult failure to thrive	00101
Risk for spiritual distress	00067	Feeding self-care deficit	00102
Readiness for enhanced spiritual well-being	00068	Impaired swallowing	00103
Ineffective coping	00069	Ineffective breast-feeding	00104
Impaired adjustment	00070	Interrupted breast-feeding	00105
Defensive coping	00071	Effective breast-feeding	00106
Ineffective denial	00072	Ineffective infant feeding pattern	00107
Disabled family coping	00073	Bathing or hygiene self-care deficit	00108
Compromised family coping	00074	Dressing or grooming self-care deficit	00109
Readiness for enhanced family coping	00075	Toileting self-care deficit	00110
Readiness for enhanced community coping	00076	Delayed growth and development	00111
		Risk for delayed development	00112
Ineffective community coping	00077	Risk for disproportionate growth	00113
Ineffective therapeutic regimen management	00078	Relocation stress syndrome	00114
Noncompliance (specify)	00079	Risk for disorganized infant behavior	00115
Ineffective family therapeutic regimen management	00080	Disorganized infant behavior	00116
Ineffective community therapeutic regimen management	00081	Readiness for enhanced organized infant behavior	00117
Effective therapeutic regimen management	00082	Disturbed body image	00118
Decisional conflict (specify)	00083	Chronic low self-esteem	00119
Health-seeking behaviors (specify)	00084	Situational low self-esteem	00120
Impaired physical mobility	00085	Disturbed personal identity	00121
Risk for peripheral neurovascular dysfunction	00086	Disturbed sensory perception (specify: visual, auditory, kinesthetic, gustatory, tactile, olfactory)	00122

Nursing diagnosis	Taxonomy II codes	Nursing diagnosis	Taxonomy II codes
Unilateral neglect	00123	Posttrauma syndrome	00141
Hopelessness	00124	Rape-trauma syndrome	00142
Powerlessness	00125	Rape-trauma syndrome: Compound reaction	00143
Deficient knowledge (specify)	00126		00144
Impaired environmental interpretation syndrome	00127	Rape-trauma syndrome: Silent reaction	00145
Acute confusion	00128	Risk for posttrauma syndrome	
Chronic confusion	00129	Anxiety	00146
Disturbed thought processes	00130	Death anxiety	00147
Impaired memory	00131	Fear	00148
Acute pain	00132	**New nursing diagnoses (effective April 2000)**	
Chronic pain	00133		
Nausea	00134	Risk for relocation stress syndrome	00149
Dysfunctional grieving	00135	Risk for suicide	00150
Anticipatory grieving	00136		
Chronic sorrow	00137	Self-mutilation	00151
Risk for other-directed violence	00138	Risk for powerlessness	00152
Risk for self-mutilation	00139	Risk for situational low self-esteem	00153
Risk for self-directed violence	00140	Wandering	00154
		Risk for falls	00155

Glossary

Accountability: obligation to accept responsibility for or account for one's actions

Accreditation: official recognition from a professional or government organization that a health care facility meets relevant standards

Advance directive: document used as a guideline for life-sustaining medical care of a patient with an advanced disease or disability, who is no longer able to indicate his own wishes; includes living wills and durable powers of attorney for health care

Barthel index and scale: functional assessment tool used to evaluate an older patient's overall well-being and self-care abilities; evaluates the ability to perform 10 self-care activities

Case management: model for management of health care facilities in which one professional — usually a nurse or a social worker — assumes responsibility for coordinating care so that patients move through the health care system in the shortest time and at the lowest possible cost

Charting by exception (CBE): charting system that departs from traditional systems by requiring documentation of only significant or abnormal findings

Core charting: charting system that focuses on the nursing process; components include a database, plan of care, flow sheets, progress notes, and discharge summary

Critical pathway: documentation tool used in managed care and case management in which a time line is defined for the patient's condition and for the achievement of expected outcomes; used by caregivers to determine on any given day where the patient should be in his progress toward optimal health

Database: subjective and objective patient information collected during your initial assessment of the patient; includes information obtained by taking your patient's health history, performing a physical examination, and analyzing laboratory test results

Diagnosis-related group (DRG): system of classifying or grouping patients according to medical diagnosis for purposes of reimbursement of hospitalization costs under Medicare

Durable power of attorney for health care: legal document whereby a patient authorizes another person to make medical decisions for him should he become incompetent to do so

FOCUS charting: charting system that uses assessment data, first to evaluate patient-centered topics (or foci of concern) and then to document precisely and concisely

Health history: summary of a patient's health status that includes physiologic, psychological, cultural, and psychosocial data

Health maintenance organization (HMO): organization that provides an agreed-upon health service to voluntary enrollees who prepay a fixed, periodic fee that's set without regard to the amount or kind of services received (people who belong to an HMO are cared for by member doctors with limited referrals to outside specialists)

Incident report: formal written report that informs hospital administrators (and the hospital's insurance company) about an incident and that serves as a contemporary factual statement in the event of a lawsuit

Incremental record: record kept according to time and occurrences

Independent practice association (IPA) model HMO: health maintenance organization that contracts with an association of doctors to provide doctor services to its members while the doctors maintain their independent practices

Informed consent: permission obtained from a patient to perform a specific test or procedure after the patient has been fully informed about the test or procedure

Interventions: nursing actions taken to meet a patient's health care needs; should reflect nurse's agreement with the patient on how to meet defined goals or expected outcomes

Joint Commission on Accreditation of Healthcare Organizations (JCAHO): private, nongovernmental agency that establishes guidelines for the operation of hospitals and other health care facilities, conducts accreditation programs and surveys, and encourages the attainment of high standards of institutional medical care; members include representatives from the American Medical Association, American College of Physicians, and American College of Surgeons

Katz index: assessment tool used to evaluate a patient's ability to perform the basic functions of bathing, dressing, toileting, transfer, continence, and feeding

Lawton scale: assessment tool used to evaluate a patient's ability to perform relatively complex tasks, such as using a telephone, cooking, managing finances, and taking medications

Learning outcomes: outcomes developed as part of a patient-teaching plan that identify what a patient needs to learn, how you'll teach him, and how you'll evaluate what he has learned

Living will: witnessed document indicating a patient's desire to be allowed to die a natural death, rather than be kept alive by life-sustaining measures; applies to decisions that will be made after a terminally ill patient is incompetent and has no reasonable possibility of recovery

Minimum data set (MDS): standardized assessment tool that must be filled out for every patient admitted to a long-term care facility as mandated by the federal government

North American Nursing Diagnosis Association (NANDA): organization responsible for developing and categorizing nursing diagnoses and examining applications of nursing diagnoses in clinical practice, education, and research

Nursing diagnosis: clinical judgment made by a nurse about a patient's responses to actual or potential health problems or life processes; describes a patient problem that the nurse can legally solve; may apply to families and communities as well as individual patients

Nursing process: systematic approach to identifying a patient's problems and then taking nursing actions to address them; steps include assessing the patient's problems, forming a diagnostic statement, identifying expected outcomes, creating a plan to achieve expected outcomes and solve the patient's problems, implementing the plan or assigning others to implement it, and evaluating the plan's effectiveness

Occurrence reporting: reporting by doctors, nurses, or other hospital staff of incidents, either when they're observed or shortly after; also called incident reporting

Occurrence screening: identification of adverse events through a review of medical records

Outcome criteria: standards by which measurable goals, or outcomes, are objectively evaluated

Outcome documentation: charting that focuses on patient behaviors and responses to nursing care; documents the patient's condition in relation to predetermined outcomes included in the plan of care

Peer review organization (PRO): basic component of a performance improvement program in which the results of health care given to a specific patient population are evaluated according to outcome criteria established by peers of the professionals delivering the care; promoted by professional organizations as a means of maintaining standards of care

Practice guidelines: sequential instructions for treating patients with specific health problems

Preadmission screening annual resident review (PASARR): form used to assess the mental status of a patient before admission to a long-term care facility; required for Medicare or Medicaid reimbursement

Problem-intervention-evaluation (PIE) charting: charting system that organizes patient information according to patient's problems; integrates the patient's plan of care into the progress notes in order to simplify the documentation process

Problem-oriented medical record (POMR): method of organizing the medical record; consists of baseline data, a problem list, and a plan of care for each problem

Performance improvement: commitment on the part of a health care facility or several health disciplines to work together to achieve an optimal degree of excellence in the services rendered to every patient (state regulatory and accrediting agencies may require health care facilities to regularly monitor, evaluate, and seek ways to improve the quality of care)

Resident assessment protocol (RAP): form required by federal mandate for use in long-term care facilities that identifies the patient's primary problems and care needs and documents the existence of a plan of care

Risk management: identification, analysis, evaluation, and elimination or reduction of risks to patients, visitors, or employees; involves loss prevention and control and the handling of all incidents, claims, and other insurance- and litigation-related tasks.

SOAP charting: structured method of recording progress notes in which data are organized into four categories: Subjective, Objective, Assessment, and Planning

SOAPIE charting: structured method of recording progress notes in which data are organized into six categories: Subjective, Objective, Assessment, Planning, Implementation, and Evaluation

SOAPIER charting: structured method of recording progress notes in which data are organized into seven categories: Subjective, Objective, Assessment, Planning, Implementation, Evaluation, and Revision

Source-oriented narrative record: method of organizing the medical record in which each discipline records information in a separate section of the medical record

Utilization review: program, initiated by reimbursing agents to maintain control over health care providers, that may focus on length of stay, treatment regimen, validation of tests and procedures, and verification of the use of medical supplies and equipment

Index

i refers to an illustration; t refers to a table.

i refers to an illustration; t refers to a table.

i refers to an illustration; t refers to a table.

i refers to an illustration; t refers to a table.